MW01365756

Current Review of Complementary Medicine

Current Review of Complementary Medicine

Edited by

Marc S. Micozzi, MD, PhD

Adjunct Professor
Department of Medicine
University of Pennsylvania
Executive Director
College of Physicians of Philadelphia
Philadelphia, Pennsylvania

With 19 contributors

Philadelphia

CURRENT MEDICINE, INC.

400 Market Street
Suite 700
Philadelphia, PA 19106

Director of Product Development: *Mary Kinsella*
Editorial Supervisor: *Susan L. Hunsberger*
Developmental Editor: *Jennifer Wood*
Editorial Assistant: *Lisa M. Janda*
Associate Art Director: *Jerilyn Bockorick*
Cover Design: *Jerilyn Bockorick*
Layout: *Stacey Caiazzo, Chris Allan*
Illustration Director: *Birck Cox*
Illustrator: *Lisa Weischedel*
Production Director: *Lori Holland*
Production: *Constance Copeland*
Marketing: *Amy Giuffi*
Indexing: *Holly Lukens*

Current review of complementary medicine / Marc S. Micozzi, editor.
    p. cm.
    Includes bibliographical references and index.
    ISBN 1-57342-129-3 (alk. paper)
    1. Alternatice medicine.   I. Micozzi, Marc S., 1953-
II. Title: Complementary medicine.
    [DNLM: 1. Alternative Medicine.   WB 890 C976 1999]
R733.C87   1999
615.5--DC21
DNLM/DLC
for Library of Congress   99-12780
                                                                             CIP

ISBN 1-57340-129-3

©1999 by Current Medicine, Inc. All rights reserved. No part of this publication may be reproduced, stored in a retrieval system, or transmitted in any form by any means electronic, mechanical, photocopying, recording, or otherwise without prior consent of the publisher.

Although every effort has been made to ensure that drug dosages and other information are presented accurately in this publication, the ultimate responsibility rests with the prescribing physician. Neither the publishers nor the author can be held responsible for errors or for any consequence arising from the use of the information contained therein. Any product mentioned in this publication should be used in accordance with the prescribing information prepared by the manufacturers. No claims or endorsements are made for any drug or compound at present under clinical investigation.

Printed in the United States by Edwards Brothers.
5 4 3 2 1

Preface

Critics of complementary medicine often say that there is no scientific evidence to indicate that these therapeutic approaches work. As recent developments indicate, this criticism is increasingly outdated. It was a review of the scientific data that led the U.S. Food and Drug Administration (FDA) to reclassify the acupuncture needle from an experimental to a therapeutic device. The agency acted because of evidence indicating that this treatment provided significant relief to those suffering from conditions such as chronic pain and asthma. In a related development that surprised many people, the U.S. Agency for Health Care Policy and Research concluded that spinal manual adjustment, as practiced by chiropractors, osteopathic physicians, and others, constitutes a more effective and cost-effective treatment for lower-back pain than either drugs or surgery. This decision was based on the kind of outcomes-based research that both advocates and critics of complementary medicine have long demanded.

In fact, so many units of the federal government are currently researching different aspects of complementary medical approaches that U.S. Senator Arlen Specter (Republican, Pennsylvania) has requested a government-wide survey documenting these efforts.

This debate is complicated by the fact that when significant research on the efficacy of complementary approaches is published in a foreign country, the research is largely ignored in the United States. A recent case in Germany provides a clear example of this challenge. For much of the past 200 years, German research set the standard for scientists around the world. When a commission established by the German government (known as Commission E) issued reports on the efficacy of hundreds of natural medicines, its work attracted little attention in the United States. The American Botanical Council, a private, nonprofit group, has now published English translations of these monographs and will be providing this information to legislators and those who make health policy. Other nations in Asia, Africa, and Latin America have also published research on natural medicines.

Conducting clinical trials or outcome-based research is a very expensive process, but guidelines may be developed to help save both the federal government and potential private funding sources considerable time and money. It is important to make a distinction between medical approaches that truly represent alternatives and those that are simply unusual. Most credible alternative approaches (*eg*, Chinese acupuncture or Ayurvedic, the medicine of India) have been passed down from generation to generation for thousands of years. They have been used by thousands of practitioners on millions of patients. From a cultural historical perspective, approaches that have no value probably would have died out a long time ago. Conversely, unusual medical therapies have no cultural traditions to speak of; typically, such approaches are associated with a few individuals who are unable or unwilling to scientifically replicate their results. To date, the complementary medical approaches that have been validated by contemporary science are generally those with long cultural histories.

Scientific validation of alternative medical approaches is important because physicians use any ethical treatment that has been proven to work. Contemporary physicians depend on clinical evidence when making decisions about appropriate treatments for their patients. Although we have decades of experience performing clinical trials, the financial resources needed to do the research are not easy to obtain.

If the federal offices conducting research continue to be hampered by small budgets, information that could help save lives might be delayed for years. Some experts believe a joint public and private initiative involving the government, foundations, universities, and corporations should help initiate the kind of comprehensive research program need to determine which complementary therapies may benefit medical practice and public health.

In the meantime, we will do our best to provide clinicians with valid information on current innovations and controversies in their field to allow a sound basis for making clinical decisions.

Marc S. Micozzi, MD, PhD

Contributors

Keith Berndtson, MD
Assistant Professor
Department of Family Medicine
Rush Medical College
Midwest Regional Medical Director
American WholeHealth, Inc.
Chicago, Illinois

Bhaswati Bhattacharya, MA, MPH, MD
Department of Family Medicine
Columbia-Presbyterian Medical Center
Richard and Hinda Rosenthal Center for
    Complementary and Alternative Medicine
New York, New York

Hyla Cass, MD
Assistant Clinical Professor
Department of Psychiatry
University of California School of Medicine
Los Angeles, California

Michael D. Cirigliano, MD
Assistant Professor
Department of Medicine
University of Pennsylvania
Philadelphia, Pennsylvania

David Edelberg, MD
Assistant Professor
Department of Internal Medicine
Rush Medical College
Chairman and Founder
American WholeHealth, Inc.
Chicago, Illinois

Joyce C. Frye, DO, MBA
Instructor
Department of Obstetrics and Gynecology
Jefferson Medical College
Founder and Director
The Women's Group
Former Chairman
Department of Gynecology
Presbyterian Medical Center
Philadelphia, Pennsylvania

Mary Lou Galantino, PhD, PT
Associate Professor
Program in Physical Therapy
Richard Stockton College of New Jersey
Pomona, New Jersey
Physical Therapy Clinical Specialist in Chronic Pain
University of Pennsylvania
Philadelphia, Pennsylvania

Steven C. Halbert, MD
Associate Clinical Director for Protocol Development
Thomas Jefferson Center for Integrative Medicine
Philadelphia, Pennsylvania

George R. Haynes, PhD
School of Education
Associate Dean
Division of Lifelong Learning
Drexel University
Philadelphia, Pennsylvania

Eric Leskowitz, MD
Instructor
Department of Psychiatry
Harvard Medical School
Senior Clinical Instructor
Department of Psychiatry
Tufts University School of Medicine
Psychiatrist
Spaulding Rehabilitation Hospital
Boston, Massachusetts

Lee Lipsenthal, MD
Vice President and Medical Director
Preventive Medicine Research Institute
Sausalito, California

Dean Ornish, MD
Professor
Department of Medicine
University of California
San Francisco, California
President and Director
Preventive Medicine Research Institute
Sausalito, California

Contributors, continued

Daniel Redwood, DC
Redwood Chiropractic and Wellness
Virginia Beach, Virginia

Annette Ridenour
President
Aesthetics, Inc.
San Diego, California

Mary Ellen Scheckenbach, MAc
Registered Acupuncturist
Thomas Jefferson Center for Integrative Medicine
Philadelphia, Pennsylvania

Andrew G. Sparber, RN, MS, CS
Psychiatric Liaison Nurse
Clinical Center
National Institutes of Health
Bethesda, Maryland

Suzanne S. Teuber, MD
Assistant Professor
Department of Internal Medicine
University of California
Davis, California

John Weeks
Publisher and Editor
The Integrator for the Business of Alternative Medicine
Seattle, Washington

Jacqueline C. Wooton, MEd
President
Alternative Medicine Foundation
Bethesda, Maryland

Contents

Chapter 1
Creating an Herbal Formulary for Clinical Practice 1
BHASWATI BHATTACHARYA

Background. 1
Creation of an Herbal Pharmacy: Goals and Purpose 2
Research 2
Reassessment. 3
Integrating Herbs into the Main Hospital Pharmacy 3
Outpatient Pharmacy Setup. 3
Implementation 3
Preparing the Space 4
Herbs to Use. 4
Education 5
Evaluation and Sustenance 6
Research 6
Legal Aspects 6
Conclusions 7

Chapter 2
Ten Most Common Herbs in Clinical Practice. 9
MICHAEL D. CIRIGLIANO

Specific Herbal Remedies. 9
Integration of Herbal Remedies into Clinical Practice 16

Chapter 3
Herbs in Women's Health Care 21
JOYCE C. FRYE

Therapeutic Use of Herbs for Gynecologic Problems. 22
Conclusions. 26

Chapter 4
St. John's Wort and Depression 29
HYLA CASS

Background. 29
An Ancient Medicine Rediscovered. 30
Depression 30
Clinical Research 32
Seasonal Affective Disorder. 33
Premenstrual Syndrome 34
Pharmacology 34
Side Effects 35
Transition from Pharmaceutical Antidepressants to St. John's Wort . 36
Formulation. 37
Combinations. 37
Diet and Lifestyle 37
Conclusions. 37

Contents, continued

Chapter 5
Food Allergy: Myths and Realities 39
SUZANNE S. TEUBER

Definition of Adverse Reactions to Foods 39
Evaluation of Adverse Reactions to Foods 39
Unproven Methods in Diagnosis or Therapy 41
Conclusions 41

Chapter 6
Integrative Treatment of Fibromyalgia and Chronic Fatigue/Immune Dysfunction Syndrome 45
KEITH BERNDTSON

Conventional versus Integrative Medicine 45
Integrative Treatment Issues 47
Conclusions 52

Chapter 7
Acupuncture 57
MARY ELLEN SCHECKENBACH

National Institutes of Health Consensus Report 58
Efficacy of Acupuncture Compared with
  Placebo Acupuncture and Standard Care 59
Role of Acupuncture in the Treatment of Various Conditions in
  Comparison or Combination with Other Interventions 60
Biological Effects of Acupuncture 60
Issues to Address Before Acupuncture is
  Incorporated into the Current Health-Care System 61
Directions for Future Research 62
Conclusions 62
New Research 62
Studies of Biologic Mechanisms 63
Discussion of Research Issues 64
Conclusions 65

Chapter 8
Spinal Adjustment for Low Back Pain 69
DANIEL REDWOOD

Contemporary Chiropractic 69
Primary Care Physicians 70
Screening the Patient 71
Research on Manual Adjustment for Low Back Pain 72
Acute versus Chronic Low Back Pain 72
Evidence for Manual Methods in Chronic Cases 72
Preventing Acute Cases from Becoming Chronic 73
Low Back Pain with Leg Pain 74
Other Considerations When Referring Patients to Chiropractors . . . 74
Choosing the Individual Chiropractor 76

Contents, continued

Chapter 9
Current Controversies in Therapeutic Touch 79
ERIC LESKOWITZ

- Overview of Alternative Medicine. 79
- Subtle Energy. 80
- History of Therapeutic Touch 80
- The Technique of Therapeutic Touch 81
- Relevant Research. 81
- Clinical Applications 82
- A Recent Controversy 82
- Conclusions. 83

Chapter 10
Chelation Therapy: Cardiovascular Cure or Heavy Metal Hype? 85
STEVEN C. HALBERT

- History. 85
- Mechanisms of Action 86
- Clinical Applications of Chelation Therapy 87
- Contraindications and Toxicity. 87
- Treatment Protocol 88
- Conclusions. 88

Chapter 11
Intensive Lifestyle Intervention for Coronary Artery Disease: Alternative Medicine or Common Sense? 91
LEE LIPSENTHAL AND DEAN ORNISH

- Heart Disease in the United States 92
- Revascularization Procedures. 92
- Cholesterol-Lowering Therapy 93
- Lifestyle Modification. 93
- Diet. 93
- Exercise 94
- Psychosocial Risk Factors 94
- Stress and the Heart 95
- Stress Management 95
- Conclusions. 96

Chapter 12
Complementary Therapy in HIV Disease: Living Long and Living Well 101
MARY LOU GALANTINO

- Addressing Pain Syndromes Through Complementary Interventions 101
- Energy-Based Systems. 102
- Movement Therapies in HIV Disease 103
- Movement Therapy 104

Contents, continued

Chapter 13
Insurance Coverage for Alternative Therapies 107
JOHN WEEKS

Overview 107
Forces Behind the Coverage Movement 107
Current Extent of Complementary and
   Alternative Medicine Intervention 110
Selecting and Defining a Complementary and
   Alternative Medicine Benefit 111
Complementary and Alternative Medicine:
   Grafting or Health Creation? 118

Chapter 14
Business Aspects of Building an Integrative Medical Practice 121
DAVID EDELBERG

Alternative Medicine 121
The Integrated Practice 122
The Future of Integrated Medicine 123
Problems and Financial Aspects of the Integrated Practice 123

Chapter 15
Designing a Healing Clinical Office Environment: Creating Healing Spaces 125
ANNETTE RIDENOUR

Background 125
Creating a Business Plan 125
Design 125
Conclusions 128

Chapter 16
Continuing Educational Opportunities in Complementary Medicine 131
GEORGE R. HAYNES

Chapter 17
Surveys of Complementary and Alternative Medicine .. 139
JACQUELINE C. WOOTON AND ANDREW G. SPARBER

Methodology 140
General Social Trends in the Use of
   Complementary and Alternative Medicine 140
Use of Cancer Therapies 142
Use of Therapies for HIV/AIDS 144
Use of Complementary and Alternative
   Medicine for Miscellaneous Health Categories 147

Contents, continued

    Physician Involvement in Complementary
        and Alternative Medicine 148
    Federal Surveys and Initiatives 150
    Conclusions and Recommendation 150

Chapter 18
Herbs or Homeopathy: What's the Difference? 155
JOYCE C. FRYE

    Background 155
    Indications for Use 156
    Preparation of the Homeopathic Remedy 156
    Dosage 156
    More Information 157

Index 159

Creating an Herbal Formulary for Clinical Practice

Bhaswati Bhattacharya

Setting up and sustaining an herbal formulary in a clinical practice site oriented to conventional medicine requires ambition, patience, and a well-composed toolbox of resources. It is also a tremendous opportunity for providers and patients to learn about the clinical benefits of herbs and to develop a closer relationship during the journey toward better health, things often not emphasized with the prescription of drugs. This project can be one of the most exciting ways for a physician to manifest interest in and commitment to complementary medicine and also educate fellow physicians and health care providers about the applications and prevalence of herbal use among their patients.

BACKGROUND

Most MDs trained in the past two decades were left ignorant of herbal pharmacology during medical school. No training was provided in botany or in the uses, popularity, or clinical research of medicinal herbs. Foxglove, willow bark, and the Pacific yew tree were simply plants from which drugs were formulated. These attitudes still prevail in most medical schools although it is known that most current drugs originated from plants [1].

Logically, most doctors in practice after such training are skeptical about and uncomfortable with using agents they have not been trained to use. The limits of medical programs thus leave us disconnected from the actual health practices of our patient population and create an attitude of arrogance and ignorance that prevents us from learning about our patients and their lives. This attitude also closes us to the possibilities of natural treatment resources around us.

The desire to overcome this limited perspective has led several medical doctors to reorient their practices to include herbal formularies. It has also led to the ongoing education of students and residents about holistic medicine in programs such as the two at Beth Israel Medical Center in New York: the Phillips Family Practice/Institute for Urban Health, which has a Chinese herbal formulary on site, and the Center for Integrative Health Care, which is working to set up a formulary integrated with the hospital under the guidance of Benjamin Kligler. The Program in Integrative Medicine at the University of Arizona is also setting up an herbal pharmacy for use by its fellows and physicians under the guidance of Andrew Weil. In New Mexico, Tieraona Low Dog, an herbalist and midwife before her medical training, has set up a formulary and a video teaching series to accompany herbal practice. Montefiore Medical Center in New York has an active herbal pharmacy created by Marcey Shapiro in the early 1990s and now directed by Ellen Tattelman, who precepts residents and teaches patients and providers while managing the formulary.

Creation of an Herbal Pharmacy: Goals and Purpose

The first step in creating an herbal pharmacy is to establish a well-stated purpose and a set of goals as well as a timeline. The initial purpose of the pharmacy should be stated simply and clearly to the proposal review group:

> to provide a modality of medicinally active products under consultation and with support to a group of patients, some of whom may already be using herbs.

Goals for the pharmacy include providing high-quality, cost-effective herbs to well-informed populations; increasing communication between providers and patients regarding frontier methods of healing chronic medical conditions that have not been helped by conventional methods; supplying patients with safe herbs supplied by investigated companies; creating immense research potential for faculty using herbs clinically; furnishing medical education opportunities for students, residents, and faculty; and increasing the interface between the philosophies and modalities of healers in the community and the world of conventional clinical practice.

The committee that defines the purpose and goals should include the medical director of the site, the nursing supervisor, the residency program director if the project is at a teaching site, a pharmacist consulted frequently by the clinic, and an expert in the practice of herbs. Creation of an adjunct consultation committee should be considered; this would be composed of nonclinical experts who can lend insight and objectivity and may be available to teach. Table 1-1 lists types and examples of specialists that would be valuable members of such a committee.

Types of herbs used in the pharmacy will depend on the background and experience of committee members. The setup and practice of the program will necessarily differ depending on the herbal therapy implemented—Chinese versus Western herbs, Ayurvedic, Native American, homeopathic, or mixed formulations. The philosophy of use will also depend on the practitioners. Some members may envision herbs as a natural substitute for drugs and may use only isolated formulations. Others may view herbs as an extension of the spiritual energy of healing, as herbalists do, and may use them to restore harmony and balance to people with diseases. The philosophy, whether pharmacologic or spiritual, should be clarified, understood, and agreed on by group members so that the setup and formulations can be optimized by the practitioners. If the group is inexperienced with herbs, Western herbs should be tried first and formulations of herbs from another philosophy or medical tradition should be introduced as clinical situations indicate.

Finally, the logistics of setting up and running the pharmacy should be discussed to ascertain whether key resources are available for undertaking the project. How will the herbs be prescribed? Who will be in charge of managing the pharmacy? How will payments be made? Who will be in charge of reordering herbs? Where will the herbs be kept—in the main pharmacy or in a space at the clinic from which they will be dispensed? Who can send an order to the pharmacy? Where will initial funding come from?

Research

After the proposal has been formulated and presented to a local group of key people who support the project vision, project leaders should investigate the environment outside the practice. As with any good research project, homework is necessary. Whose support is required to make the pharmacy happen? Does a strong group of practitioners exist in the area who are absolutely close-minded to the value of herbs in modern clinical practice? The influence of such a group on the project should be assessed shrewdly.

In addition, too many research and clinical projects are initiated in the field of "alternative medicine" that are ignorant of previous research. This is often because mainstream investigators do not know how to access non-mainstream work. Frequently, investigators are also ignorant about what is happening locally, either within the same medical center or the same geographic locale. In addition, some researchers do not have the resources to connect with other researchers' efforts. The most successful clinical projects will be those that are well connected and aware of their social environment.

Consulting with area providers, apothecaries, and herbal pharmacies is the best way to begin. Find out if there is a similar pharmacy in the area and who directs it. If a well-run, reliable, doctor-friendly herbal pharmacy is already established in the area, it may be unproductive to initiate another. In

TABLE 1-1. Types of Specialists to Consult in Setting Up an Herbal Pharmacy

Naturopaths
  Carlo Calabrese (Bothell, WA)
  Michael Murray (Portland, OR)
  Mary Bove (Bridgeport CT)
Pharmacognosists
  Norman Farnsworth (Chicago, IL)
  James A. Duke (Fulton, MD)
  Varro Tyler (West Lafayette, IN)
Pioneers/Clinical Researchers
  Marcey Shapiro (Oakland, CA)
  Andrew Weil (Tucson, AZ)
  Fredi Kronenberg (New York, NY)
Herbalists
  Tieraona Low Dog (Albuquerque, NM)
  Mark Blumenthal (Austin, TX)
  Rob McCaleb (Boulder, CO)
Ethnobotanists
  Michael Balick (New York, NY)
Chinese Herbalists
  Harriet Beinfeld (San Francisco, CA)
  Ted Kaptchuk (Boston, MA)
  Jeffrey Yuen (New York, NY)
  Kevin Ergil (New York, NY)

addition, look in your own medical center's outpatient pharmacy. Pharmacies at many health-care facilities stock Echinacea, St. John's wort (*Hypericum capsulatum*), garlic, saw palmetto, and vitamins, and can order various additional products easily.

Seek out physicians in the area to learn who might support your efforts. Call physicians who have set up herbal pharmacies and find out what obstacles they had to overcome to continue successfully. Try to ascertain whether physicians in your medical center would be open or eager to refer patients to this new formulary for select herbs. Learn about other groups with high concentrations of physicians experienced in the clinical use of herbs, such as the Special Interest Group in Complementary/Alternative Medicine of the American Association of Medical Colleges; the Society of Teachers of Family Medicine; the Interest Group on Alternative and Complementary Practices of the American Public Health Association; the American Holistic Medical Association; and the Humanistic Medicine group of the American Medical Student Association. Nonphysician groups include the American Herbalist Guild, the American Botanical Council, the Herb Research Foundation, and naturopathic schools such as Bastyr University near Seattle, Washington.

Be aware of what is happening in herbal medicine on a national level. The National Institutes of Health (NIH) National Center for Complementary & Alternative Medicine, formerly known as the Office of Alternative Medicine, started in 1992 and proceedings from its founding conference have been published [2]. The center has built a website (http://altmed.od.nih.gov/nccam/), operated an information clearinghouse, and sponsored dozens of conferences. In addition, it has funded the start of 10 specialty centers, several of which are exploring clinical trials of herbs for particular conditions.

REASSESSMENT

After completing field research, the pharmacy's purpose and goals should be reexamined. The effort required to maintain the pharmacy privately in a clinic setting or as an addition to the hospital formulary should be assessed. After initial research and assessment, ascertain whether the pharmacy would provide a needed service to the community of providers and patients. Does a mechanism exist for the pharmacy to sustain itself within the environment? Are there people in the clinical arena who will strongly support or oppose the setup of an herbal pharmacy?

When assessing the goals and purpose of the pharmacy, the project committee must assess the projected profile of the people using the pharmacy. What population of people will use the herbs dispensed? Will medical center personnel be able to purchase from the supply, or will it be available only to patients? Inpatient versus outpatient access should be discussed. Where will the herbs be stored to ensure that only the target population receives them? What does the hospital formulary allow, suggest, or stipulate about herbal treatments being dispensed at your clinic?

If the medical practice is part of a larger medical center, much of the initial effort must be focused on finding allies and supporters of the project. These may be members of the Board of Trustees, select administrative heads, or influential professors. They should be people whose belief in the mission will help overcome future obstacles and who may help locate experts or funding needed for the project.

INTEGRATING HERBS INTO THE MAIN HOSPITAL PHARMACY

Inpatient herb use should include a formal mechanism enabling providers to access and order the herbs. The simplest way to arrange this is to include the herbs as a part of the inpatient pharmacy. The formulary committee most likely already stocks substances such as vitamins and minerals that are medically indicated. The project committee should therefore approach the pharmacy with medical indications for additional vitamins and selected herbs and ask the members to review and evaluate the data. References should be provided from standard medical journals, recent updates, and classic pharmacologic references. Appendices should include naturopathic texts with data on herbs in clinical practice.

OUTPATIENT PHARMACY SETUP

Most practitioners with plans to create an herbal pharmacy setup envision an outpatient setup in their clinical practice group. This endeavor requires greater attention to detail, administrative issues, management, and sustenance of physical space. First, a location should be chosen that is both convenient and secure. A pantry or coat closet that can be locked is ideal. Airflow and moisture in the space should be minimized. An area should be created for drop-down counter space and shelf space. Free wall space can be used to display posters and charts. Anticipate using the space as densely as possible so that the pharmacy can expand without outgrowing the space. Extras include a laptop computer for tracking and accessing information and herbal databases while in the pharmacy area.

Pharmacy logistics must be discussed. Which patient base will be able to use the herbs? Who will manage the pharmacy space and usage? Who will reorder herbs? Where will dispensation tracking be done? Who will collect the monies from payment? Which practitioners can order from the pharmacy? How will prescribing guidelines be conveyed to prescribers, by newsletter, E-mail, or bulletin?

IMPLEMENTATION

After a comprehensive plan and setup have been established and the project is fully supported, it is important to contact the formulary and institution formally and communicate your intention. By this time, the points of resistance, if any, will be known and the committee will have proposed solutions. Common areas of resistance include: closed-mindedness of "scientific" doctors, opposition of nonpharmaceutically pure agents, support for the drug industry, and opponents of alternative medicine in general. These issues are best handled individually using as many evidence-based clinical studies as possible. Appealing to an openness for clinical research positions the pharmacy within the movement toward accumulating good clinical data on the efficacy of herbs for particular clinical conditions.

Administrative criteria must be fulfilled for the pharmacy to meet all the medical guidelines that may concern officials. Advice and suggestions should be solicited regarding how to fulfill the requirements while still manifesting the vision of the herbal formulary. Data on projected usage, physician attitudes, and patient prevalence of use should be provided.

PREPARING THE SPACE

Herbal catalogs should be ordered. Consult experts about which companies they use and try to stick with well-known, well-reputed companies. Table 1-2 provides a list of sources. If you have previous experience with herbs, order your usual catalogs for the pharmacy and request more information about the packaging and processing of their products so that this information is readily available for the formulary committee, the Office of Occupational Safety and Health Administration (OSHA), or interested administrators. Contact the hospital pharmacy to find out which guidelines their new drugs have to meet when they order from a new vendor.

Drugs are monitored by the U.S. Food and Drug Administration. Herbs and vitamins are considered food supplements. Use of herbs in clinical practice will be judged on medical and clinical appropriateness. Therefore, mainstream articles on clinical efficacy and pharmacologic proof of efficacy should be kept on hand. A toxicology manual with chapters on herbal drugs, including an extensive area of herb–drug interactions, is also recommended [3,4].

A series of looseleaf binders can be useful for compiling and tracking information, such as a list of practitioners who can prescribe from the pharmacy and their qualifications in the botanicals/medicines approved by the committee. Another binder should contain criteria that physicians must meet to prescribe from the pharmacy, including botanical courses, rotations, completion of internships with botanists, and continuing medical education (CME) coursework. If the prescribers are all naturopathic doctors or if the clinic is not closely monitored by a mainstream medical center review board, this information may be less critical. Criteria for prescribing privileges might also include internal hands-on training from clinic personnel. A third binder should contain references for each of the herbs included in the pharmacy and current articles pertaining to mainstream clinical trials with herbs.

A binder should also be created to track the herbs prescribed, listing the patient record number, the herb provided, the amount dispensed, the condition for which the herb is dispensed, the amount paid, and the prescriber. Also track the herbs purchased by the pharmacy with dates, amounts, and costs. These basic accounting measures will eliminate many problems and minimize auditing hassles.

Finally, dispensing tools, glass jars, self-sealing plastic bags, and labels should accumulated. Preparation instructions and dosing of herbs should be explained on handouts designed for the patient. Specialized handouts on contraindications related to pregnancy and herb–drug interactions should be prepared and made available.

HERBS TO USE

Which herbs should be included? For a new pharmacy, the best approach is to start with a small formulary of 10 to 12 herbs that will be the most useful for the practice. Focus on chronic ailments for which conventional drugs are not commonly successful in relieving symptoms. Respiratory ailments, women's health problems, dermatologic care, or preventive health supplementation are excellent areas on which to focus. Start with herbs known for low toxicity and drug interactions. Use herbs that are easily available in your area. Be cognizant of the local flora and what medicinal properties they have.

Herbs that work well on the respiratory system and are popular in winter months include mullein (*Verbascum thapsus*), licorice (*Glycyrrhiza glabra*), hyssop (*Hyssopus officinalis*), cherry bark (*Prunus virginiana*), flaxseed (*Linum usitatissimum*), garlic (*Allium sativum*), hops (*Humulus lupulus*), hawthorn (*Crataegus oxyacantha* and *C. monogyna*), skullcap (*Scutellaria laterifolia*), and chamomile (*Matricaria recutita*). Infusins, decoctions, and compresses can be made by the patients to relieve the symptoms of pharyngitis, mild bronchitis, or viral illness.

Women's health issues are an increasing focus for doctors who are providing wellness care to women. Raspberry leaf (*Rubus idaeus*) infusion is a reputed tonic for dysmenorrhea and irregular monthly cycles. It has few side effects and can be easily prepared.

Treatment of dermatologic lesions, such as psoriasis, eczema, or tinea, is often frustrating with steroid preparations or antibiotic gels. Aloe is an herb well known in the southwestern United States, where its gel is used for burns, rashes, and unbroken skin

TABLE 1-2. HERB SUPPLIERS

Company	Location	Phone	Website
Frontier Cooperative Herbs	Norway, IA	319-227-7991	http://www.frontierherb.com
Nature's Way Herbs	Springville, UT	—	http://www.naturesway.com
Tieraona's Herbals	Albuquerque, NM	505-256-3951	—
K'an Herb Company	Scotts Valley, CA	800-543-5233	—
Metagenics	San Clemente, CA	800-692-9400	http://www.metagenics.com

lesions. Turmeric is an herb reputed in the Ayurvedic tradition for its antimicrobial properties and soothing effect. Arnica, especially in the homeopathic formulation, is a common remedy that is widely used in Europe for burns and local inflammation.

Immunostimulants, such as Echinacea, and modulators, such as milk thistle (Silybarum) and Ginkgo biloba, are commonly used in preventive health care. In addition, recent pilot studies stemming from the original National Health and Nutrition Examination Survey [5,6] trial data have shown that vitamins C and E may be helpful in preventing exacerbation of childhood asthma.

EDUCATION

Learn the clinical evidence for herbs used in the pharmacy and develop a sense of how herbalists use those herbs. Begin with a search for recent literature on efficacy and precautions, checking not only in MEDLINE but also in other electronic databases (Table 1-3) [7]. Scan the Internet for relevant information. Find one or two good reference books and read them. Periodicals devoted to the clinical efficacy of herbs and journals covering botanical medicine are increasing. Devise a filing system for collecting and organizing these articles, such as the binder system previously mentioned.

A regular source of education is essential for incoming practitioners who will be using the pharmacy. Courses for physicians are available around the country, either as live CME conferences or on videotape. Recommended readings and self-education methods should be listed. For example, the clinic could organize a self-learning curriculum for physicians that includes reading a selection of introductory articles, watching a series of videos, visiting the local botanical garden, and shadowing an experienced herbalist or attending an herbal preparation workshop [8]. Basic herbal language and terminology should be covered. All practitioners should learn how to prepare herbs as tinctures, decoctions, infusions, teas, salves, and suppositories as part of the practice of herbal medicine. A deeper understanding of the different formulations of natural herbs compared with pills and tinctures is essential for explaining herbal use to patients.

As of 1998, more than 70 conventional medical education programs in the United States provided course offerings focusing on alternative medicine [9]. Many focus on or provide an overview of herbal medicines, thus providing more and more medical students with perspective on other treatment philosophies. As the number of doctors so trained increases, the opportunities for learning how to integrate herbals into clinical practice will also increase. A library of reference books should be set up, perhaps in the pharmacy space or in a reference book room, and should include the classic texts listed in Table 1-4. Software programs that focus on herbs are increasingly available for clinical use. One of the best known is IBIS (*see* Table 1-3), designed by naturopaths for clinical reference and simultaneous tracking.

When dispensing herbs, provide patients with handouts on the herbs prescribed that list the guidelines for their preparation and use and advice about adverse effects. In addition, patients should receive a standard evaluation and assessment form for tracking symptoms and effects of their prescribed herbs.

Educational planning for the pharmacy should include a multidisciplinary consultation committee, which provides a

TABLE 1-3. HERBAL RESEARCH DATABASES

Database	Organization	Website/Email Address
MEDLINE/PubMed	U.S. National Library of Medicine	http://www.ncbi.nlm.nih.gov
IBIS (Interactive BodyMind Information System)	AM'RTA	http://www.teleport.com/~ibis (for demo)
CINAHL (Cumulative Index for Nursing and Allied Health)	CINAHL Information Systems	http://www.cinahl.com/CDir_CDB.html
Planetree Health Resource Center	N/A	http://www.planetreesanjose.org
Toxline	U.S. National Library of Medicine	http://igm.nlm.nih.gov
Herb Research Foundation Library	Herb Research Foundation	http://www.sunsite.unc.edu/herbs/hrinfo.html
AMED: Alternative and Allied Medicine Database	British Medical Library	http:www.krinfo.ch/www/rs/ds/OLD/AMED.html
NAPRAlert	University of Illinois, Chicago Department of Pharmacognosy (Norman Farnsworth)	http://www.fiz-karlsruhe.de/napraler.html
EmBase	Elsevier Science	usembase-f@elsevier.com
American Indian Ethnobotany Database	University of Michigan (Daniel E. Moerman, PhD)	http://www.umd.umich.edu/cgi-bin/herb
CISCOM (Centralized Information Service for Complementary Medicine)	Research Council for Complementary Medicine	rccm@gn.apc.org
Cochrane Collaboration Database of Systematic Reviews	Research Council for Complementary Medicine	rccm@gn.apc.org

Data from Wooton [7].

strong way to enforce quality and investment in the project. This group of qualified personnel should function to advise on herbs, troubleshoot, and lend suggestions particular to your setup. Keep the formulary committee informed and educated as well, as members may be ignorant about the clinical use of herbs. Respect institutional requirements but also challenge rules selectively with the hope of expanding patient care. Keep local pharmacies current on the use of herbs in your clinic.

Common fears regarding herb use will have to be addressed. Explaining herbal pharmacology may validate its use to other physicians. Patients who are open to (or against) using herbs will indicate this immediately when herbal remedies are suggested. If a scientific explanation of herbal versus pharmaceutical use is needed, the following pharmacologic receptor model can be used:

> Pharmaceutical products are formulated using one isolated chemical compound. Most act as ligands that occupy receptors on different tissues of the body, creating pharmacologic effects, which are the desired effective action, and side effects, which are the undesired actions. Herbs contain one or several putative active chemical molecules but also contain precursors and postcursors of those compounds that are directly related chemically to the active compound. These precursors are thought to occupy those receptors in vivo, producing pharmacologic actions that are considered to be side effects. Because they occupy the same pharmacotherapeutic niche but do not have as potent an effect as the active molecule, the side effects are lessened. The active compound can then use the receptors to create the desired actions.
>
> A common example of this principle is the use of carbidopa/levodopa in Parkinsonism. Carbidopa occupies and inhibits the enzyme that converts levodopa outside the central nervous system (CNS) so that levodopa can penetrate the CNS at higher levels and be converted there to the active compound dopamine.

Remember that ongoing training courses are now available for physicians and should be attended regularly by someone in the group for training in botanicals, vitamins, nutritionals, and homeopathy. Much of this training will be in the biomedical pharmaceutical model, but it will also contain clinical practice guidelines essential for ongoing education and practice.

TABLE 1-4. RECOMMENDED TEXTS

Trease and Evans' Pharmacognosy [9]
The Honest Herbal [10]
Botanical Influences on Illness [11]
PDR for Herbal Medicines [12]
The Complete German Commission E Monographs: Therapeutic Guide to Herbal Medicines [13]

EVALUATION AND SUSTENANCE

After dispensing herbs for a given period, monitor usage patterns and make sure that patients are preparing and using the herbs as prescribed. Proper preparation ensures that the appropriate pharmacologic compounds are being included in the substances used by the patients.

Use follow-up surveys and daily symptom diaries to determine actual patient benefit. In addition, periodic follow-up is an excellent way to discover which side effects a patient is experiencing without assessing his or her entire complement of medications. The tracking program should be included in the patient's chart and cross-referenced by medical record number in the pharmacy's dispensation logbooks. Also consider surveying the patient population for usage patterns and the prescribing practitioners for what they actually use. In this way, you can keep the herbs in the clinic well-correlated with the needs of the users.

An excellent tracking system study is underway using participants of the CME course *Botanical Medicine in Modern Clinical Practice* [15]. A team of researchers is compiling actual indications, side effects, and usage patterns as determined by physicians. In addition, participants belong to a "listserv," or email group list, that sends queries and responses regarding botanicals used in ongoing practice.

Maintaining the pharmacy will require ongoing educational efforts and training of other members of the clinical practice. Logbooks should be kept current and key faculty members who will commit to the project for a projected time period should be identified. Resources should be made available to update and continually enrich the knowledge base of these members so that the practice can sustain the regular use of herbs. Encouraging staff and clinic members to obtain their herbals from the pharmacy will educate members, increase turnover of herbal supplies to maintain freshness, and help sustain the financial base of the pharmacy.

RESEARCH

In the same way that we learn about the profile of a new drug through its use in a wider population of patients, we can also expect to learn about herbs and how they can benefit our patients. In addition to the research projects being done through the NIH National Center for Complementary and Alternative Medicine and the appointed specialty centers, dozens of medical centers have now opened a department, center, or project focusing on alternative medicine. Networking with these other groups by exploring their sites on the Internet and attending select conferences and CME programs is an important part of understanding the evolving clinical knowledge base.

LEGAL ASPECTS

Physicians in the United States are licensed by individual states to practice medicine according to the particular rules of the state [16,17]. There is an openness in the legal terminology that physicians may use any tools they need to diagnose, treat, or alleviate suffering. This ambiguity allows physicians the freedom to use herbs judiciously as food supplements. It is important to check state requirements or restrictions and to be aware of the privileges and responsibilities involved in creating an herbal pharmacy.

Financial issues should also be discussed by the committee. Learn which insurance groups cover vitamins, minerals, and food supplements when prescribed by a physician, and inform patients and encourage them to ask their insurance providers. Make sure you have an understanding with your patient about payment for herbs. Accept checks and give receipts for purchases.

Fear of legal repercussions can be handled by including references that support your use of a particular herb regimen in the patient's chart. Highlight and include relevant materials. Track carefully which herbs were prescribed and correlate this information with the master log that lists the lot numbers and dates of all herbs purchased.

CONCLUSIONS

This project is an exciting undertaking for a clinical practice group where clinicians in different areas of the health-care provider spectrum are interested. Herbal medicines will connect your practice with your patients, many of whom are already using these "food supplements." It will also connect practitioners with a gentle healing art and, potentially, the same ecologic, holistic attitude that herbalists have toward using botanicals for healing the human system.

REFERENCES AND RECOMMENDED READING

Recently published papers of particular interest have been highlighted as:
• Of interest
•• Of outstanding interest

1. Grifo F, Newman D, Bhattacharya B, *et al.*: The origins of prescription drugs. In *Biodiversity and Human Health*. Edited by Grifo F, Rosenthal J. Washington, DC: Island Press; 1997:131–163.

2. National Institutes of Health Office of Alternative Medicine: Herbal medicine. In *Alternative Medicine: Expanding Medical Horizons*. Bethesda, MD: National Institutes of Health; 1994:183–206.

3. D'Arcy PF: Adverse reactions and interactions with herbal medicines, part 2: drug interactions. *Adverse Drug React Toxicol Rev* 1993, 12:147–162.

4. Leikin JB, Paloucek FP: *Poisoning and Toxicology Compendium with Symptoms Index: Perspectives on the Safety of Herbal Medicines*. Cleveland: Lexi-Comp, Inc; 1998.

5. Schwarz J, Weiss ST: Dietary factors and their relation to respiratory symptoms: the second National Health and Nutrition Examination Survey. *Am J Epidemiol* 1990, 132:67.

6. Bucca C, Rolla G, Oliva A, Farina JC: Effect of vitamin C on histamine bronchial responsiveness of patients with allergic rhinitis. *Ann Allergy* 1990, 65:311.

7. Wooton J: Directory of databases for research into alternative and complementary medicine. *J Altern Complement Med* 1997, 3:179–190.

8. Girard-Couture C: Integrating natural medicines into allopathic hospital pharmacies. *Altern Complement Ther* 1998, 5:241–251.

9. Bhattacharya B: MD programs in the United States with complementary and alternative medicine education: an ongoing listing. *J Altern Complement Med* 1998, 4:325–335.

10. Evans WC: *Trease and Evan's Pharmacognosy* edn 14. Philadelphia: WB Saunders; 1996.

11. Tyler VE: *The Honest Herbal*. Binghamton, NY: Haworth Press; 1993.

12. Werbach MR, Murray MT: *Botanical Influences on Illness: A Sourcebook of Clinical Research*. Tarzana, CA: Third Line Press; 1994.

13. *PDR for Herbal Medicine* edn 1. Montvale, NJ: Medical Economics Company; 1998.

14. Blumenthal M, Busse WR, Goldberg A, *et al.*: *The Complete German Commission E Monographs: Therapeutic Guide to Herbal Medicine*. Boston, MA: Integrative Medicine Communications; 1998.

15. *Botanical Medicine in Modern Clinical Practice*. CME coursebook. New York: Columbia University, 1998.

16. Cohen MH: *Complementary and Alternative Medicine: Legal Boundaries and Regulatory Perspectives*. Baltimore: Johns Hopkins University Press; 1998.

17. Pinco RG: The evolving status of herbals and phytomedicines in the United States. In *Medicinal Plants: Their Role in Health and Biodiversity*. Edited by Tomlinson TR, Akerele O. Philadelphia: University of Pennsylvania Press; 1998.

Ten Most Common Herbs In Clinical Practice

Michael D. Cirigliano

In recent years, the use of herbal remedies by the public has increased dramatically, which has made it imperative that health-care providers be knowledgeable about these products, including their uses and potential side effects. Many have become widely accepted and used by the public, whereas others have remained in obscurity. In the recently released English translation of the German Commission E Monographs [1••], a survey of the most popular herbal remedies as indicated by annual herbal supplement sales in natural food stores in the United States was undertaken by Richman and Witkowski [2]. Table 2-1 illustrates their findings. The herbal products listed are those with the highest levels of sales in the health-food market based on survey questionnaires from 100 stores and reflecting sales from 1996 projected on the first 2 months of 1997 [1••]. Since this study was published, several herbs have increased in popularity and moved up the list while others have become less popular.

In this chapter, the ten herbal treatments most likely to be encountered by the practicing health-care provider are reviewed. In addition, those herbal remedies that show the greatest promise from a clinical perspective are also discussed. Although this overview is not exhaustive, the more essential characteristics of each herbal treatment are covered and a discussion of clinical usage and guidelines follows to assist the clinician when making decisions about the integration of herbal treatments into practice. Although much needed research has begun on the proper clinical use and efficacy regarding herbal remedies, further needed study will, it is hoped, occur to allow a scientific and rational approach to the use of herbal remedies in the coming years.

SPECIFIC HERBAL REMEDIES

Echinacea

As noted in Table 2-1, Echinacea is the most popular herb in the United States and has generated $300 million in sales annually [3]. Echinacea is native to Kansas, Nebraska, and Missouri [4••]. Historically, Echinacea has been used for topical wound-healing and to stimulate the immune system [4••]. Current thought holds that the major active components of Echinacea include a glycoside (echinacoside) and high-molecular-weight polysaccharides, which may account for its wound-healing and immunostimulant properties [5]. These extracts appear to exert their effects by stimulating phagocytosis and by increasing cellular respiratory activity and the mobility of leukocytes [5]. One component of Echinacea, arabinogalactan, was effective in activating macrophages to cytotoxicity and inducing macrophages to produce tumor necrosis factor, interleukin-1 (IL-1), and interferon β-2 [5]. Despite these findings, no single compound appears to be responsible for the plant's activity [4••].

In recent years, a great deal of study has been devoted to the immunostimulant activity of Echinacea. In vivo immunostimulant activity in mice has been documented for Echinacea, noted by enhancement of phagocytosis and by increased serum elimination of carbon particles (*ie*, carbon clearance test) [6]. In vitro immunostimulant activity has been noted with phagocytosis enhancement and tumor necrosis factor secretion stimulation in human macrophages and lymphocytes, which is believed to be the reason for its nonspecific T-cell activation [7]. Immunostimulant properties are thought to result partly from binding of the polysaccharide fractions to carbohydrate receptors on the cell surface of T-cell lymphocytes, which results in nonspecific T-cell activation [8].

In humans, Echinacea has been used for its action on cell-mediated immunity. In one study, administration of a single dose subcutaneously resulted in stimulation of cell-mediated immunity, when given with a 1-week "free" interval after administration [9]. In contrast, this same study demonstrated that daily administration depressed the immune system. Unfortunately, many human trials that were done in the past were not randomized, controlled, double-blind trials. In other human studies, Echinacea was evaluated for its effects on upper respiratory tract infections; statistically significant decreases in symptoms and duration of flulike illness were noted [10]. These effects appeared to depend on dosage. In yet another human study, 108 volunteers with a history of recurrent upper respiratory infections had less frequent and less severe recurrences when taking Echinacea [11,12]. Almost all human studies, unfortunately, have been flawed by poor study design and quality. Melchart *et al.* [13] published a meta-analysis of 26 controlled trials on the immunostimulant effects of Echinacea.

Unfortunately, none of the trials is of sufficient methodological quality to be conclusive [14•]. In one of these studies, Dorn [15] studied 100 patients with acute flulike infections who were taking 30 mL of Echinacea preparation compared with placebo. Seven cold symptoms (*eg*, lethargy, limb pain, headache, rhinitis, cough, sore throat, and pharyngeal redness) were rated; those taking Echinacea for 8 days were found to have a statistically significant decrease compared with those in the placebo group. Dorn suggested that, based on these data, taking a suitable Echinacea preparation when symptoms first appear can, "in favorable cases," shorten the duration of a common cold by 25% to 33% (Figure 2-1) [15].

Echinacea has been approved by the German Commission E [1••] for adjunct therapy for influenza-like infections, colds, chronic infections of the respiratory tract and lower urinary tract, and topically for poorly healing wounds and chronic ulcerations.

Side effects appear to be rare. Some may experience short-term fever, nausea, and vomiting, and allergic reactions are possible. According to the German Commission E [1••], use of Echinacea should not exceed 8 continuous weeks of use. Patients with a history of tuberculosis, autoimmune disorders such as multiple sclerosis, and those with HIV infection should not use Echinacea because of its immunomodulating properties. No known drug interactions involving Echinacea have been documented, but some studies suggest possible depletion

TABLE 2-1. TOP HERB SUPPLEMENTS SOLD IN NATURAL FOOD STORES IN THE UNITED STATES IN 1997

1997	1996
1. Echinacea	1
2. Garlic	2
3. Ginkgo biloba	4
4. Goldenseal (*Hydrastis canadensis*)	5
5. Saw palmetto	9
6. (tie) Aloe	12
(tie) Asian Ginseng (*Panax ginseng*)	3
7. Cat's claw	14
8. *Astragalus*	27
9. Cayenne	11
10. Siberian ginseng (*Elutherococcus senticosus*)	7
11. Bilberry	23
12. Cranberry	18
13. Dong quai (*Angelica sinensens*)	17
14. Grapeseed extract	15
15. Cascara sagrada (*Rhamnus carolinia*)	10
16. St. John's wort	n/a
17. Valerian	13
18. Ginger	18
19. Feverfew (*Chrysanthemum parthenium*)	23

Adapted from Richman and Witkowski [2]; with permission.

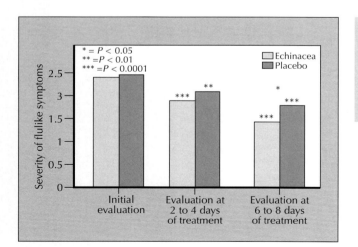

FIGURE 2-1. In a randomized, double-blind study, 100 patients with acute flulike symptoms were evaluated comparing an Echinacea preparation with placebo. Seven cold symptoms were rated for severity using a semiquantitative scoring system. These symptoms included lethargy, limb pain, headache, rhinitis, cough, sore throat, and pharyngeal redness. Each column represents mean values for 50 patients. (*Adapted from* Dorn [15].)

of vitamin E stores. Concurrent use of a multivitamin may be prudent. Because hepatotoxic effects may be associated with persistent use, Echinacea should not be taken with other known hepatotoxic drugs (anabolic steroids, amiodarone, methotrexate, or ketoconazole) [16•]. Because the safety of Echinacea has not been established in pregnancy and lactation, use of Echinacea during pregnancy should be avoided.

In summary, although animal studies support some of the uses for Echinacea, further well-designed clinical studies using standardized preparations and larger numbers of patients are needed to verify its safety and efficacy. The German Commission E [1••] recommends a daily dose of 6 to 9 mL of the expressed juice or 2 to 5 g of dried root.

Garlic

Garlic is one of the most studied herbal remedies likely to be encountered in clinical practice. Historically, it has been used to treat leprosy, to cure deafness, and for treatment of earaches, flatulence, and scurvy [4••]. More recently, medical interest has focused on its potential lipid-lowering qualities, antihypertensive effects, and antiplatelet activity. Allicin, formed from the dimerization of 2-propenesulfenic acid, is believed to be responsible for some of the pharmacologic activity of the plant [4••]. This component of garlic is thought to act as an antioxidant by increasing the levels of catalase and glutathione peroxidase, both of which are antioxidant enzymes. In addition, diallyl disulfide, which represents a breakdown product of allicin, has been shown in animal studies to lower cholesterol [17]. Garlic is thought to lower serum cholesterol and triglycerides along with increasing fibrinolysis [18]. The lipid-lowering effects attributed to garlic are thought to result from a reduction in triacylglycerol biosynthesis through a reduction in tissue concentrations of NADPH and from inactivation of enzymes involved in lipid synthesis through an interaction with enzyme thiol groups [17,19].

Recently, several randomized, placebo-controlled trials have studied the efficacy of garlic in lowering cholesterol. Two meta-analyses of numerous randomized placebo-controlled trials found cholesterol levels decreased by as much as 9% to 12% and triglyceride levels decreased from 8% to 27% with use of garlic [20,21]. In two other randomized, controlled trials, no influence on serum lipoproteins, cholesterol absorption, or cholesterol synthesis was noted with used of garlic supplements [22,23]. Unfortunately, these studies were both small and some controversy exists regarding the particular garlic supplements used in the studies. In addition to its lipid-lowering effects, some data also suggest that garlic may have mild hypotensive effects with use [24]. Antithrombotic activity has also been noted; studies show a decreased serum fibrinogen concentration and inhibition of platelet aggregation [24,25].

Garlic has been approved by the German Commission E [1••] as adjunct therapy to diet in lowering levels of lipids in blood and for preventative measures in age-dependent vascular changes.

Although garlic is considered relatively safe, adverse effects have occurred with use including nausea, vomiting, and diarrhea. In addition, use with warfarin sodium and other "antiplatelet" drugs may increase the risk of bleeding. One case report exists in the literature noting a spontaneous spinal epidural hematoma in an 87-year-old man using garlic [26]. Other reports exist regarding elevated INRs in patients recently started on garlic [16•]. Garlic may reduce blood glucose levels and therefore should be used with caution in patients on hypoglycemic agents.

In summary, despite conflicting data regarding efficacy, garlic appears to have potential uses for lowering cholesterol and for modest lowering of blood pressure. Usual dosages are 300 mg, taken two to three times daily, standardized to 1.3% allicin.

Ginkgo

The ginkgo tree is the world's oldest surviving tree species and its medicinal use goes back at least 5000 years [5]. Historically, it has been used to treat asthma and chilblains (*ie*, swelling of the hands and feet from exposure to damp cold)[4]. More recently, a concentrated, standardized extract of ginkgo leaves known as Egb 761 has been marketed and used in numerous studies [27]. Two groups of active constituents are felt to be most responsible for the positive effects of ginkgo. These are the terpene lactones and ginkgo flavone glycosides [28], which are thought to have inhibitory effects on platelet aggregation and platelet activation factor. They have antioxidant properties and are thought to improve circulatory perfusion by dilating arteries and capillaries [28]. Noted antioxidant properties appear to require the synergistic action of the flavonoids, terpenoids, and organic acids, which are all found in the extract Egb 761 [29].

Many clinical trials have reported diminished symptoms of cerebrovascular insufficiency with use of Egb 761 [30,31]. In addition to cerebrovascular effects, improved peripheral circulation has been observed in patients using this extract [32]. In a large study done in 1997 and published in the *JAMA*, Egb 761 was studied in a placebo-controlled, double-blind, randomized trial for 1 year with positive findings in the treatment of dementia [33]. In this study, cognition and social functioning in patients with mild to moderate dementia secondary to Alzheimer's disease or multi-infarct dementia were stabilized and in some cases improved with the use of ginkgo extract. Other studies have noted an improvement in mountain sickness in patients taking ginkgo extract [34] and it has also been used with some success in patients with depression [35].

Ginkgo extract has been approved by the German Commission E [1••] for symptomatic treatment of disturbed performance in organic brain syndrome, including primary degenerative dementia and dementia attributed to vascular causes. It is also approved in Germany for use in peripheral arterial occlusive disease and for vertigo and tinnitus.

Ingestion of ginkgo extract has not been associated with severe side effects [4••]. In fact, adverse events from clinical trials did not differ from those in placebo groups. Some may experience headache, dizziness, heart palpitations, and gastrointestinal upset [4••]. Case reports have noted spontaneous hyphema in a man aged 70 years and spontaneous bilateral subdural hematomas secondary to use of ginkgo extract [36,37]. Given this, use with warfarin sodium and other nonsteroidal anti-inflammatory drugs

(NSAIDs) should be avoided until further study confirms its safe concomitant use.

In summary, significant numbers of studies show promise for the use of ginkgo extract Egb 761 in the treatment of dementia, cerebrovascular insufficiency, peripheral vascular disease, and even mountain sickness. A daily dosage of 120 mg/d in two or three divided doses standardized to contain 6% terpene lactones and 24% ginkgo flavone glycosides of Egb 761 extract have been used.

Saw Palmetto

Saw palmetto has been used for many years to treat genitourinary problems including increases in sperm production, in breast size, and in sexual vigor [4••]. It has also been used historically as a mild diuretic and against prostatic enlargement. More recently, interest has focused on saw palmetto and its effects on benign prostatic enlargement. It is currently thought that sterol components (including beta-sitosterol, campesterol and stigmasterol) are most important with regard to saw palmetto's activity on the prostate [38]. Additional components of importance include free fatty acids and long-chain alcohols. The mechanism of action for saw palmetto is thought to result from a significant decrease in prostatic nuclear androgen and estrogen receptors [39]. Saw palmetto extract inhibits the enzyme 5-α-reductase, thus blocking the conversion of testosterone to dihydroxytestosterone [40]. In addition, saw palmetto blocks uptake of testosterone and dihydroxytestosterone by the prostate. Saw palmetto has also been shown to inhibit the formation of phospholipase A_2 and 5-lipoxygenase enzymes, thus decreasing production of arachidonic acid [41].

In recent years, numerous studies have been undertaken to evaluate the efficacy of saw palmetto for the treatment of benign prostatic enlargement (Figure 2-2) [42]. In a recent systematic review in *JAMA*, Wilt *et al.* [43•] reviewed 18 randomized, controlled trials involving 2939 men. They concluded that use of saw palmetto extract improved urologic symptoms and flow measures and that, compared with finasteride, saw palmetto produced similar improvement in urinary tract symptoms and urinary flow and was associated with fewer adverse treatment events [43•]. One study compared therapy with finasteride to that with saw palmetto for 6 months and found similar significant improvements in the International Prostate Symptom Score, quality of life, and peak urinary flow rate [44]. Notably, saw palmetto extract did not appear to cause impotence or alter prostate-specific antigen levels. In another study however, α-1 antagonists appeared to be more effective than saw palmetto extract [45].

Saw palmetto has been approved by the German Commission E [1••] for urination problems associated with benign prostatic hyperplasia.

Adverse side effects with use of saw palmetto appear to be minimal and usually involve only mild gastrointestinal upset [46]. The recommended dosage is 160 mg twice daily of extract standardized to contain between 85% and 95% fatty acids and sterols [14].

Ginseng

Ginseng in its various species represents one of the most popular herbal remedies in the world. It has been estimated that as many as 6 million Americans use this herbal treatment for its reported beneficial effects [4••]. For more than 2000 years, various forms of this plant have been used for medicinal purposes [4••]. In fact, the ginseng genus *Panax* derives from the Greek word "all healing" and has been used throughout the centuries to help with aging, cancer, and bleeding disorders [4••]. Most recently, ginseng has been touted as an "adaptogen" that provides protection from mental and physical stress and fatigue, enhances sexual performance, and improves other age-related complaints [5].

Several different species of ginseng exist, including *Panax quinquefolius* (American ginseng), *Panax ginseng* (Korean or Chinese ginseng), and *Eleutherococcus senticosus* (Siberian ginseng). Different species possess different properties; the clinician should be aware of the effects of each species. The most important active constituents of ginseng are likely the triterpenoid saponins, collectively known as ginsenosides [47]. The many properties attributed to ginseng appear to be related to its ability to augment adrenal steroidogenesis through an indirect action on the pituitary gland [4••]. Ginseng is thought to have "adaptogenic" qualities that promote a nonspecific increase in resistance to the noxious effects of physical, chemical, or biologic stress [4••]. Ginseng is thought to increase muscle stimulation by nerve impulses, modify brain-wave tracings, and affect the hypothalamic–pituitary–adrenal axis, which may be responsible for its reported antifatigue activity [47]. In addition, ginseng

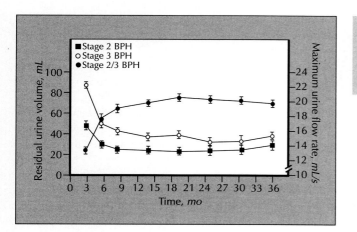

FIGURE 2-2. In a study by Bach [42], saw palmetto was administered to three cohorts of patients with varied degrees of benign prostatic hypertrophy (BPH) over a 3-year period and measures of residual urine volume and maximum flow rate were obtained. (*Adapted from* Bach [42]; with permission.)

appears to promote sparing of glycogen use in exercising muscle [48]. Many believe that ginseng exerts a balancing effect on the hypothalamic–pituitary–adrenal axis [47]. Ginseng's ability to promote secretion of adrenocorticotropic hormone (ACTH) appears to be the means by which it exerts this balance [47]. Recent research has led to the conclusion that ginseng may promote release of nitric oxide, thus leading to enhanced antioxidant activity and vasodilatory effect [49]. Ginseng also appears to have the ability to lower blood sugar levels [16•].

Unfortunately, much of the literature involving ginseng in human trials is of poor methodological quality and offers little value. Several studies, including a 3-month randomized, controlled trial showing a significant increase in "quality of life" scores in users of ginseng [50], have shown benefit from the use of ginseng. In another study, volunteers who took ginseng had a statistical improvement in their ability and speed when performing mathematical calculations [51]. Other studies have noted increased physical performance and reduced fatigue in patients taking ginseng [52].

In one study, 30 patients undergoing bypass surgery received a cardioplegic solution containing ginseng extract. Enhanced recovery of cardiac hemodynamic performance and significantly reduced mitochondrial swelling during the period of ischemia was noted [53]. Additionally, ginseng has shown positive results in a double-blind, placebo-controlled study of 36 newly diagnosed patients with diabetes [54].

Ginseng has been approved by the German Commission E [1••] for use as a tonic for invigoration and fortification in times of fatigue and debility and for declining capacity for work and concentration [2].

Side effects noted include hypertension, insomnia, headache, and skin eruptions [4••]. Several case reports have suggested that ginseng may possess estrogenic activity and may cause vaginal bleeding and even mastalgia with diffuse breast nodularity [55,56]. Use in patients with hormonally driven tumors should be questioned because of this theoretical concern. Because ginseng may possess some antiplatelet activity, it should be avoided in patients taking warfarin sodium or other NSAIDs [16•]. Patients on hypoglycemic agents should be cautioned about use of ginseng and its possibility of lowering serum glucose. Because of its stimulant activity, ginseng has been reported to exacerbate the symptoms of manic depression.

In summary, some studies appear to support the beneficial effects of ginseng. Certainly, more well-designed clinical studies are needed to verify these findings. The German Commission E [1••] recommends a daily dose of 1 to 2 g of root or equivalent preparations. Preparations should be standardized to provide 10 mg of ginsenosides [5].

St. John's Wort

Although St. John's wort has always been a popular herbal remedy, it was not until 1997, when St. John's wort was featured in an article in *Newsweek* magazine and later on the ABC News program *20/20* that sales skyrocketed. As a result, sales of the herb that year totaled $47.8 million [1••]. Since then, St. John's wort has become one of the most popular herbal remedies in the country. It has been used since the Middle Ages primarily for its anti-inflammatory and healing properties [4••]. Current interest is focused on its antidepressant and anxiolytic properties (*see* Chapter 4). In 1993, 2.7 million prescriptions were written for St. John's wort in Germany [57]. In fact, physicians in Germany prescribe it four times more often than fluoxetine hydrochloride [58]. Although much interest has been focused on hypericin and pseudohypericin as being the most important constituents, recent study has addressed other components, including flavonoids and xanthones [57].

The exact mechanism of action in St. John's wort for treatment of depression is not known. Originally, it was thought that its major action was as a monoamine oxidase (MAO) inhibitor. This, however, has recently been challenged and some clinicians suggest that St. John's wort may in fact possess more activity as a selective serotonin reuptake inhibitor (SSRI) [59]. In humans, numerous studies have noted a positive effect in treatment of depression with St. John's wort extract (Figure 2-3) [60]. In one meta-analysis, 23 randomized trials evaluating over 1700 patients with mild to moderate depression compared St. John's wort to placebo and other conventional antidepressants [61]. These results found St. John's wort to be significantly superior to placebo and "similarly effective" as conventional antidepressants. Fewer side effects were noted in patients taking St. John's wort when compared with those taking more standard treatments.

St. John's wort has been approved by the German Commission E [1••] for psychovegetative disturbances, depressive moods, anxiety, and nervous unrest.

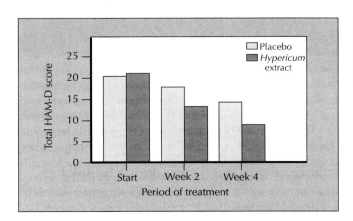

FIGURE 2-3. In a placebo-controlled, double-blind study in 101 depressed patients, *Hypericum* extract was administered daily and compared with placebo for 4 weeks. (*Adapted from* Hänsgen and Vesper [60].)

Side effects associated with use of St. John's wort extract appear to be mainly related to its association with photosensitivity. Patients should avoid excessive sun exposure while taking St. John's wort. In addition, although its exact mechanism of action remains unknown, some believe that St. John's wort possesses MAO inhibitor properties. Thus, use with other psychoactive agents including SSRIs or other MAO inhibitor agents should be avoided due to the theoretical risk of precipitating serotonin syndrome, which can lead to mental status changes, muscle rigidity, hyperreflexia, hyperthermia, and tachycardia. No dietary restrictions seem necessary while using St. John's wort. In controlled trials, no side effects were noted (including abnormalities on electroencephalograms or in laboratory studies) after 6 weeks of treatment [4••]. Usual dosage is 300 mg, three times daily of an extract standardized to 0.3% hypericin [14].

Valerian

For centuries, valerian has been used as a sedative. Approximately 50 tons of valerian are sold yearly in France [4••]. It is thought that the active components of valerian are the valepotriates and valeric acid [47]. In addition to its use as a sedative, valerian has been used for migraine headaches, insomnia, hysteria, fatigue, and intestinal cramps [47]. Valerian's actions are considered secondary to inhibition of the enzyme system responsible for the catabolism of gamma aminobutyric acid (GABA) in the brain [62]. Increased GABA concentrations are associated with a decrease in central nervous system (CNS) activity [46]. Components of valerian also bind to the same receptors as benzodiazepines, but with less affinity and milder clinical effects [63]. In human trials, several placebo-controlled crossover trials have noted improved sleep quality and decreased sleep latency with use of valerian [64,65].

Valerian has been approved by the German Commission E [1••] for restlessness and sleeping disorders based on nervous conditions.

Side effects and toxicity appear to be low with use of valerian. Several side effects have been noted, however, including headaches, excitability, uneasiness, and cardiac disturbances [4••]. Recommended dosages are between 150 and 300 mg of valerian extract standardized to 0.8% valeric acid [47].

Ginger

Another herbal remedy with centuries of use throughout the world is ginger. It has been used as a flavoring agent, an aid to digestion, and to treat motion sickness and relieve nausea [4••]. Current interest involves use of ginger for the treatment of motion sickness, hyperemesis gravidarum, and arthritis. The active components of ginger are thought to include volatile oils composed of shogaol and gingerols [4••]. Gingerols and shogaol are noted to have cardiotonic activity [5]. Gingerols are noted to have analgesic, sedative, and gastrointestinal tract motility effects [66].

In human trials, mixed results have been noted with the use of ginger for motion sickness. In one study, it was reported to be effective as a prophylactic against seasickness [67]. A group of 80 naval cadets was given either ginger or placebo and maintained symptom reports. After 4 hours, 1 g of ginger was found to be superior to placebo in reducing vomiting, cold sweating, nausea, and vertigo. In another controlled trial, ginger was found to be more effective for motion sickness than dimenhydrate [68]. In that study, 36 patients used 100 mg of dimenhydrate or ginger and were then placed in a motorized revolving chair. Although those patients taking either placebo or dimenhydrate could only remain in the chair for less than 6 minutes, one half of those patients who took ginger were able to remain on the revolving chair until the end of the study [68]. In other studies, ginger was used for the treatment of hyperemesis gravidarum with positive results. Several studies however, refute positive claims regarding motion sickness and its improvement with ginger intake.

Ginger has been approved by the German Commission E [1••] for dyspepsia and for prevention of motion sickness.

Ginger has very few noted side effects. No reports of severe toxicity in humans have been published [5]. According to the German Commission E [1••], use of ginger should not be considered in patients with gallstones due to its possible cholagogic properties. Because of its demonstrated in vitro antiplatelet action and its hypoglycemic activity, use in patients on anticoagulation therapy or patients taking hypoglycemic agents should be avoided [4••].

In summary, studies appear to support the use of ginger for the treatment of motion sickness and nausea. Dosages of ginger range from 250 mg to 1 g of powdered root several times per day [14].

Kava

Kava and its medicinal uses were first described in Western literature by the crew of Captain James Cook in 1768 during their travels to the Pacific [47]. The kava plant is indigenous to the islands of the South Pacific [4••]. It has been used in that region as a ceremonial drink that promotes relaxation [4••]. Other historic uses for kava include for treatment of uterine inflammations, headaches, colds, and rheumatisms. It has also been used as a sedative and aphrodisiac [4••]. Current indications are that the most pharmaceutically active components of kava are the kava lactones [47]. Other compounds within the plant may also be responsible for the sedative and anxiolytic activities of kava [47].

The mechanism of action of kava is not fully understood. Studies in animals have shown that kavalactones modify receptor domains rather than interact specifically with receptor-binding sites [47]. It is also thought that the kavalactones may act primarily on the limbic system to produce its effects [47]. Studies have demonstrated that GABA-A receptors are upregulated by kava use [69]. Notably, animal studies have demonstrated no loss of effectiveness with continued use, unlike other standard pharmaceutical anxiolytics [47].

Numerous trials in humans have shown a positive effect on anxiety and insomnia with the use of kava, which has led to its being one of the most popular sleeping aids in Europe [70]. In one randomized, placebo-controlled, double-blind trial, patients were given standardized kava extract or placebo [71]. Those treated with kava had a significant reduction of symptoms after 1 week of therapy as noted by the Hamilton Anxiety Scale (HAM-A) [71]. More than six controlled, double-blind studies have been published on the therapeutic efficacy of kava in patients [72]. In a study comparing kava extract with standard benzodiazepine therapy over 6 weeks, no statistically significant differences were noted in the degree of improvement achieved (Figure 2-4) [73] with all three agents used.

Kava has been approved by the German Commission E [1] for treatment of conditions of nervous anxiety, stress and restlessness.

Side effects with use of kava were evaluated in an observational study looking at 4049 patients who took 105 mg/d of extract standardized to 70% kavalactones. An incidence of 1.5% side effects was noted and involved mainly gastrointestinal complaints and allergic skin reactions [74]. Prolonged use of kava can cause a transient yellow discoloration of the skin known as kava dermopathy [4••]. This condition is reversible with discontinuation of kava. Case reports of extrapyramidal side effects have also been reported in the literature with use of kava; however, no lasting side effects were seen after discontinuation of use [75]. Use of kava should be avoided in patients already taking prescription anxiolytic agents. One case report notes coma in a patient using kava while also taking alprazolam [76]. Caution should also be used in patients who drink alcohol and take barbiturates. The German Commission E [1••] recommends limiting use to no more than 3 months without medical advice. Kava has the potential to adversely affect motor reflexes and judgment for patients when driving or operating heavy machinery [2]. Intake of higher-than-recommended dosages of kava should be discouraged.

In summary, several studies in humans support use of kava for anxiety-related conditions. As with most herbal remedies, however, more well-designed clinical research is needed to confirm its safety and efficacy, especially with long-term use. Most studies used dosages of between 60 and 120 mg of kavalactones daily [72].

Milk Thistle

Milk thistle has been used as an herbal remedy for almost 2000 years [77•]. Long used as a remedy for liver disorders, recent studies indicate significant interest and use by the general public [78]. Currently, many use milk thistle for disorders of the liver including chronic conditions such as hepatitis C and cirrhosis. It is believed that the most active ingredient of milk thistle is silymarin, which consists of four isomers: silybinin, isosilybinin, silydianin, and silychristin [72]. Silybinin (the most biologically active component) is thought to have antioxidant properties [77•]. It inhibits lipid peroxidation of hepatocyte, microsomal, and erythrocyte membranes in rats and protects against injury by suppressing hydro-gen peroxide and super oxide anions [77•]. Silybinin also increases hepatocyte protein synthesis by stimulating ribosomal RNA polymerase [79].

Animal studies have noted that silymarin protects the liver against hepatotoxins, including drugs, mushroom poisoning, viruses, and radiation [14]. In one randomized, double-blind, placebo-controlled trial in humans, the 4-year mortality rate decreased by 30% in patients treated for 2 years with silymarin. These benefits appeared to be most apparent in patients with alcohol-related cirrhosis [80]. In another study, patients with chronic active hepatitis who received 1 week of therapy with silymarin were noted to have decreased levels of serum transaminases and bilirubin values [81].

Milk thistle has been approved by the German Commission E [1••] for use in toxic liver damage and for supportive treatment in chronic inflammatory liver disease and hepatic cirrhosis.

No contraindications or side effects with use of milk thistle have been published. Some reports of mild diarrhea, allergic reactions, and urticaria have been noted. Use in patients with severe or decompensated cirrhosis should be avoided [82]. In addition, patients with diabetes should monitor blood sugar levels carefully, because silymarin may lower blood sugar levels [83].

In summary, silymarin appears to be effective in treating acute and chronic viral and drug-, alcohol-, and toxin-induced hepatitis [76]. More study is needed, however, because of the quality of many of the studies involved with this herbal remedy. Common dosages of silymarin involve 140 mg capsules, standardized to 70% silymarin, two or three times daily [14].

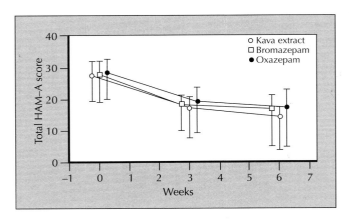

FIGURE 2-4. Kava extract compared with standard benzodiazepine therapy over a 6-week period using the Hamilton Anxiety Scale (HAM-A). (*Adapted from* Woelk *et al.* [73]; with permission.)

INTEGRATION OF HERBAL REMEDIES INTO CLINICAL PRACTICE

As knowledge of herbal remedies becomes more readily available to practicing clinicians, guidelines for their use must be developed to aid in the judicious use of these treatments. Recently, several clinical guidelines were published in *JAMA* [84•]. Although general in nature and not evidence-based, these guidelines represent an initial attempt to aid the clinician in helping patients make rational decisions regarding their own care and especially with regard to the integration of herbal treatments. As time passes, pharmaceutical companies and major drug manufacturers are beginning to market standardized herbal preparations. This will undoubtedly make the job of the physician much easier when using herbal remedies in clinical practice. Unfortunately, many sources of herbal products are still subject to lack of quality control and substandard manufacturing. Patients must be aware that the herbal remedies that they currently buy may, in fact, contain contaminants and *not* contain the herbal ingredients desired.

For example, in Table 2-2, 23 ginseng preparations were analyzed and total panaxoside concentrations were measured [85]. In 10 preparations, no panaxoside was detected. The varied concentrations of panaxoside indicate the need for more rigid control and quality assurance.

Although many of the herbal remedies already mentioned have significant amounts of human data and studies to back up claims made in support of their use, it is quite evident that more well-designed studies are needed to confirm safety and efficacy for clinical use. Table 2-3 illustrates several key points important to the physician regarding herbal treatment use. These guidelines, although conservative, are warranted if we as clinicians follow the principle of "first do no harm."

Herbal treatments have significant potential for adding to the existing armamentarium of therapeutic agents. Clinicians must be aware that due to a lack of adequate information on efficacy and toxicity, advice will remain imperfect and a matter of judgment [86•]. Advice should be given in such a fashion that is congruent with the patient's personal needs and in the physician's best judgment given available knowledge. As new clinical trials come to light, physicians will have an ever-increasing knowledge base allowing the prudent use of herbal remedies in clinical practice.

TABLE 2-2. COMPARISON OF INDIVIDUAL AND TOTAL PANAXOSIDE CONTENT OF ROOTS AND COMMERCIAL PRODUCTS

Sample	Individual Panaxoside Concentration, mg									Total Panaxoside Concentrations per 250-mg Sample, mg
	Ro	Rb1	Rb2	Rc	Rd	Re	Rf	Rg1	Rg2	
Root	—	0.79	—	0.58	0.50	0.29	0.53	—	0.57	3.26
Root	—	1.2	3.7	—	—	1.5	—	1.2	—	7.6
Root	—	1.8	—	2.2	0.38	.067	1.8	—	—	6.86
Root	None	None	None	None	None	None	None	None	None	
Root	0.49	0.28	—	0.29	0.42	0.13	0.19	—	—	1.78
Root	0.36	0.8	0.18	0.32	—	—	0.27	—	—	1.93
Soft gelatin capsule	—	0.86	—	.069	—	—	—	—	0.31	1.86
Soft gelatin capsule	—	0.30	—	—	0.77	—	0.32	—	—	1.39
Tablet	None	None	None	None	None	None	None	None	None	
Tablet	None	None	None	None	None	None	None	None	None	
Tablet	None	None	None	None	None	None	None	None	None	
Dry-filled capsules	0.42	0.46	0.10	0.26	—	0.17	0.40	—	—	1.8
Dry-filled capsules	0.42	0.22	—	0.44	0.31	0.10	0.17	—	—	1.66
Extracts	None	None	None	None	None	None	None	None	None	
Extracts	None	None	None	None	None	None	None	None	None	
Extracts	—	0.15	0.16	0.16	0.10	0.10	0.30	—	—	0.97
Granules and powders	None	None	None	None	None	None	None	None	None	
Granules and powders	—	0.36	—	—	—	0.28	—	—	0.29	0.91
Granules and powders	None	None	None	None	None	None	None	None	None	
Granules and powders	0.33	0.27	—	—	0.27	—	—	—	—	0.87
Granules and powders	—	0.26	—	—	—	—	—	—	—	0.28
Granules and powders	—	0.46	—	—	—	0.58	—	—	—	1.03
Granules and powders	—	—	—	—	—	0.26	—	—	—	0.26
Ginseng-containing soap	—	—	—	—	—	0.60	—	—	—	0.6

(Adapted from Liberti and der Marderosian [85]; with permission.)

Table 2-3. Advising Patients About Herbal Therapies

All patients should be asked about use of herbal therapies and dietary supplements.
"Natural" does not necessarily mean safe.
Herbal/pharmaceutical interactions do occur, therefore avoid combined use.
Lack of standardization of herbal agents may result in variability among manufacturers in herbal's content and efficacy.
Lack of quality control and regulation may result in contamination during manufacture and potential misidentification of plant species.
Herbal treatments should not be used if the patient is contemplating pregnancy or during pregnancy or lactation because of lack of long-term clinical trials proving safety.
Herbal treatments should not be used in dosages higher than that recommended.
Herbal treatments should not be used for more than several weeks due to a lack of studies proving long-term safety.
Herbal treatments with known adverse effects and toxic effects should be avoided.
Infants, children, and the elderly should not use herbal treatments.
An accurate diagnosis and discussion of proven treatment options are essential before considering herbal treatments.
Adverse effects should be documented in the patient's chart and therapy discontinued.

Adapted from Cirigliano and Sun [84•]; with permission.

References and Recommended Reading

Recently published papers of particular interest have been highlighted as:
- Of interest
- •• Of outstanding interest

1.•• Blumenthal M, Rister R, Goldberg A, et al.: *The Complete German Commission E Monographs: Therapeutic Guide To Herbal Medicines.* Boston, MA: Integrative Medicine Communication; 1998.
This a complete herbal reference.

2. Richman A, Witkowski JP: *Herbs by the Numbers: Whole Foods' Third Annual Natural Herbal Product Sales Survey.* Austin, TX: Whole Foods; 1997.

3. Canedy D: Real medicine or medicine show? Growth of herbal sales raises issues about value. *The New York Times* July 23, 1998:C1.

4.•• *The Review of Natural Products.* St. Louis, MO: Facts and Comparisons; 1997.
This a another complete herbal reference.

5. der Marderosian A: *New Ideas in Herbal Therapy.* New York: Power-Pak Communications; 1998.

6. Wagner H: Immunostimulating polysaccharides (heteroglycans) of higher plants. *Arzneim-Forsch* 1985, 35:1069–1075.

7. Vomel T: Der einfluss eines pflanzelischen Immunostimulans auf die Phagozytose von Erythozyten durch das retikulohistozytare System der isoliert perfundierten Rattenleber. *Arzneim-Forsch* 1985, 35:1437–1439.

8. Mose J: Effect of echinacin on phagocytosis and natural killer cells. *Med Welt* 1983, 34:1463–1467.

9. Westendorf J: Carito- in-vitro Untersuchungen zum Nachweiss spasmolytischer und kontraktiler Einflusse. *Therapiewoche* 1982, 32:6291–6297.

10. Braunig B, Dorn M, Limburg E, et al.: Enhancement of resistance in common cold by Echinacea purpurea. *Z Phytother* 1992, 13:7–13.

11. Hobbs C: Echinacea, a literature review: botany, history, chemistry, pharmacology, toxicology, and clinical uses. *HerbalGram* 1994, 30:33–47.

12. Schoneberger D: Influence of the immunostimulating effects of the pressed juice of Echinaceae purpurae on the duration and intensity of the common cold: results of a double-blind clinical trial. *Forum Immunol* 1992, 2:18–22.

13. Melchart D, Linde K, Worku F, et al.: Immunomodulation with Echinacea a systematic review of controlled clinical trials. *Phytomedicine.* 1994, 1:245–254.

14.• O'Hara M, Kiefer D, Farrell K, et al.: A review of 12 commonly used medicinal herbs. *Arch Fam Med* 1998, 7:523–536.
This an excellent review.

15. Dorn M: Milderung grippaler Effekte durch ein pflanzliches Immunstimulans. *Naturund Ganzheitsmedizin* 1989, 2:314–319.

16.• Miller LG: Herbal medicinals: selected clinical considerations focusing on known or potential drug–herb interactions. *Arch Int Med* 1998, 158:2200–2211.
This an excellent review.

17. Adoga GI: The mechanism of the hypolipidemic effect of garlic oil extract in rats fed on high sucrose and alcohol diets. *Biochem Biophys Res Comm* 1987, 142:1046–1052.

18. The action of garlic in the pathogenesis of atherosclerosis: selected abstracts from the fourth International Congress on Phytotherapy. *Eur J Clin Res* 1992, 3A:1–12.

19. Lau BHS: Allium sativum (garlic) and atherosclerosis: a review. *Nutr Re:* 1983, 3:119–128.

20. Warshafsky S, Kamer R, Sivak S: Effect of garlic on total serum cholesterol. *Ann Intern Med* 1993, 1:599–605.

21. Silgay C, Neil A: Garlic as a lipid-lowering agent: a meta-analysis. *J R Coll Physicians Lond* 1994, 28:2–8.

22. Berthold HK, Sudhop T, von Bergmann K: Effect of a garlic oil preparation on serum lipoproteins and cholesterol metabolism: a randomized controlled trial. *JAMA* 1998, 279:1900–1902.

23. Isaacsohn JL, Moser M, Stein EA, et al.: Garlic powder and plasma lipids and lipoproteins: a multicenter, randomized, placebo-controlled trial. 1998, 158:1189–1194.

24. Symposium on the chemistry, pharmacology and medical applications of garlic. *Cardiol Pract* 1989, 7:1–15.

25. Apitz-Castro A: Effects of garlic extract and of three pure components isolated from it on human platelet aggregation, arachidonate metabolism release reaction and platelet ultrastructure. *Thromb Res* 1983, 32:155–169.

26. Rose KD, Croissant PD, Parliament CF, *et al.*: Spontaneous spinal epidural hematoma with associated platelet dysfunction from excessive garlic ingestion: a case report. *Neurosurgery* 1990, 26:880–882.
27. DeFeudis FV: *Ginkgo Biloba Extract (Egb 761): Pharmacological and Clinical Applications.* Paris: Elsevier; 1991.
28. Brown D, Gaby A, Reighert R, *et al.*: *Clinical Applications of Natural Medicine Dementia and Age-Related Cognitive Decline.* Seattle: Natural Product Research Consultants; 1997.
29. Packer L, Haramaki N, Kawabata T, *et al.*: Ginkgo biloba extract (Egb 761). *Effect of Ginkgo Biloba Extract (Egb 761) on Aging and Age-Related Disorders.* Paris: Elsevier; 1995:23–47.
30. Hopfenmuller W: Evidence for a therapeutic effect of Ginkgo biloba special extract: meta-analysis of 11 clinical trials in patients with cerebrovascular insufficiency in old age. *Arzneim Forsch* 1994, 44:1005–1013.
31. Kleljnen J, Knipshild P: Ginkgo biloba for cerebral insufficiency. *Br J Clin Pharmacol* 1992, 34:352–358.
32. Ernst E: Ginkgo biloba extract in peripheral arterial diseases: a systematic research based on controlled studies in the literature. *Fortsch Med* 1996, 114:85–87.
33. Le Bars PL, Katz MM, Berman N, *et al.*: A placebo-controlled, double-blind, randomized trial of an extract of ginkgo biloba for dementia. *JAMA* 1997, 278:1327–1332.
34. Roncin J, Schwartz F, D'Arbigny P: Egb 761 in control of acute mountain sickness and vascular reactivity to cold exposure. *Aviat Space Environ Med* 1996, 67:445–452.
35. Schubert H, Halama P: Depressive episode primarily unresponsive to therapy in elderly patients: efficacy of ginkgo biloba extract (Egb 761) in combination with antidepressants. *Geriatr Forsch* 1993, 3:45–53.
36. Rosenblatt M, Mindel J: Spontaneous hyphema associated with ingestion of ginkgo biloba extract [letter]. *N Engl J Med* 1997, 336:1108.
37. Rowin J, Lewis SL: Spontaneous bilateral subdural hematomas associated with chronic ginkgo biloba ingestion have also occurred. *Neurology* 1996, 46:1775–1776.
38. Brown D, Austin S, Reichert R: *Clinical Applications of Natural Medicine Benign Prostatic Hyperplasia and Prostate Cancer Prevention.* Seattle: Natural Product Research Consultants; 1997.
39. Di Silverio F, D'Eramo G, Lubrano C, *et al.*: Evidence that *Serenoa repens* extract displays an antiestrogenic activity in prostatic tissue of benign prostatic hypertrophy patients. *Eur Urol* 1992, 21:309–314.
40. Sultan C, Terraza A, Devillier C: Inhibition of androgen metabolism and binding by a liposterolic extract of *Serenoa repens B* in human foreskin fibroblasts. *J Steroid Biochem* 1984, 20:515–519.
41. Breau W, Hagenlocher M: Antiphlogistic activity of an extract from Sabal serrulata fruits prepared by supercritical carbon dioxide: in vitro inhibition of the cyclooxygenase and 5-lipoxygenase metabolism. *Arzneim-Forsch Drug Res* 1992, 42:547–551.
42. Bach D: Medikamentöse Langheitbehandlung der BPH. Ergebnisse einer prospektiven 3-Jahres Studie mit dem Sabalextrakt IDS 89. *Urologe* 1995, 35:178–183.
43.• Wilt TJ, Ishani A, Stark G, *et al.*: Saw palmetto extracts for treatment of benign prostatic hyperplasia: a systematic review. *JAMA* 1998, 280:1604–1609.

This an excellent review.

44. Carraro J, Raynaud J, Koch G: Comparison of phytotherapy (permixon) with finasteride in the treatment of BPH: a randomized international study of 1098 patients. *Prostate* 1996, 29:231–240.
45. Grasso M, Montesano A, Buonaguidi A, *et al.*: Comparative effects of alfuzosin versus *Serenoa repens* in the treatment of symptomatic benign prostatic hyperplasia. *Arch Esp Urol* 1995, 48:97–103.
46. Newall C, Anderson L, Phillipson J: *Herbal Medicines: A Health-Care Professionals.* London: Pharmaceutical Press; 19
47. Murray MT: *The Healing Power of Herbs-The Enlightened Person Guide to the Wonders of Medicinal Plants* edn 2. Rocklin, CA: Prima Publishing; 1995.
48. Avakia EV, Evonuk E: Effects of *Panax* ginseng extract on tissue glycogen and adrenal cholesterol depletion during prolonged exercise. *Planta Medica* 1979, 36:43–48.
49. Gillis CN: *Panax* ginseng pharmacology: a nitric oxide link? *Biochem Pharmacol* 1997, 54:1–8.
50. Marasco C, Vargas R, Salas V, *et al.*: Double-blind study of a multivitamin complexes supplemented with ginseng extract. *Drugs Exp Clin Res* 1996, 22:323–329.
51. D'Angelo R, Grimaldi M, Caravaggi M, *et al.*: A double-blind, placebo-controlled clinical study on the effect of a standardized ginseng extract on psychomotor performance in healthy volunteers. *J Ethnopharmacol* 1986, 16:15–22.
52. Shibata S, Tanaka O, Shoji J, *et al.*: Chemistry and pharmacology of Panax. In: *Economic and Medicinal Plant Research* vol 5. Edited by Wagner H, Hikino H, Farnsworth NR. New York: Academic Press; 1985:217–284.
53. Zhan Y, Xu XH, Jiang YP: Effects of ginsenosides on myocardial ischemia/reperfusion damage in open-heart surgery patients. *Med J China* 1994, 74:626–628.
54. Sotaniemi EA, Haapakkoski E, Rautio A: Ginseng therapy in non-insulin dependent diabetic patients. *Diabetes Care* 1995, 18:1373–1375.
55. Hopkins MP, Androff L, Benninghoff AS: Ginseng face cream and unexplained vaginal bleeding. *Am J Obstet Gynecol* 1988, 159:1121–1122.
56. Palmer BV, Montgomery ACV, Monteriro JCMP: Ginseng and mastalgia. *Br Med J* 1978, 1:1284.
57. Linde K, Ramirez G, Mulrow CD, *et al.*: St. John's wort for depression: an overview and meta-analysis of randomized clinical trials. *Br Med J* 1996, 313:253–238.
58. National Institutes of Health: NIH to explore St. John's wort. *Science* 1997, 276:391.
59. Brown DJ: European phytomedicines: research updates on chemistry, pharmacology, and clinical applications: selected highlights of the two day symposium on phytomedicines at the 212th American Chemical Society Meeting, Orlando, Florida, August 27–28, 1996. *Q Rev Nat Med* 1997, VOL:23–30.
60. Hänsgen KD, Vesper I: Antidepressive Wirksamkeit eines hochdosierten Hypericum-Extrakfes. *Med Wochenschr* 1996, 138:29–33.
61. Linde K, Gilbert R, Murlow C, *et al.*: St. John's wort for depression: an overview and meta-analysis of randomized clinical trials. *Br Med J* 1996, 313:253–257.
62. Riedel E: Inhibition of gamma-aminobutyric acid catabolism by valerenic acid derivatives. *Planta Medica* 1982, 48:219–220.
63. Mennini T, Bernasconi P, Bombardelli E, *et al.*: In vitro study of the interaction of extracts and pure compounds from Valeriana officinalis roots with GABA, benzodiazepine and barbiturate receptors in rat brain. *Fitoterapia* 1993, 534:291–300.
64. Leatherwood P, Chauffard F, Heck E, *et al.*: Aqueous extract of valerian root (*Valeriana officinalis L*) improves sleep quality in man. *Pharmacol Biochem Behav* 1982, 17:6541.
65. Lindahl O, Lindwell L: Double-blind study of a valerian preparation. *Pharmacol Biochem Behav* 1989, 32:1065–1066.
66. Mascolo N, Jain R, Jain S, *et al.*: Ethnopharmacologic investigations of ginger (Zingiber officinale). *J Ethnopharmacol* 1989, 27:129–140.
67. Grontved A: Ginger root against seasickness: a controlled trial on the open sea. *Acta Otolaryngol* 1988, 105:45–49.
68. Mowrey DB, Clayson DE: Motion sickness, ginger, and psychophysics. *Lancet* 1982, 1:655–657.

69. Jussofie A, Schmiz A, Hiemke C: Kavapyrone enriched extract from Piper methysticum as modulator of the GABA binding site in different regions of rat brain. *Psychopharmacology* 1994, 116:469–474.

70. Bruneton J: *Pharmacognosy, Phytochemistry, Medicinal Plants.* Paris: Lavoisier Publishing; 1995.

71. Kinzler E: Effect of a special kava extract in patients with anxiety, tension, and excitation states of nonpsychotic genesis. *Arzneimittelforsch* 1991, 41:584–588.

72. Schulz V, Hansel R, Tyler VE: *Rational Phytotherapy: A Physicians' Guide to Herbal Medicine.* Berlin, Germany: Springer Verlag; 1997.

73. Woelk H, Kapoula O, Lehrl S, *et al.*: Treatment of patients suffering from anxiety. *Z Allg Med* 1993, 69:271–277.

74. Hansel R, Keller K, Rimpler H, *et al.*: *Hagers Handbuch der Pharmazeutischen Praxis* edn 6. Berlin, Germany: Springer Verlag; 1994.

75. Schelosky L, Raffauf C, Jendroska K, *et al.*: Kava and dopamine antagonism. *J Neurol Neurosurg Psych* 1995, 58:639–640.

76. Almeida JC, Grimsley EW: Coma from the health food store: interaction between kava and alprazolam. *Ann Intern Med* 1996, 125:940–941.

77.• Flora K, Hahn M, Rosen H, *et al.*: Milk thistle (*Silybum marianum*) for the therapy of liver disease. *Am J Gastroenterol* 1998, 93:139–143.

This an excellent review.

78. Flora KD, Rosen HR, Benner KG: The use of naturopathic remedies for chronic liver disease. *Am J Gastroenterol* 1996, 91:2654–2655.

79. Takahara E, Ohta S, Hirobe M: Stimulatory effects of Silibinin on the DNA synthesis in partially hepatectomized rat livers: nonresponse in hepatoma and other malignant cell lines. *Biochem Pharmacol* 1986, 35:538–541.

80. Pares A, Planas R, Torres M, *et al.*: Effects of silymarin in alcoholic cirrhosis of the liver: results of a controlled, double-blind, randomized, and multicenter trial. *J Hepatol* 1998, 28:615–621.

81. Buzzelli G, Moscarella S, Glusti A, *et al.*: A pilot study on the liver protective effect of silybin-phosphatidylchlorine complex (IdB 1016) in chronic active hepatitis. *Int J Clin Pharmacol Ther Toxicol* 1993, 31:450–460.

82. Beckwith J: Herbal Medicine. Prescriber's Letter. 1997; Document no. 131033.

83. Velussi M, Carnigoi A, Viezzoli L, *et al.*: Silymarin reduces hyperinsulinemia, malondialdehyde levels and daily insulin need in cirrhotic diabetic patients. *Curr Ther Res* 1993, 53:533–545.

84.• Cirigliano MD, Sun A: Advising patients about herbal therapies. *JAMA* 1998, 280:1565–1566.

This paper discusses integration of complementary medicine into practice.

85. Liberti LE, der Marderosian A: Evaluation of commercial ginseng products. *J Pharma Sci* 1978, 67:1487–1489.

86. Eisenberg DM: Advising patients who seek alternative medical therapies. *Ann Intern Med* 1997, 127:61.

This paper also discusses integration of complementary medicine into practice.

Herbs in Women's Health Care

Joyce C. Frye

Plants are truly nature's medicine. They have been used from time immemorial to aid in healing illness. Our pets innately chew on them in our yards for apparently specific effects, and numerous commonly used prescription medicines are derived from or are synthesized to be like the "active ingredients" found in plants. This activity of attempting to reduce the medicinal value of the plant to a single agent is sometimes known as "reductionist" medicine. Advocates of returning to the use of the original herbs maintain that the whole plant or plant part is able to work more gently and effectively because of synergism with other constituents in the plant that increase its activity or ameliorate the side effects of the primarily active ingredient.

Although it may be true that there are certain advantages to the use of herbs, it is important to remember that medicinal herbs are medicines, and should be regarded with the same respect and skepticism accorded conventional agents. They should be used for specific indications only after a diagnosis has been made and for limited periods of time. Any condition that does not improve within the anticipated timeframe for the condition being treated should be reassessed for the accuracy of both the diagnosis and the treatment. Adverse reactions should be watched for diligently and use of the herb should be stopped if any such contraindications seem to appear. Conversely, the practitioner must not be too hasty in determining that an herb does not work. Because of their gentle action, 2 to 3 months are often required to see an effect.

The medicinal activity of specific herbs can vary greatly. Differences in the age of the plant, the quality of soil, the time of harvest, and methods of cleaning, drying, and storing contribute to the variable quality of the end product under the best of conditions. Under worse conditions, contamination with pesticides, fungi, and outright substitution of less expensive or more easily obtained substances is a real concern. To the extent possible, the consumer should be satisfied that these considerations have been controlled in the products chosen.

Combination herbal and herbal/nutritional supplements present a separate set of problems. Unexpected drug interactions can occur with combinations of herbs just as they do with prescription medicines. Combining should be left to the experts. But in the unregulated marketplace in the United States, manufacturers and marketers should not be assumed to be experts. Thus, patients considering the use of herbal combinations should be sufficiently well informed to know the reason each ingredient is included in a given product. In addition, they should be extremely cautious about combining separate herbal formulations recommended for different conditions, *eg,* one combination for sleep and another for menopause, if potentially unforeseen interactions or overdoses are to be avoided.

A great deal of folklore supports the use of various plants for specific ailments. Additionally, many herbal medicine texts give recipes for combinations of herbs to be used to treat various conditions such as menopause or dysmenorrhea. Unfortunately, they frequently do little to distinguish individual differences in etiology or symptomatology that might warrant use of one herb or combination over another. They do even less, in most cases, to explain the potential physiologic mechanisms involved in producing the medicinal effect.

Available English-language information about herbs was expanded greatly in 1998 with the publication of the translation of the German Commission E Monographs [1], which give safety and efficacy profiles for over 300 herbs. In this chapter, recommendations from leading herbalists are compared with the Commission E herb profile to find independent support for recommendations and safety. Information from randomized, controlled trials is scarce for many herbs, but is included where available. An attempt is also made to explain the biologic reason for choosing one herb over another for a particular problem when possible.

THERAPEUTIC USE OF HERBS FOR GYNECOLOGIC PROBLEMS

Medical problems of the female reproductive system can be divided into two basic categories: problems related to the hormonal cycle and problems related to infections. The basic physiology is discussed first, followed by a review of the available scientific data for some of the most popular herbs to see how the data contribute to an appropriate application of the herbs' potential use. Herbs are listed by their common names (shown in bold) as well as their Latin name.

The Female Hormonal Cycle

In the normal ovarian cycle, the lining of the uterus proliferates and ovarian follicles mature under the influence of follicle-stimulating hormone (FSH) secreted by the pituitary gland, which in turn causes rising ovarian production of estrogen (primarily β-estradiol). This first half of the menstrual cycle is known as the follicular phase. Toward the end of the follicular phase, luteinizing hormone (LH) surges, resulting in ovulation and the production of progesterone for the remainder of the cycle. Progesterone converts the endometrium to a secretory state during the resulting luteal phase. This lasts for approximately 14 days (assuming no pregnancy has occurred) at which point estrogen and progesterone levels fall and the endometrium breaks down, resulting in menses.

Secretion of FSH and LH from the pituitary is under the control of releasing factors (RF) that originate in the hypothalamus and respond to an elaborate feedback mechanism from the ovary. Prolactin, thyroid, adrenal, and growth hormones are also controlled through the hypothalamus and pituitary with the result that disturbance in those systems can also distrupt the menstrual cycle. Disturbances of the menstrual cycle occur when hormones are increased, decreased, or out of balance. Additionally, the hypothalamus seems to be involved in generating emotions, such as rage and fear, which may explain why stress seems to contribute to menstrual irregularity in some women [2].

Choosing the Correct Herb

Choosing the correct herb for menstrual irregularities is much easier with an understanding of the underlying problem. For example, amenorrhea (prolonged missed menses) occurs for many reasons. Numerous factors can interfere with normal hormonal cyclicity. An elevated prolactin might well respond to vitex. Low estrogen levels secondary to low body weight or approaching menopause might respond to **red clover** (*Trifolium praetense*) or **black cohosh** (*Cimicifuga racemosa*). Polycystic ovary (PCO) syndrome might also respond to black cohosh, although this syndrome is often accompanied by excess body weight. Amenorrhea due to low levels of hypothalamic or pituitary hormones or due to thyroid hormone abnormalities may not respond to any of these. Thus, if the reason for any irregularity of the menstrual cycle is unknown, it is best to start with hormonal evaluation and diagnosis under the supervision of a physician.

Estrogen-like Herbs

Phytoestrogens are useful for hormonal regulation because of their estrogen-like effects. Chemically, they are phenols rather than steroids, but they have the ability to bind to and activate estrogen receptors. In vivo, they have 0.1% to 15% of the estrogenic potency of estradiol, the primary premenopausal estrogen [3]. Clinically, phytoestrogens may enhance estrogen function in the body if the underlying condition is estrogen deficiency, or inhibit estrogen through competitive binding if the underlying condition results from estrogen excess. Many foods also contain phenolic phytoestrogens; soybeans are a particularly rich source. Bean sprouts, alfalfa sprouts, and flax seeds also have large quantities. Studies of urine and blood levels reveal that vegetarians have considerably higher levels of phytoestrogens than those who consume traditional Western diets.

Red clover leaves contain the richest source of isoflavone (a subclass of phenol phytoestrogens) among herbs. James Duke, a retired U.S. Department of Agriculture ethnobotanist recommends red clover tea for both hot flashes and menstrual cramps [4]. Herbalist Susun Weed also recommends infusions for hot flashes and other menopausal symptoms as well as to produce the other benefits of estrogens, such as protection from bone loss [5]. Weed also indicates that red clover acts as a blood thinner and thus should be avoided when heavy menses are part of the problem.

The Commission E Monographs [1] do not include an analysis of red clover. It has been known, however, to cause abortion in sheep and cattle overgrazing on it [6]. Thus, it is prudent for anyone attempting pregnancy to avoid using it. Also of concern are laboratory tests in which red clover stimulated estrogen receptor (ER)-positive breast cancer cell growth almost as strongly as estradiol [7].

Black cohosh is recommended for its estrogenic effects by Duke [4] and Weed [5] as well as by noted naturopath Michael Murray [8] and herbalist Varro Tyler [9]. It is perhaps the best studied of the herbs with estrogen-like effects, although the mechanism of action has not yet been fully elucidated. The drug is made from the dried roots of wild plants harvested in North America after the fruit has appeared [10]. Commercial formulations include capsules, solutions, tablets, and tinctures. In animal studies, black cohosh has been observed in mice to increase circulation to the genitals and to increase uterine and ovarian weight—a sign of stimulation. In ovariectomized rats, black cohosh decreased serum cholesterol and bone loss [11]. However, other researchers found no uterotropic or vaginotropic effects and proposed that the therapeutic effects occurred because of an interference with neurotransmitters rather than through a direct estrogenic action [12].

In vitro, a *Cimicifuga* extract inhibited human breast cancer cell proliferation. Numerous clinical studies (primarily published in Germany) have used various self-evaluation scales and Kupperman's Menopause Index as well as objective assessment of vaginal cytology in comparison with both placebo and with estriol, conjugated estrogens, and combined estrogen and progesterone. Therapeutic efficacy was generally found to be equivalent to various estrogen preparations.

The Commission E Monographs [1] list black cohosh root as an approved herb for use in premenstrual discomfort, dysmenorrhea (menstrual cramps), and climacteric (menopausal) neurovegetative ailments. The biologic effects listed are estrogen-like action, LH suppression, and binding to ERs. With these actions, the benefit in reducing menopausal symptoms due to ER binding in the pituitary is obvious.

It is less clear why black cohosh should be helpful for premenstrual symptoms and dysmenorrhea. Conventional wisdom has suggested that a relative deficiency of progesterone relative to estrogen is the reason for this effect. However, defective luteal phase progesterone production is often preceded by a follicular phase in which there has been a poor preovulatory estrogen rise. Thus, the additional estrogen effect early in the menstrual cycle may contribute to this benefit.

The significance of LH suppression by black cohosh is interesting to consider. Menopausal hot flashes are generally considered to be associated with elevated levels of both LH and FSH, but, curiously, relief can be attained by reducing only LH. However, another clinical entity associated with elevated LH in relation to FSH is PCO, characterized by excess ovarian estrogen production in the first half of the menstrual cycle with resulting irregular or absent ovulation and irregular menses. The ER-binding capacity of black cohosh combined with its ability to lower LH levels suggests a potential role in the treatment of this syndrome that deserves further investigation.

The recommended dose of black cohosh is 40 mg/d, although some studies have been conducted with 40 mg twice daily. Between 4 and 8 weeks of treatment are often needed before benefit is observed. Occasional gastric discomfort is the only listed side effect; no interactions with other drugs have been described. However, recommended duration of administration according to the Commission E Monographs [1] is limited to 6 months. The reason for this warning remains unclear. After a more recent extensive review of the literature, Gruenwald [13] has indicated that he believes that it can be safely used for several years.

Dong quai (*Angelica sinensens*) is one of the most popular of the herbs used to regulate the menstrual cycle and control hot flashes. Unfortunately, its historical use comes primarily from traditional Chinese medicine, and little in the Western literature supports it. Tyler [9] does not include dong quai in his *Herbs of Choice*, and the Commission E Monographs [1] do not mention it, although another species of *Angelica* is included for its therapeutic effect on the gastrointestinal system.

A randomized, controlled trial comparing dong quai with placebo failed to demonstrate any difference between the two in relief from hot flashes [14]. However, in traditional Chinese medicine, dong quai is used primarily as a blood tonic (R. Freedman, personal communication, 1997). It would only be given to "chilly" people, not to those who were constitutionally warm. Weed [5] echoes this philosophy, indicating that for those who are "hot much of the time anyway...ingestion may make you flash all the more." Thus, another study comparing dong quai with placebo in women who are generally chilly *except* for their hot flashes would be worthwhile.

Weed [5] also counsels against using dong quai while bleeding heavily, in the presence of fibroids, if taking other blood-thinning agents such as aspirin (if bloated), or in the presence of diarrhea. These restrictions notwithstanding, she does recommend it to relieve hot flashes, regulate menses, relieve uterine pain, increase vaginal secretions, restore youthful complexion, reduce headaches, relieve water retention, eliminate palpitations, ease menopausal insomnia, restore emotional calm, relieve menopausal rheumatism, and restore liver tone.

Duke [4] also refers to dong quai as one of the most widely used herbs in Chinese women's medicine. In addition to its reputation as a "sex enhancer," it is used for treatment of amenorrhea, premenstrual syndrome, menstrual cramps, and menopause. Pregnancy is the only contraindication to its use. Murray and Pizzorno [8] list dong quai among herbs with proven estrogenic activity, citing several general sources [15–18]. Little additional explanation for its physiologic effects has been determined.

Other Estrogenic Herbs

In the list of herbs with proven estrogenic activity, Murray and Pizzorno [8] also include **licorice** (*Glycyrrhiza glabra*), **fennel** (*Foeniculum vulgare*), **unicorn root** (*Aletris vulgare*), and **false unicorn root** (*Helonius opulus*). A separate set of in vitro tests for hormonal effects demonstrated estrogen receptor binding by licorice as well as by red clover, **mandrake** (*Mandragora autumnalis*), and **thyme** (*Thymus vulgaris*) [7]. The Commission E Monographs [1] include licorice, fennel, and thyme as approved herbs for respiratory and gastrointestinal indications, but there is no specific mention of estrogenic properties.

However, licorice does contain phytosterols. Duke [4] indicates that glycyrrhizin, the active ingredient in licorice, acts like an isoflavone and clinically increases or decreases estrogen activity depending on the underlying state. A note of caution, however—with extensive use, glycyrrhizin may cause retention of sodium and water and loss of potassium, thus resulting in hypertension. Deglycyrrhizinated forms are available but do not appear to be useful for any estrogenic effect. Use of the whole root is contraindicated in pregnancy, and doses should not exceed 15 g of root nor should therapy be continued for longer than 6 weeks without medical supervision. Licorice is also widely used in formulas in traditional Chinese medicine.

Unicorn root, false unicorn root, and mandrake are not listed in the Commission E Monographs [1]. Weed [5] and Duke [4] both include false unicorn root in their lists of herbs that are useful for menopause. However, Weed gives its botanical name as *Chamaelirium luteum* [5]. Duke indicates that its active ingredient, anethole, is less estrogenic than glycyrrhizin [4].

Other Herbs with Hormonal Effects

Chasteberry (*Vitex agnus-castus*) has been in use since the Middle Ages as a menstrual regulator [5,9]. A powder or tincture of the fresh or dried mature fruit is used. Only recently has a mechanism of action been proposed. In vitro studies with cultures of anterior pituitary cells from mice and rats have demonstrated significant inhibition of prolactin secretion both in the basal state and after thyroid releasing hormone (TRH) stimulation, which is similar to the action of dopamine [19,20]. Duke [4] reports that vitex also increases LH and decreases FSH (compared with black cohosh, which decreases LH).

In a randomized, double-blind, controlled trial described by Böhnert [21], women with menstrual irregularities, luteal phase defect, and "latent prolactinemia" (prolactin elevated to 70 and 120 ng/mL at 15 and 30 minutes after TRH stimulation) were treated for 3 months with 20 mg of a vitex preparation or placebo. Results included a significant ($P < 0.0001$) reduction in prolactin release, increased luteal phase of 5 days on average, increased midluteal progesterone levels, and reduction in symptoms of premenstrual syndrome (PMS) [22]. In another study, vitex compared favorably with vitamin B_6 in the treatment of PMS in a dose of 3.5 to 4.2 mg/d [23].

The Commission E Monographs [1] recommend doses between 30 and 40 mg of vitex for irregularities of the menstrual cycle, premenstrual complaints, and mastodynia (painful breasts). Occasional itching is the only known side effect. Interaction with dopamine-receptor antagonists is likely. Thus, use of this herb appears to be safe for those who are not receiving therapy with psychoactive drugs.

Other Menstrual Cycle Aids

Goldenrod (*Solidago sp.*) is the most effective and safest of the herbal diuretics, according to Tyler [9]. This therapeutic effect may be beneficial for some forms of premenstrual syndrome in which fluid retention and breast tenderness are prominent symptoms. Herbal diuretics generally cause increased excretion of water without the accompanying excretion of sodium and potassium seen with conventional diuretics. Thus, they are not appropriate for the treatment of true edema as in hypertension and heart failure. The Commission E Monographs [1] list its use for irrigation of the lower urinary tract and prophylaxis against urinary calculi. The recommended dose is the equivalent of 6 to 12 g of the herb.

Duke [4] also lists **Dandelion** (*Taraxacum officinale*) as a safe and potent diuretic, and the Commission E Monographs [1] endorse it. However, Tyler [9] does not agree, stating that there is no significant documented proof of its pharmacologic activity.

Shepherd's purse (*Bursae pastoris*) is approved by the Commission E Monographs [1] for the treatment of mild-to-moderate menorrhagia (heavy bleeding) with no known side effects or drug interactions. It appears to increase the strength of uterine contractions (as well as cardiac contractions). The dose is 10 to 15 g/d, typically in the form of a tea that is consumed throughout the day rather than all in one dose. Weed [5] is enthusiastic in her endorsement of this herb for uterine hemorrhaging. She recommends putting the tincture under the tongue by the dropperful when flooding is severe, with the expectation of seeing results within a few hours.

Persistent heavy bleeding and any midcycle bleeding should always necessitate diagnostic evaluation by a physician. However, this herb generally acts quickly and may be used in an emergency until diagnosis is made and until other slower-acting, cycle-regulating measures have a chance to work.

Ginkgo (*Ginkgo biloba*) has been found to have numerous pharmacologic effects, particularly in relation to circulation. The active ingredient is extracted from leaves of the ginkgo tree. The extraction method seems to make a difference in the pharmaceutical quality of the extract. The type known as EGb 761 appears to be most therapeutically effective [24].

The circulatory effect of ginkgo may be beneficial for the treatment of decreased libido—a frequent complaint among menopausal women. Although this problem undoubtedly has multiple causes with relational and emotional issues playing a large role, decreasing blood circulation to the genital area with attendant decreasing estrogen levels may be a factor. Duke [4] cites several studies in men in which ginkgo was shown to improve erectile dysfunction. In an open trial, both men (84%) and women (91%) found ginkgo to be successful in relieving sexual dysfunction associated with antidepressants [25]. Several months are often required to notice an effect. The dose is 120 to 240 mg/d with hypersensitivity the only apparent contraindication.

Wild yam (*Diascorea villosa*) is included here to clarify some of the controversy surrounding it and because of its extremely widespread use. Diosgenin, the active ingredient in wild yam, is used by pharmaceutical companies as the precursor for approximately 50% of the production of steroids, including estrogen and progesterone [26]. However, no scientific evidence indicates that this conversion can be made in vivo. Many commercially produced yam creams have additional progesterone added to them, resulting in what some have referred to as the "yam scam." Duke [4] points out that much less diosgenin is present in wild yam than in many other herbs. Nonetheless, herbalists such as Weed [5] often recommend it. If any activity exists, it would come from the peeled root, which Duke [4] indicates could be made into a paste and added to creams or vaginal lubricants [4]. The Commission E Monographs [1] do not include it.

Infections of the Female Reproductive Tract

Female gynecologic infections are among the most common reasons that patients visit a physician. These include common vulvo/vaginal infections such as yeast, bacterial vaginosis, *Trichomonas*, and Herpes Simplex virus; bladder or urinary tract infections; and more serious pelvic infections of the uterus, fallopian tubes, and surrounding tissues.

Many women confuse normal vaginal secretions with infections, and thus douche or seek treatment when none is needed. Normal vaginal secretions change in character throughout the menstrual cycle. Most women have fairly minimal secretions for a few days after completion of menses. As they approach midcycle and ovulation, the secretions tend to become more profuse and have a clear, mucus-like consistency (good for transporting sperm through the cervix to facilitate conception; the observation of this change is the basis for natural family planning). Following ovulation, the secretions become more creamy white in nature and progressively heavier until onset of menses. In women taking oral contraceptives, the secretions may be more like premenstrual secretions throughout the cycle due to the effect of progestagen in the pill. Local irritants, such as deodorant soaps and sprays and bubble baths, can also cause vulvar redness and burning, which are difficult to distinguish from that of some infections.

Vaginal infections are typically characterized by increased vaginal secretions that are burning, itching, discolored, and malodorous. Many women inaccurately associate all such changes with yeast infections. The diagnosis is important because some infections related to *Trichomonas*, *Chlamydia*, and *Neisseria gonorrheae* are sexually transmitted and potentially more serious. If a woman has any question about the cause of the infection or if it does not resolve promptly with herbal treatment, a diagnostic visit with a women's health-care practitioner should be made.

Bladder infections typically involve symptoms of increased urgency and frequency of urination with small quantities of urine that may burn as it is passed. Some women also confuse this burning with yeast infections in which the irritated skin burns as the urine comes in contact with it. Again, an accurate diagnosis is important to choose the appropriate treatment. The best prevention for bladder infections is to drink adequate quantities of water at all times and to void promptly after sexual intercourse.

Upper urinary tract infections are characterized by fever and pain in one or both kidneys (at the side of the back just above the level of the waist). Pelvic infections often start during menses and cause crampy menstrual-like pain that persists. If unattended, pain is typically progressive and fever develops. Professional medical evaluation should be carried out promptly at the first sign of any of the above.

Anti-infective Herbs

American or purple coneflower (*Echinacea angustifolia*) is a general immune-system booster that may be started at the first sign of any kind of infection. According to Richman and Witkowski [27], Echinacea was the top-selling herb in the United States in 1996 and 1997. An extensive list of actions of Echinacea as demonstrated in human and animal experiments includes increased immune effects as a result of increasing leukocytes and spleen cells, increased capacity for phagocytosis by human granulocytes, and increased body temperature, activation of the alternative complement pathway, T-cell activation, interferon secretion, and antibody binding.

Clinical studies have demonstrated therapeutic effects. In one study, women with recurrent vaginal yeast infections were treated with a standard imidazole drug used for yeast infections either alone or in combination with one of several forms of Echinacea. Those treated with combination therapy had significantly fewer recurrences [28]. Duke [4] cites a report concerning rapid resolution of *Herpes genitalis* outbreaks when Echinacea therapy begins at the first sign of an outbreak.

The Commission E Monographs [1] list contraindications to the use of Echinacea that include progressive systemic disease, such as tuberculosis and multiple sclerosis, and pregnancy (for reasons that are not specified). Side effects may be allergic reactions as well as nausea and vomiting, although these effects are rare. No interactions with other drugs are known. In Europe, delivery modalities include injectable as well as oral forms that contain expressed juice of the fresh, above-ground parts harvested in flower with a daily dose of 6 to 9 mL. In the United States, tinctures and capsules are the most readily available forms. Duke [4] recommends a teaspoon of tincture three times daily in tea or juice. The Commission E Monographs [1] recommend that intake be limited to 8 weeks at a time.

Bearberry (*Arctostaphylos uva ursi*) is the most effective antibacterial herb for urinary tract infections, according to Tyler [9]. Its active ingredient, arbutin, is converted into hydroquinone in the intestine, which is metabolized in alkaline urine to compounds that have antibacterial activity in vitro against many bacteria commonly associated with urinary tract infections. The Commission E Monographs [1] specifically list *Escherichia coli*, *Proteus vulgaris*, *Pseudomonas aerginosa*, *Enterococcus faecalis*, *Staphylococcus aureus*, *Ureaplasma urealyticum*, *Mycoplasma hominis*, and *Streptococcus strains*.

Uva ursi is contraindicated in pregnancy, lactation, and in children under 12 years of age. It should not be used in combination with agents that may acidify the urine. Tyler [9] notes that substances such as milk, tomatoes, fruits, and potatoes help to alkalinize the urine, as does taking 6 to 8 g (about 1/4 oz) of baking soda. However, infected urine tends to be more alkaline in any case. Theoretically, it may be that a smaller effect of the herb is needed as the body heals itself.

The dose of uva ursi is the equivalent of 3 g of dried leaves in an infusion with 150 mL (approximately 2/3 cup) of water three times daily. Murray and Pizzorno [8] warn that excess doses should not be taken because toxic effects have occurred with as little as 15 g. Signs of toxicity include ringing in the ears, nausea and vomiting, shortness of breath, delirium, and convulsions.

Cranberry (*Vaccinium macrocarpon*) and its botanical relative **Blueberry** also contain arbutin, according to Duke [4]. More important is that they have been recognized as containing a substance that prevents adherence of bacteria to the bladder wall. This has now been identified as proanthocyanidin [29]. Although cranberry juice requires large amounts of added sugar to be palatable and thus, in adequate amounts, is high in calories, the capsule form can be standardized to this active ingredient and taken on a preventative daily basis by those who suffer from recurrent bladder infections.

Garlic (*Allium sativa*) is attributed with both antibacterial and antimycotic actions in the Commission E Monographs [1]. Tyler [9] indicates that garlic has been studied extensively since ancient times and that over 1000 scientific papers have been published just in the past 20 years. Much of this investigation concerns garlic's cholesterol-lowering and antiplatelet effects when taken internally. However, it has also been studied as a topical application. In the laboratory, it worked as well as ketoconazole against many various skin fungus isolates [30]. Allicin from fresh garlic seems to be the primary active ingredient for both anti-infective and cardiovascular benefits. Unfortunately, many commercial preparations lose their allicin in the manufacturing process, so fresh garlic works best.

For vaginal infections, Weed [5] suggests wrapping a peeled clove of garlic (being careful not to pierce the inner skin because the juice burns) in gauze with a string attached; this can be inserted like a tampon nightly for up to 6 nights. If this procedure lacks appeal, Duke [4] suggests adding a teaspoon of fresh garlic juice to yogurt and soaking a tampon in it or using it as a douche. For an exhaustive description of the research and uses of garlic, see *Garlic: The Science and Therapeutic Application of Allium Sativum and Related Species* by Koch and Lawson [31].

Aloe (*Aloe vera*) has been widely used historically for the treatment of acute skin conditions, burns, and wound healing. The fresh gel from the inner plant is the effective agent. According to Tyler [9], studies using the fresh material have demonstrated facilitation of the attachment and growth of new cells. It also appears to have antibacterial, antifungal, and analgesic properties. However, the active ingredient (which has yet to be identified) appears to be lost in many commercial preparations, which have not been demonstrated to be effective in many cases. An aloe plant can be kept in the bathroom, a piece of leaf broken off, and the juice extruded to apply to local irritations until the more specific agent has time to work.

Lemon balm (*Melissa officinalis*) is a member of the mint family. It has been demonstrated to contain various substances that have antiviral activity, making it a useful treatment for Herpes lesions in both the oral and genital regions [9]. Duke [4] explains that these substances block receptor sites on the cell, which render it impossible for the virus to attach itself and the for infection to spread. In a randomized, placebo-controlled study, subjects applying a 1% lemon-balm cream within 72 hours of a suspected outbreak had significantly smaller lesion area and faster healing time. Side effects were minimal but included occasional local burning and itching [32].

The Commission E Monographs [1] do not mention this use of lemon balm. However, they list its use for sleep disorders and gastrointestinal complaints, and for these, it has no contraindications. The fresh or dried leaf is used to make a tea that can be blotted on herpetic lesions. A pharmaceutical cream containing *Melissa officinalis* is marketed in Europe for this use.

CONCLUSIONS

Thousands of medicinal plants grace our planet. Many have multiple uses, and undoubtedly, many more than have been listed here could have similar application. As with learning the use of conventional drugs such as antibiotics or antihypertensives, experience has taught that the best way to approach them is to take a few at a time. These can be learned well and used for specific indications, which is equally useful but far less confusing than trying to learn them all at once and then have little basis to choose between them when the time comes to use one. It is hoped that this chapter has provided the reader with reasonable grounds for choosing a single herb for most common women's reproductive health problems.

REFERENCES AND RECOMMENDED READING

Recently published papers of particular interest have been highlighted as:
- Of interest
- Of outstanding interest

1. Blumenthal M, Rister R, Goldberg A, *et al.*: *The Complete German Commission E Monographs* Boston, MA: Integrative Medicine Communications; 1998.
2. Deutsch J, Deutsch D: *Physiological Psychology.* Homewood, IL: Dorsey Press; 1966.
3. Kelly G, Husband A, Waring M: Phenolic phytoestrogens. *Q Rev Nat Med* 1998, 5:63–77.
4. Duke J: *The Green Pharmacy.* Emmaus, PA: Rodale Press; 1997.
5. Weed S: *Menopausal Years the Wise Woman Way.* Woodstock, NY: Ash Tree Publishing; 1992.
6. Braden A, Thain R, Shutt D: Comparison of plasma phytoestrogen levels in sheep and cattle after feeding on fresh clover. *Austral J Agricul Res* 1971, 22:663–670.
7. Zava D, Dollbaum C, Blen M: Estrogen and progestin bioactivity of foods, herbs, and spices. *Proc Soc Exp Biol Med* 1998, 217:369–378.
8. Murray M, Pizzorno J: *Encyclopedia of Natural Medicine.* Rocklin, CA: Prima Publishing; 1991.
9. Tyler V: *Herbs of Choice: The Therapeutic Use of Phytomedicinals.* New York: Haworth Press; 1994.
10. Fisher J: From China to Peru. In *Origins of Garden Plants.* London: Constable; 1982.
11. Beurscher N: *Cimicifuga racemosa L.*-Black cohosh. *Q Rev Nat Med* 1996, 3:19–27.
12. Einer-Jensen N, Ahao J, Andersen K, *et al.*: Cimicifuga and Melbrosia lack oestrogenic effects in mice and rats. *Maturitas* 1996, 25:149–153.
13. Gruenwald J: Standardized black cohosh (*Cimicifuga*) extract [clinical monograph]. *Q Rev Nat Med* 1998, 2:117–125.
14. Hirata J, Swiersz L, Zell B, *et al.*: Does dong quai have estrogenic effects in postmenopausal women? A double-blind, placebo-controlled trial. *Fertil Steril* 1997, 6:981–986.
15. Duke J: *Handbook of Medicinal Herbs.* Boca Raton, FL: CRC Press; 1985.
16. Leung A: *Encyclopedia of Common Natural Ingredients Used in Food, Drugs, and Cosmetics.* New York: John Wiley & Sons; 1980.
17. *British Herbal Pharmacopoeia.* West Yorks: British Herbal Medical Association; 1983.
18. Elghamry M, Shihata I: Biological activity of phytoestrogens. *Planta Medica* 1965, 13:352–357.
19. Jarry H, Leonhardt S, Wuttke W, *et al.*: *Agnus castus* as a dopaminergic active principle in Mastodyn N. *Z Phytother* 1991, 12:77–82.
20. Sliutz G, Speiser P, Schultz A, *et al.*: *Agnus castus* extracts inhibit prolactin secretion of rat pituitary cells. *Hormone Metab Res* 1993, 25:253–255.

21. Böhnert K: The use of *Vitex agnus castus* for hyperprolactinemia. *Q Rev Nat Med* 1997, 4:19–21.
22. Miulewicz A, Gejdel E, Sworen H, *et al.*: *Vitex agnus castus* extract for the treatment of menstrual irregularities due to latent hyperprolactinemia. *Arzneim-Forsch Drug Res* 1993:752–756.
23. Lauritzen C, Reuter J, Repges R, et al.: Treatment of premenstrual tension syndrome with *Vitex agnus castus*: controlled double-blind study versus pyridoxine. *Phytomed* 1997, 4:183–189.
24. Reichling J, Saller R: Quality control in the manufacturing of modern herbal remedies. *Q Rev Nat Med* 1998, 5:21–28.
25. Cohen A, Bartlik B: *Gingko biloba* for antidepressant-induced sexual dysfunction. *J Sex Marital Ther* 1998, 24:139–145.
26. Weiss R: *Herbal Medicine*. Gothenburg, Sweden: Ab Arcanum; 1988.
27. Richman A, Witkowski JP: *Herbs by the Numbers: Whole Foods' Third Annual Natural Herbal Product Sales Survey*. Austin, TX: Whole Foods; 1997.
28. Cowugniet E, Kuhnast R: Recurrent candidiasis: adjuvant immunotherapy with different formulations of Echinacin. *Therapiewoche* 1986, 36:3352–3358.
29. Howell A, Vorsa N, Der Maderosian A, *et al.*: Inhibition of the adherence of P-fimbriated Escheria coli to uroepithelial-cell surfaces by proanthocyanidin extracts from cranberries. *N Engl J Med* 1998, 339:1085–1086.
30. Venugopal P, Venugopal T: Antidermatophytic activity of garlic (*Allium sativum*) in vitro. *Int J Derm* 1995, 34:278–279.
31. Koch H, Lawson L: *Garlic: The Science and Therapeutic Application of Allium Sativum and Related Species*. Baltimore, MD: Williams and Wilkins; 1996.
32. Wobling R, Leonhardt K: Local therapy of herpes simplex with dried extract of *Melissa officinalis*. *Phytomed* 1994, 1:25–31.

St. John's Wort and Depression

Hyla Cass

Public demand for the use of natural medicines is increasing, with a major focus on herbs in general and on St. John's wort (Hypericum perforatum) in particular. Its sales in the United States increased 20-fold between 1995 and 1996, from $10 million to $200 million annually. Estimated retail sales from May 1997 through May 1998 were $400 million [1]. Known to healers for thousands of years, its use for the treatment of depression has been validated by modern-day research, the majority of which has been conducted in Germany. Indeed, this herb is routinely prescribed there as an antidepressant. The U.S. National Institutes of Health has also begun a major three year study on the use of St. John's wort for depression.

St. John's wort is generally well tolerated, with minimal side effects, especially compared with those produced by prescription antidepressants. At higher doses, heightened photosensitivity is possible. Contrary to earlier information, it has been determined that this herb is not a significant monoamine oxidase (MAO) inhibitor, and thus has no related dietary or drug restrictions.

In this chapter, I discuss the uses, effectiveness, and actions of St. John's wort as well as adverse effects, length of time of onset, and long-term effects, and how it compares with pharmaceutical antidepressants. There is also a review of recent research to determine what conclusions can be drawn regarding the future clinical promise of this herb.

BACKGROUND

The traditional medicines of various cultures are experiencing a timely resurgence. In 1996, over 100,000 deaths and over 1 million hospitalizations were attributed to prescription medications *that were used as prescribed*. In contrast, practically no mortality risk exists with herbs, and the side effects are generally mild. Far less likely to cause harm, they are even safer when prescribed appropriately by knowledgeable professionals.

In my own practice of orthomolecular psychiatry, I have incorporated the use of natural products whenever possible, with excellent overall results. Pharmaceuticals are generally aimed at relieving symptoms. In contrast, herbs, vitamins, minerals, and amino acids serve more to support metabolic processes and restore balance. It may be wise to follow the example of our European medical colleagues who study phytomedicine, the medical use of herbs, as part of their pharmacology education, and thus dispense herbs more freely. In fact, in Germany, where doctors can prescribe either phytomedicines or pharmaceuticals with insurance reimbursement, the prescriptions of St. John's wort outnumber those for all other antidepressants combined. Of course, there are cases where pharmaceuticals remain the treatment of choice.

An Ancient Medicine Rediscovered

St. John's wort is a perennial leafy herb with yellow, five-petaled flowers. Native to Europe, western Asia, and northern Africa, it now also thrives in Pacific Northwest in the United States. Its name comes from its flowering on St. John's Day, June 24, and "wort" is Old English for plant. The leaves have a perforated appearance owing to translucent oil glands, giving it the species name *perforatum*. The herb has a long history of use; it is described by Dioscorides, the Greek herbalist, Pliny, the Roman naturalist in the 1st century, as well as by Hippocrates and Paracelsus. The herbalists of ancient times used St. John's wort for a wide variety of ailments, many still relevant in folk medicine today. These include kidney and lung ailments, wound healing, insomnia, and depression. When the first European colonists arrived in North America, they found that the Native Americans were already familiar with the herb, using it for diarrhea, fevers, snakebite, wounds, and other skin problems. It later served as a valuable medicine for treating soldiers' wounds during the Civil War and was prescribed by homeopathic practitioners of the period for diverse ailments.

Unfortunately, toward the end of the 19th century, the medical establishment in the United States turned its back on traditional folk remedies. Medical authorities established what we now term as "conventional medicine," focusing their attention on medical and surgical techniques and on manufactured drugs. They lobbied Congress and the various state legislatures for the prohibition of herbal medicine, which had a chilling impact on the legitimate use of herbs to promote health. Teachings that had been passed down through the ages were dismissed as primitive superstition, and the medical profession lost touch with these gifts of the natural world. Current laws continue to restrict the use of specific healing claims on herbal medicine labels. Only recently has conventional medicine begun to explore once again the potential contributions that herbs can make to health.

Depression

Depression is one of the most common of all psychiatric disorders and is not only disruptive to the lives of its sufferers and its families, but has great economic impact worldwide. In 1990, the direct and indirect costs related to major depressive disorder amounted to over $40 billion. Major depression occurs in 10% to 20% of the world's population in the course of a lifetime. Women are more often affected than men, by a ratio of 2:1 and are at particular risk during periods of hormonal flux, such as prior to menstruation and following childbirth. About 2% of the population may suffer from a depressive personality.

Classification of Depression

Depression can be classified into several main groups, following the guidelines of the Diagnostic and Statistical Manual of Mental Disorders (the clinical guide that describes and categorizes mental disorders) [2]. These classifications are listed in Table 4-1. Symptoms of depression are listed in Table 4-2.

Major Depressive Disorder

Major depressive disorder is defined as having at least five of the symptoms in Table 4-2 for a minimum of 2 weeks, with one of these being depressed mood or loss of interest. It includes a diminution in ability to function as before. The standard psychiatric treatments for major depressive disorder include medication and psychotherapy.

Adjustment Disorder with Depressed Mood

Adjustment disorder, sometimes referred to as reactive depression, results from an identifiable stressor that has occurred within the preceding 3 months, such as the loss of a job, a divorce, or a disaster, such as an earthquake or fire. It impairs the individual's ability to function in school or at work and also affects his or her relationships. The depression clears with time, generally within 6 months.

Dysthymia

The term *dysthymia* comes from the Greek and literally means "bad mood." Though not as severe and disabling as a major depressive disorder, for those suffering from dysthymia, or mild to moderate depression, life is mostly "just going through the motions." In most cases, it is chronic, or long-term, in nature. By definition, the individual has at least three of the

TABLE 4-1. CLASSIFICATION OF DEPRESSION

Major depressive disorder
Dysthymia
Adjustment disorder with depressed mood
Bipolar disorder
Seasonal affective disorder (SAD)

Data from The Diagnostic and Statistical Manual of Mental Disorders [2].

TABLE 4-2. SYMPTOMS OF DEPRESSION

Persistent sad, anxious, or "empty" mood
Pessimism or feelings of hopelessness
Loss of interest or pleasure in usual activities, including sexual intercourse
Insomnia, early-morning awakening, or excessive sleeping
Agitation
Significant change in weight
Decreased energy, fatigue, or a sense of being "slowed down"
Low self-esteem, feelings of worthlessness, or excessive or inappropriate guilt
Difficulty in concentrating, remembering, or making decisions
Recurrent thoughts of death or suicide, a suicide attempt, or a specific suicide plan

symptoms listed in Table 4-2 and no history of a major depressive episode in the first 2 years of the disturbance.

Seasonal Affective Disorder

Another form of depression is seasonal affective disorder (SAD), which is especially prevalent in countries at the extreme northern and southern latitudes where there is reduced daily sunlight during the winter months. A disturbed circadian rhythm leads to symptoms such as marked decrease in energy, increased need for sleep, and carbohydrate cravings. Treatment consists of antidepressant therapy, light therapy, or a combination of both.

Bipolar Disorder

Far less common than other forms of depressive disorders, bipolar disorder, or manic-depressive illness, involves cycles of depression and elation, or mania. Sometimes the mood switches are dramatic and rapid, but in most cases they are gradual.

Causes of Depression

Depression has a strong genetic component. For example, it is estimated that 50% to 60% of all persons with unipolar depression have a first-degree relative who suffers from some form of affective disorder. In bipolar disorder, the concordance rate in identical twins (monozygotic) is 69% and for fraternal or dyzygotic only 13%, which demonstrates the power of "nature" over "nurture." Psychologic causes also play a part (in some depressions more than others). For example, most studies agree that the likelihood of a depressive episode is five to six times greater 6 months after a stressful life incident.

Depression is thought to be mediated by brain neurotransmitters, most importantly norepinephrine, serotonin, and, to a lesser extent, dopamine. The biogenic amine hypothesis of depression postulates an impairment in serotonin or norepinephrine activity: a deficient supply of catecholamines to specific neuroreceptor sites in the brain, or dysfunction in the latter.

Brain biochemistry is disrupted by toxic pollution of the air and water, combined with inadequate diet and excessive stress. For adequate function, the complex biochemistry of neurotransmitter production requires adequate raw materials and coenzymes, including amino acids, essential fatty acids, vitamins, and minerals. Thus, nutritional deficiencies that are caused by inadequate intake, toxic overload that diverts nutrients, or stress affect mood. Among the basic requirements for mental and physical health are clean air, healthful food, adequate exercise, and a low-stress lifestyle.

Indications

St. John's wort is indicated primarily for patients with dysthymia. A commonly used research tool for measuring levels of depression is the Hamilton Depression Index (the HAM-D). The examiner assigns a numeric value to each of a variety of depressive symptoms, such as feelings of fear or sadness, sleep disturbance, or impaired concentration. These scores are then totaled; a higher score indicates a more severe depression. Mild to moderate depression is represented by a score below 25. While debilitating, such depression is generally not incapacitating or dangerous.

St. John's wort is effective in approximately 55% of patients. Although results can often be seen immediately, the full effects may take up to several weeks to develop. St. John's wort can also be used in the treatment of seasonal affective disorder (SAD) [6], premenstrual syndrome (PMS), chronic insomnia, and anxiety. However, St. John's wort is not appropriate in cases of severe anxiety or depression, with attendant inability to function, or when accompanied by suicidal ideation. It is also not recommended in bipolar disorder, for fear of precipitating a manic episode. In actual practice, this effect is unusual, and with appropriate monitoring, can be avoided [7]. It has been used in obsessive compulsive disorder, but no studies to this effect have been published to date. A summary of indications for St. John's wort is listed in Table 4-3.

Other Possible Causes Of Depression

Before beginning pharmaceutical or herbal treatment, certain medical conditions must be ruled out, including chronic fatigue syndrome, anemia, hypothyroidism, and hypoglycemia. St. John's wort may be especially useful in treating chronic fatigue syndrome related to chronic, relapsing viral infection (Epstein-Barr virus, cytomegalovirus, herpes) because it has been shown to have immune-enhancing properties as well. Moreover, it has been found to alleviate symptoms of fibromyalgia, a chronic pain syndrome that often accompanies chronic fatigue syndrome. The pain of fibromyalgia is in part due to low levels of serotonin. One of the key findings in patients with fibromyalgia is a reduction in REM sleep, as well as in the deeper levels (stage III and IV). This does not permit the necessary nightly restoration to the mind and body (including the immune system), resulting in people with fibromyalgia waking up tired and in pain. Improved sleep leads to an improvement in symptoms. St. John's wort extract (300 mg, 0.3% hypericin content), especially in combination with magnesium (200 to 250 mg), both three times daily, enhances sleep and reduces pain, likely by restoring serotonin levels [8].

Clinical Research

A great deal of research has been conducted on St. John's wort. In 1994, the *Journal of Geriatric Psychiatry and Neurology* [9] devoted an entire issue to the subject. The issue involved 17 studies and was a prelude to the meta-analysis by Linde *et al.* [10••] that brought the most attention to the herb. Published in the *British Medical Journal* in 1996, the article reviewed 23

TABLE 4-3. SUMMARY OF INDICATIONS
Mild to moderate depression
Anxiety associated with depression
Seasonal affective disorder (SAD)
Insomnia associated with depression– promotes restful sleep and enhanced dreaming
Premenstrual syndrome
Sleep disorders

controlled studies involving 1757 depressed patients. The researchers concluded that St. John's wort is three times more effective than a placebo, and as effective as prescription antidepressants, but without the side effects. Fifteen studies compared the herb with a placebo, and eight compared it with conventional antidepressants. Most trials were carried out with the compound LI160 (Jarsin300), a St. John's wort extract containing 0.3% hypericin, available in many pharmacies under the brand name Kira (Lichtwer Pharma, Berlin, Germany).

The 4- to 8-week placebo-controlled studies, performed in the private practices of various psychiatrists, internists, and general practitioners, showed St. John's wort to be significantly superior to placebo. The daily dosage levels ranged from 350 mg to 1000 mg of standardized hypericum extract, or 0.4 mg to 2.7 mg per day of hypericin. An average of 55% of the hypericum users responded to the treatment, which is much higher than the 22% response rate measured in the placebo group. In both groups, individual depression levels were measured by the HAM-D. Scores of the groups receiving St. John's wort were 4.4 points lower at the end of the study than the scores of those receiving the placebo, indicating a greater improvement. Only 0.4% of the persons taking St. John's wort dropped out of the study because of side effects, compared with 1.6% of placebo users. This higher drop-out rate may be due to the patients' (mis)perceiving their clinical symptoms as being caused by the substance rather than by their underlying illness.

The Linde et al. [10••] meta-analysis also looked at studies comparing St. John's wort with several antidepressant drugs, including maprotiline hydrochloride, imipramine hydrochloride, bromazepam, amitriptyline hydrochloride, and desipramine hydrochloride. Extract dosages ranged from 500 mg to 900 mg daily. These studies showed that St. John's wort did slightly better (63.9%) than the antidepressants (58.5%) in eliciting a positive response. In addition, only 0.8% of subjects taking the herb dropped out of the study because of side effects, whereas 3.0% of those on drug treatment ended their participation early.

St. John's Wort versus Placebo

Harrer and Sommer [9] conducted a 4-week, double-blind study examining the effectiveness of St. John's wort extract in treating mild to moderate depression in which 105 outpatients were given either 300 mg of LI 160 or a placebo three times daily. Members of both groups started out with nearly identical HAM-D scores. After 2 weeks, the average HAM-D score of the group taking the herb dropped from 15.81 to 9.64 and, at 4 weeks, to 7.17. The placebo group, conversely, dropped from 15.83 to 12.28 by the second week, and to 11.30 by the fourth week. Overall, 67% of the active group had HAM-D scores that showed a response to treatment, whereas only 28% of the placebo group responded. In other words, two thirds of the St. John's wort users had a significant reduction in their depressive symptoms in only 4 weeks. There were improvements in the symptoms of depression, such as feelings of sadness, hopelessness, helplessness, and uselessness, in addition to reductions in insomnia, fear, headache, cardiac symptoms, and exhaustion. There also were no reported side effects. The researchers concluded that, "Hypericum extract is therefore a low-risk antidepressant for treatment of mild and moderate depression, with the advantage of reliable antidepressant efficacy and a minimum of side effects" (Figure 4-1).

A 6-week double-blind study by Hänsgen et al. [11] reached the same conclusions. They selected 72 patients, aged 18 to 70 years, who had been depressed from a minimum period of 2 weeks to a maximum of period of 6 months and who met the criteria for major depression but were not psychotic or suicidal. Each patient received either 300 mg of St. John's wort extract (LI 160) or a placebo three times daily. After 4 weeks, the study participants all received St. John's wort for an additional 2 weeks. This crossover procedure allowed researchers to observe the hypericum group when they continued treatment for 14 additional days while also measuring the response of the former placebo group to a short trial of St. John's wort.

Although the active group started with an average HAM-D score slightly higher than that of the control group (21.2 versus 20.4), those taking the herbal extract experienced substantially greater reductions in their depressive symptoms during the first 4 weeks. The HAM-D scores of the St. John's wort recipients dropped to 9.2, whereas the average score of the placebo group declined to only 14.7.

During the fifth and sixth weeks, the hypericum group continued to improve. Their average HAM-D score declined another 32% to 6.3, for a total drop of 70% in 6 weeks. Those who switched from the placebo to St. John's wort for the last 2 weeks experienced similar improvements. Only 3 patients

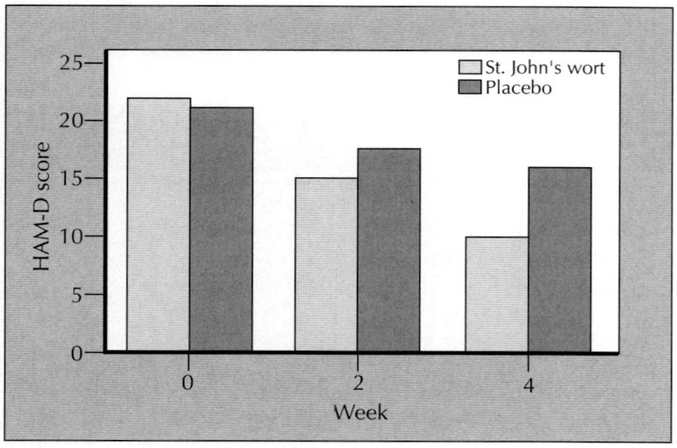

Figure 4-1. Hamilton Depression Scale (HAM-D) scores during 6-week treatment period with imipramine or St. John's wort shows no significant difference in their efficacy. (*Adapted from* Harrer and Sommer [9].)

reported mild side effects, two of whom were actually taking the placebo (Figure 4-2).

St. John's Wort versus Tricyclics

Ten trials compared St. John's wort to tricyclic antidepressants in 1997 [10••,12,13], showing the herb to be as effective as the drug, with much better tolerance. Notably, all but one study used lower doses of medication than are used in the United States (for example, imipramine, 25 mg three times daily) [14]. However, the German investigators who performed this study intentionally chose the lower dose, which in Germany is considered sufficient for outpatients with depression. A higher dose would produce noticeable side effects that would break the double blind.

One study in patients with severe depression (HAM-D scores above 25) used clinical doses of imipramine (150 mg/d) compared with St. John's wort, 1800 mg [15]. A total of 209 patients were followed for 6 weeks in a randomized, double-blind, multicenter trial. The results showed that St. John's wort was nearly as effective as 150 mg of imipramine, but with far fewer side effects. Harrer et al. [16] compared St. John's wort with a synthetic antidepressant, maprotiline, in a 4-week, 102-patient double-blind study. Results showed equivalent effectiveness in the two products. HAM-D scores for those receiving hypericum dropped by 49% compared with a 51% reduction for maprotiline. However, hypericum produced 43% fewer side effects than the synthetic drug.

Vorbach et al. [14] compared LI 160 with imipramine hydrochloride (25 mg three times daily) in a randomized, double-blind study with 135 patients over a period of 6 weeks. Although the St. John's wort group started with a slightly higher HAM-D score, patients using the herb had a better response to treatment. Their scores dropped by 56%, from 20.2 to 8.8, while those of the imipramine users declined 45%, from 19.4 to 10.7. The St. John's wort group also had greater improvements in the severity of their illnesses, according to the Clinical Global Impressions (CGI) scale, another measure of depression. Nearly 82% of patients on the herb were classified as having improved, compared with only 63% of those using imipramine. Moreover, two patients on imipramine became more depressed. In addition to being more effective, St. John's wort also had half as many side effects, of which all but one were mild. Patients using imipramine, on the other hand, indicated that one third of their side effects were either moderate or severe (Figure 4-3).

Seasonal Affective Disorder

Patients with SAD suffer depressive symptoms in the autumn and winter months due to a lack of light exposure, which can trigger hormonal changes in the brain. Symptoms include fatigue, depressed mood, anxiety, reduced activity, increased appetite and sleep requirements, and reduced libido. Light therapy has become the standard treatment. It now appears that St. John's wort is effective as well.

To determine the effectiveness of St. John's wort in treating SAD, Martinez et al. [6] studied 20 patients aged 29 to 63 years with initial HAM-D scores of at least 20. Test subjects were divided into two groups. One group received standard light therapy (3000 lux for 2 hours each day), whereas the

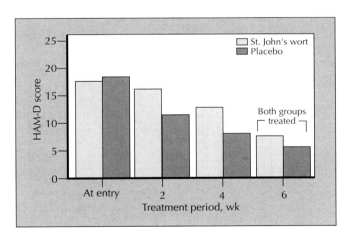

FIGURE 4-2. Hamilton Depression Scale (HAM-D) scores during 6-week treatment period with St. John's wort or placebo shows significant difference at weeks 2 and 4. During weeks 5 and 6, when both groups received St. John's wort, the placebo group improved significantly. (Adapted from Hänsgen et al. [11].)

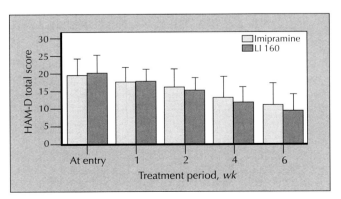

FIGURE 4-3. Symptom survey results on 3250 patients with depression before and after treatment with St. John's wort. (Adapted from Vorbach et al. [15].)

other group was treated with dim light (less than 300 lux for the same time period). Both groups were given 900 mg of herbal extract LI 160 per day (equal to 2.7 mg of hypericin daily). The researchers then measured the changes in HAM-D scores during the 4-week experiment.

The group that received bright light showed a 72% drop in their average HAMD score (to 6.1), whereas the group treated with dim light had a drop of 60% (to 8.2). Therefore, the researchers concluded that St. John's wort is almost as effective as light therapy, although the combination of hypericum and light therapy is still likely to be superior. St. John's wort can offer more convenient relief to people with SAD, making the need for light therapy less critical.

These and other studies reflect St. John's wort's effectiveness in the treatment of mild to moderate depression and SAD. Research continues on this valuable herb, including trials in the United States. Recently, a $4.3 million U.S. federal government-funded large-scale study was launched by the National Institutes of Health's Office of Complementary and Alternative Medicine, together with the National Institute of Mental Health (NIMH) and the Office of Dietary Supplements. It will compare the effectiveness of St. John's wort in subjects with severe depression (HAM-D score above 19) with that of sertraline (a serotonin reuptake inhibitor) and a placebo. The study will be conducted on 336 patients, who will be re-evaluated at 8 weeks to determine efficacy. There will be an 18-week continuation for those who have responded to treatment. Rates of response, clinical efficacy, and relapse rate will be evaluated. This will be the first study using a selective serotonin reuptake inhibitor in the standard clinical doses used in American medicine for severe depression.

PREMENSTRUAL SYNDROME

Premenstrual syndrome is a common complaint that produces both physical and mental symptoms. Because some of its mental symptoms are similar to those experienced during depression, including irritability, tension, and restlessness, it should come as no surprise that St. John's wort can help. For centuries, herbalists have recognized the herb's value in treating discomforts associated with the menstrual cycle, and it remains one of the most widely used natural treatments for PMS as well as for menstrual cramps. The latter effect likely results from the herb's ability to reduce uterine levels of prostaglandins, substances that can promote inflammation. Women's tonics often contain St. John's wort in combination with other ingredients that function in a similar manner .

PHARMACOLOGY

Active Ingredients

The active ingredients in St. John's wort are found in its buds, flowers, and distal leaves, optimally gathered when the flowers just begin to open. Constituents include the naphthodianthrones (<0.1% to 0.15%), such as hypericin, pseudohypericin, flavonol glycosides (2% to 4%), quercitin, quercitrin, isoquercitrin, hyperoside, and rutin; phloroglucinols, specifically hyperforin; and phenylpropanes, biflavones, tannins, and volatile oils [13–17]. The various properties and actions of these have been researched, but much remains to be learned.

Often, medical researchers have considered most of the complex chemical constituents of a plant to be extraneous. Now, of course, we realize these "extras" are often the ingredients that hold the secret to a plant's strength and healing power, rather than its being a specific "active ingredient." Most herbs work as a synergistic whole, and St. John's wort is likely no exception. Although hypericin has received most of the attention in scientific research, it is not likely the main antidepressant component [18]. It continues to be used as a marker for standardized extractions and is the constituent believed responsible for the herb's photosensitizing effect.

A recent issue of *Pharmacopsychiatry* [19•] suggests that hyperforin, a phlorglucinol, may be the main antidepressant ingredient in St. John's wort. An animal study showed hyperforin to be a significant reuptake inhibitor of the antidepressant neurotransmitters serotonin, dopamine, and norepinephrine [20].

A human study showed further proof of this action [21]. In a randomized, double-blind, placebo-controlled study, 142 subjects with mild to moderate depression were given one of three compounds three times daily: a placebo, 300 mg of hypericum extract WS 5573 containing 0.5% hyperforin, or 300 mg of WS 5572 containing 5.0% hyperforin. Tested at intervals over 42 days using the HAM-D, the high hyperforin group had significantly greater relief of symptoms, whereas the placebo and low hyperforin groups were comparable in their lack of improvement. This points toward the therapeutic effect of St. John's wort varying according to its hyperforin content. As is true for many herbs, however, until we have a definitive answer, it would appear a number of constituents contribute synergistically to the antidepressant effect.

Pharmacologic Breakdown

One study in healthy volunteers found a plasma half-life of 24.8 to 26.5 hours and a peak concentration time (Tmax) of 5.2 hours. Steady state appears to be achieved after 4 days [22].

Actions

Many sources have warned about a "tyramine" or "cheese" effect with St. John's wort, necessitating certain food restrictions. These have proven unnecessary, according to further evidence. Despite in vitro evidence [23], there is no evidence of this occurring in vivo nor have any reports been issued of an MAO inhibitor-based hypertensive crisis in those taking St. John's wort.

St. John's wort appears to affect multiple neurotransmitters. It acts as a serotonin reuptake inhibitor, similar to fluoxetine hydrochloride, and also raises levels of the stimulant neurotransmitters norepinephrine and dopamine [24]. It also has an affinity for the gamma aminobutyric acid (GABA) receptors, the site of action of the calming benzodiazepines [18] and appears to inhibit the cytokine, interleukin-6 (IL-6), which thereby reduces the stress hormone, cortisol. St. John's wort also raises nighttime plasma melatonin levels, which would explain its sleep-enhancing effect. Changes in sleep measured by electroencephalography (EEG) have also been noted in healthy volunteers: stage 3/4 (slow-wave) sleep was enhanced by high doses (300 mg three times daily) of the extract [25].

Dosage

The standard dosage of St. John's wort is 300 mg, three times daily of an alcohol and water extract standardized to contain 0.3% hypericin. An alternate dosing schedule is 450 mg twice daily. It should be taken with food because of the possible incidence of gastrointestinal disturbances. However, this restriction can be adjusted to suit individual needs. Doses higher than 1800 mg daily are not recommended because side effects can occur without an increase in clinical effects. The dosage is generally reduced proportionately for children.

Many commercial sources supply St. John's wort in tablet, capsule, or tincture formats. The form depends on individual preference, although tinctures are absorbed more rapidly. Similar to antidepressant medication, it may take several weeks for the full therapeutic effect to occur. The recommended length of treatment is individual, usually a minimum of 3 to 6 months. Prolonged use of the herb appears safe, based on years of use in Europe.

SIDE EFFECTS

Tricyclic Antidepressants

A serious problem with the tricyclics, particularly in patients over age 65 years, is the high incidence of side effects. These include postural hypotension, arrhythmias, dry mouth, blurred vision, confusion, weight gain, flulike symptoms, sweating, rashes, nausea, constipation or diarrhea, difficulty with urination, impotence or impaired erection in men, inhibited orgasm in women, nightmares, anxiety, and sedation. This last is particularly problematic for those who are driving as well as elderly people who are high risk for falling and other accidents.

Selective Serotonin Reuptake Inhibitors

Fluoxetine hydrochloride was the first selective serotonin reuptake inhibitor (SSRI) put on the market in 1987. Sales accounted for $1.2 billion in 1995, and over 6 million Americans use it regularly. Its success has spawned other SSRIs, including sertraline hydrochloride and paroxetine hydrochloride.

The SSRIs work by desensitizing the serotonin receptors, which leads to a greater supply of serotonin within the synapse. Higher levels of serotonin enhance mood and reduce depressive symptoms. However, the SSRIs can exact a high price for their benefits. They are considered better than the older drugs because "only" 17% of those who try them have to stop because of negative experiences, compared with nearly one third (31%) of patients receiving tricyclic drugs. The reported side effects of fluoxetine hydrochloride, listed by percentage of incidence, include nausea (21%), headaches (20%), anxiety and nervousness (15%), insomnia (14%), drowsiness (12%), diarrhea (12%), dry mouth (9%), loss of appetite (9%), sweating and tremors (8%), and rashes (3%). From my own practice and the reports of others, I believe these percentages are far too low, and that the true incidence of side effects is much higher. This discrepancy is likely due to the limited time span in the initial studies (only 4 to 6 weeks), and to the relatively small number of subjects studied.

The SSRIs also reduce sex drive [26]. Studies that looked specifically at sexual dysfunction found that 34% of all men and women using fluoxetine hydrochloride had a drop in libido or difficulty in attaining orgasm. Again, in my clinical experience, the figure is much higher. Why the discrepancy? There are several possible explanations. It is possible that many patients do not mention this side effect for various reasons, including embarrassment, sex simply not being important, or the doctor not asking about these problems. I have had patients on SSRIs who became upset when they learned that their sexual dysfunction could be due to their medication, and that their doctor had failed to tell them so. They are relieved to find that when discontinuing the product, usually an SSRI, function is restored.

For many patients, the side effects experienced are so intense that they prefer to stop their medication altogether. In many cases, synthetic antidepressants also produce subtle emotional results, with complaints of flatness or dulling of emotional responses. St. John's wort, in contrast, produces none of these side effects. It may enhance sexual feelings, and appears to allow a natural brightness of emotion and sharpness of mental functioning to emerge.

St. John's Wort

St. John's wort is generally well tolerated. Side effects are usually mild and include gastrointestinal symptoms and fatigue. No median lethal dose of standard St. John's wort extract was identified in studies of mice, rats, and dogs treated for 26 weeks, even at dosages as high as 5000 mg/kg. No mutagenic effects were noted. In the extensive German experience with St. John's wort as a treatment for depression, no reports of serious adverse consequences or drug interactions have been published [13].

A drug-monitoring study of 3250 patients receiving St. John's wort extract for 4 weeks revealed an overall incidence of side effects of 2.4% (Figure 4-4) [25]. The most common were mild stomach discomfort (0.6%); allergic reactions, primarily rash (0.5%); tiredness (0.4%); and restlessness (0.3%). Only 1.5% of the patients dropped out of the study because of adverse reactions. By comparison, about 17% of patients receiving fluoxetine hydrochloride and 31% of patients given tricyclics stopped taking the drug because of side effects [27]. Furthermore, as many as one in three patients on SSRIs develop symptoms of sexual dysfunction. In the meta-analysis by Linde *et al.* [10••], the overall incidence of side effects in the double-blind studies comparing St. John's Wort with placebo was 4.1%.

Anxiety and irritability may occur in some patients receiving St. John's wort, which is possibly related to the herb's serotonin-enhancing effect. A reduction in dosage may help, or the effect may attenuate over time. However, this simply may not be the treatment of choice for the individual.

Severe phototoxicity has occurred in sheep and cattle that graze on St. John's wort. However, this side effect has not been reported among humans taking oral St. John's wort at usual doses. One study exposed subjects to measured amounts of ultraviolet radiation after taking hypericin, which resulted in an increase in erythema in the study subjects' exposed area [28]. A study of sun-sensitive patients given twice the normal dose of the herb for 2 weeks showed a minimal decreased time to erythema on exposure to UV radiation [29]. Severe phototoxicity has been seen in AIDS patients given intravenous synthetic hypericin at a dose about 10 to 20 times the normal daily dose of St. John's wort [13]. Patients using St. John's wort should not subject themselves to artificial ultraviolet radiation and should take normal precautions against sunburn. In general, photosensitivity reactions are mild and transient, disappearing within a few days of drug discontinuation.

No drug interactions with St. John's wort are known. However, formal drug interaction studies have not been performed. Safety for young children, pregnant or nursing women, or those with severe liver or renal disease has not been established. According to one report, overdoses yielded an annual rate of 30.1 deaths per 1 million prescriptions of antidepressant, whereas there has not been a single reported death from an overdose of St. John's wort. Other advantages of St. John's Wort over antidepressants are listed in Table 4-4.

Transition from Pharmaceutical Antidepressants to St. John's Wort

For mild depression, the following protocol is suggested. With SSRIs and tricyclics, add 300 mg of St. John's wort while cutting the antidepressant dose by 50%. For example, if the patient is currently receiving 40 mg of fluoxetine hydrochloride daily, reduce the dose to 20 mg daily. A 20-mg dose is reduced to 10 mg. Because fluoxetine hydrochloride has a long half-life, 20 mg every other day will have an effect similar to 10 mg daily. If no apparent problems develop after 1 week, add another 300 mg of St. John's wort. At 2 weeks, a third dose is added, bringing the daily total to a full 900 mg. By the end of that week, the patient can discontinue the antidepressant.

This is usually a smooth process, with positive results. With more serious depression, leave the antidepressant at half strength for 1 month in combination with the St. John's wort and then reevaluate the patient, tapering off the medication as the full antidepressant effect of the herb is felt. This protocol is generally well tolerated. No reports have been published of serotonin syndrome or any other significant adverse effects. It is theoretically possible that combining St. John's wort with other serotonin-enhancing agents could produce this syndrome. The result of excessive serotonin activity, it is characterized by confusion, shivering, sweating, fever, diarrhea, and muscle spasms. Thus, when prescribing St. John's wort in combination with standard antidepressant drugs, patients should be monitored closely for any suggestive symptoms, and taken off one of the treatments if this occurs.

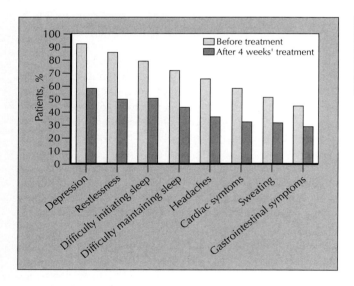

Figure 4-4. Hamilton Depression Scale (HAM-D) scores during 4-week treatment period with St. John's wort or placebo shows statistically significant improvement in the depressive symptoms at 2 weeks, with additional increase after 4 weeks. (*Adapted from* Harrer and Sommer [9].)

Table 4-4. Advantages of St. John's Wort Compared with Antidepressant Drugs

Side effects of St. John's wort are generally mild and infrequent; drug side effects include headaches, nausea, sexual dysfunction, insomnia, sedation, "drugged" feeling, agitation, heart arrhythmias, weight changes, short term memory loss, and rashes

St. John's wort is nonhabituating; nonaddictive, with no withdrawal symptoms on discontinuing use

St. John's wort does not interefere with rapid eye movement (REM) sleep; enhances sleep and dreaming

St. John's wort has no adverse effects when mixed with alcohol or most drugs (exception: monoamine oxidase [MAO] inhibitors, phenelzine sulfate, and tranylcypromine sulfate)

St. John's wort does not cause drowsiness or agitation

Cost of St. John's wort is approximately one tenth that of selective serotonin reuptake inhibitors

Changing from an MAO inhibitor to St. John's wort requires a 4-week washout period between stopping the drug and starting the herb, because we are uncertain of the mode of action of St. John's wort.

FORMULATION

Wide variation exists in the quality and content of commercially available St. John's wort preparations. This variability can affect clinical results, including the side effect profile. Patients may do well on one brand, then switch to another (on their own) with diminished effects. There may also be increased side effects, such as gastrointestinal irritation, in poorer brands. It is important to use standardized extracts to a level that permits a daily dose of approximately 2.7 mg of hypericin, the dose used in research studies. This is so even though hypericin, the marker in St. John's wort, is not likely the active antidepressant. The preparation should also include all of the other naturally occurring substances found in St. John's wort. The better manufacturers assay for these. The American Herbal Products Association (AHPA), which is the national trade association of the herbal products industry, has created standards for its members that reflect quality and reliability (the AHPA is dedicated to education, legislation, and standards in the herbal products industry, and can be reached in the Washington, DC area at (310) 951-3204 or at AHPA@ix.netcom.com). An increasing number of St. John's wort products are standardized to hyperforin, in addition to 0.3% hypericin.

COMBINATIONS

Kava

St. John's wort works well in combination with other herbs and nutrients. In my own practice, I often combine it with kava, particularly in cases of mixed anxiety and depression. St. John's wort may take 2 to 6 weeks to begin working, which some may find discouraging. The rapid response of kava, which acts on the anxiety and insomnia component, provides needed relief in the meantime [30••].

A ritual herb used for centuries in South Pacific Island ceremonies, kava has a tradition as a nonalcoholic, nonaddictive mood and social enhancer. Kava promotes mental and physical relaxation with reduction in muscle tension, without causing the drowsiness of benzodiazepines such as diazepam and alprazolam. In fact, research has shown it to *enhance* alertness and concentration.

One German study found it to be successful in treating menopausal symptoms of depression, anxiety, and insomnia [31]. The usual dose for anxiety and tension is 70 mg of standardized kavalactones, three times daily. It is generally supplied as 150 to 250 mg of kava containing 30% kavalactones (45 to 75 mg kavalactones). In higher doses, it is used to treat insomnia, enhancing rather than suppressing rapid eye movement (REM) sleep, with no morning hangover. For sleep, the dose is double or triple the daytime dose. Kava is particularly useful in older individuals, for whom the benzodiazepines can be dangerous, contributing to falls and other accidents.

Ginseng

A formula that is particularly useful in treating stress combines St. John's wort with Siberian ginseng (eleutherococcus) or Panax ginseng. These are adaptogens, which by definition act to regulate and balance the system. In particular, ginseng supports and replenishes the adrenal glands, an essential part of the stress-fighting system. These glands often become depleted in those suffering from anxiety and depression, and this nutritional support helps to restore their function [32].

Ginkgo Biloba

One of the widest-researched herbs used in Europe, ginkgo is also one of the oldest. Used extensively in Europe and increasingly in North America, it increases blood supply to the brain with improved mental functioning [33]. Studies have shown it to be an effective antidepressant when compared with placebo [34], with few and mild side effects. Dosage is 24% ginkgo flavonglycosides, 40 to 80 mg, two to three times daily. Response occurs between 2 and 12 weeks after initiation.

Elderly patients who appeared withdrawn and barely functioning may come out of their shells and interact normally after a few weeks of ginkgo treatment. These gains are lost if the program is not maintained, and will return when the ginkgo is resumed.

Other Combinations

Some formulas combine St. John's wort and kava with vitamins B_6 and B_{12}, important cofactors in the treatment of depression. Other formulas even add the amino acid tyrosine, another natural antidepressant precursor to norepinephrine. Because depression is many-faceted, with a number of underlying causes, these combinations treat more than one deficiency concurrently.

DIET AND LIFESTYLE

Correct dietary and lifestyle choices can enhance the effectiveness of St. John's wort and round out this natural approach to depression, along with various nutritional supplements that help correct underlying chemical imbalances.

CONCLUSIONS

With its low side effects and high efficacy, there is good reason to consider St. John's wort a reasonable substitute for the pharmaceutical antidepressants in the treatment of mild to moderate depression. We await the results of the NIMH study comparing it with the SSRIs and testing it for use in more severe forms of depression. In the meantime, we as physicians should recall our Hippocratic oath—"First do no harm"—in selecting the optimal treatment plan for our patients.

REFERENCES AND RECOMMENDED READING

Recently published papers of particular interest have been highlighted as:
- Of interest
- • Of outstanding interest

1. St. John's wort now top selling herb in America. *Nutrition Business Journal* 1998:1.
2. *The Diagnostic and Statistical Manual of Mental Disorders*. Washington, DC: American Psychiatric Association; 1994.
3. Stoudemire A: *Clinical Psychiatry for Medical Students* edn 2. New York: JB Lippincott; 1994.
4. Leonard BE: New approaches to the treatment of depression. *J Clin Psychiatry* 1996, 57(suppl):26–33.
5. Werbach M: *Nutritional Influences on Mental Illness*. Tarzana, CA: Third Line Press; 1991.
6. Martinez B, Kasper S, Ruhrman S, et al.: Hypericum in the treatment of seasonal affective disorders. *J Geriatr Psychiatry Neurol* 1994, 7(suppl):S29–S33.
7.•• Cass H: *St. John's Wort: Nature's Blues Buster*. Garden City Park, NY: Avery Publishing; 1998.

Combining clinical experience with a review of the scientific literature, this book provides a practical guide to the use of St. John's wort, alone or in combination with a variety of other supplements, and provides many case examples.

8. Murray M: St. John's wort extract. *Am J Nat Med* 1997, 4:17–18.
9. Harrer G, Sommer H: Placebo-controlled double-blind study examining the effectiveness of an hypericum preparation in 105 mildly depressed patients. *J Geriatr Psychiatry Neurol* 1994, 7(suppl):S9–S11.
10.•• Linde K, Ramirez G, Mulrow CD, et al.: St. John's wort for depression: an overview and meta-analysis of randomized clinical trials. *Br Med J* 1996, 313:253–258.

This is an excellent review of the research to that point and introduced St. John's wort to the English-speaking world.

11. Hänsgen KD, Vesper J, Ploch M, Roots I: Multicenter double-blind study examining the antidepressant effectiveness of the hypericum extract LI 160. *J Geriatr Psychiatry Neurol* 1994, 7(suppl):S15–S18.
12. Ernst E: St. John's Wort, an anti-depressant? A systematic, criteria-based review. *Phytomedicine* 1995, 2:67–71.
13. Schulz V: *Rational Phytotherapy*. New York: Springer Verlag; 1998.
14. Vorbach EU, Hubner WD, Arnoldt KH: Effectiveness and tolerance of the hypericum extract LI 160 in comparison with imipramine: randomized double-blind study with 135 outpatients. *J Geriatr Psychiatry Neurol* 1994, 7(suppl):19–23.
15. Vorbach EU, Hubner WD, Arnoldt KH: Efficacy and tolerability of St. John's wort extract LI 160 vs. imipramine in patients with severe depressive episodes according to ICD-10. *Pharmacopsychiatry* 1997, 30(suppl):81–85.
16. Harrer G, Hubner WD, Pozuweit H: Effectiveness and tolerance of hypericum extract LI 160 compared to maprotiline: a multicenter double blind study with 135 outpatients. *J Geriatr Psychiatry Neurol* YEAR, 7(suppl):19–23.
17. Upton R: *Hypericum Perforatum: American Herbal Pharmacopoeia Monograph*. July 1997.
18. Cott JM: In vitro receptor binding and enzyme inhibition by Hypericum perforatum extract. *Pharmacopsychiatry* 1997, 30(suppl):108–111.
19.• Muller WEG: Hyperforin and the antidepressant activity of St. John's wort. *Pharmacopsychiatry* 1998, 31:1–60.

This study indicates that hyperforin may be "the" active ingredient in St. John's wort.

20. Muller WE, Singer A, Wonnemann M, et al.: Hyperforin represents the neurotransmitter reuptake inhibiting constituent of hypericum extract. *Pharmacopsychiatry* 1998, 31(suppl):16–21.
21. Laakman G, Schule C, Baghai T, Kieser M: St. John's wort in mild to moderate depression: the relevance of hyperforin for clinical efficacy. *Pharmacopsychiatry* 1998, 31(suppl):54–59.
22. Staffeldt B, Kerb B, Brockmoller J, et al.: Pharmacokinetics of hypericin and pseudohypericin after oral intake of the hypericum perforatum extract LI 160 in healthy volunteers. *J Geriatr Psychiatry Neurol* 1994, 7:47–53.
23. Suzuki O, Suzuki O, Katsumata Y, et al.: Inhibition of monoamine oxidase by hypericin. *Planta Med* 1984, 50:2722–2724.
24. Muller WE, Rolli M, Schafer C, Hafner U: Effects of hypericum extract (LI160) in biochemical models of antidepressant activity. *Pharmacopsychiatry* 1997, 30(suppl):102–107.
25. Woelk H, Burkhard G, Grünwald J: Benefits and risks of the hypericum extract LI 160: drug monitoring study with 3250 patients. *J Geriatr Psychiatry Neurol* 1994, 7(suppl): S34–S38.
26. Balon R, Yeragani VK, Pohl R, Ramesh C: Sexual dysfunction during antidepressant treatment. *J Clin Psychiatry* 1994, 54:209–212.
27. Stokes PE: Fluoxetine: a five-year review. *Clin Ther* 1993, 15:216–243.
28. Brockmoller J, Reum T, Bauer S, et al.: Hypericin and pseudohypericin: pharmacokinetics and effects on photosensitivity in humans. *Pharmacopsychiatry* 1997, 30(suppl):94–101.
29. Gulick R, Liu H, Anderson R, et al.: *Human Hypericism: A Photosensitivity Reaction to Hypericin (St. John's Wort), Proc.VIII*. Amsterdam: International Conference on AIDS, 1992.
30.•• Cass H, McNally T: *Kava: Nature's Answer to Stress, Anxiety, and Insomnia*. Rocklin, CA: Prima Publishing; 1998.

This is a review of the physiology, diagnosis, and treatment of stress, anxiety, and insomnia and the use of St. John's wort in their treatment. Clinical cases, together with the history and politics of herb use in the United States give added dimension.

31. Warnecke G: Psychosomatic dysfunctions in the female climacteric: clinical effectiveness and tolerance of kava extract WS 1490. *Fortschr Med* 1991, 109:119–122.
32. Foster S: Three ginsengs: Asian, American, and Siberian. *Herb Companion* 1995:75–77.
33. Eckmann F: Cerebral Insufficiency treatment with g-b extract: time of onset of effect in a double-blind study with 60 inpatients. *Fortschr Med* 1990, 108:557–560.
34. Schubert H, Halama P: Depressive episode primarily unresponsive to therapy in elderly patients: efficacy of ginkgo biloba in combination with antidepressants. *Geriatr Forsch* 1993, 3:45–53.
35.• Schulz V, Hansel R, Tyler VE: *Rational Phytotherapy*. New York: Springer Verlag; 1998.

This is a well-written, in-depth discussion of herbs in common use in Europe.

36.•• Blumenthal M, Busse W, Goldberg A, et al.: *The Complete German Commission E Monographs: Therapeutic Guide to Herbal Medicines*. Boston, MA: Integrative Medicine Communication; 1998.

This is a scientific review by a panel of experts established by the German equivalent of the FDA. It evaluates the safety and efficacy of approximately 300 herbs, providing a basic reference text in the field of phytomedicine.

Food Allergy: Myths and Realities

Suzanne S. Teuber

The term *food allergy* is an all-encompassing term to the public, whereas physicians usually use this particular term to describe individuals who have IgE-mediated reactions consisting of urticaria and related symptoms [1]. This ambiguity of definition has contributed to a public perception that traditional medicine does not acknowledge all ailments that are believed to be related to foods, and has contributed to the explosion of unproven diagnostic and therapeutic modalities in use. Because many of these practices have no scientific basis and because adherence to the rigid diets and practices prescribed may induce degrees of malnutrition or social isolation, it is important for internists to be aware of the most popular unproven techniques in diagnosis and treatment

DEFINITION OF ADVERSE REACTIONS TO FOODS

A useful paradigm for classifying adverse reactions to foods and food additives has been developed [2]. Reactions that have been proven or are believed to be mediated by an immune mechanism are grouped under the term "food hypersensitivity" (or *food allergy*) [2], and those that are due to other mechanisms are termed "food intolerance." These groupings can be further subdivided (Tables 5-1 and 5-2).

The most common food hypersensitivity, an IgE-mediated reaction, affects approximately 1% to 3% of the adult population and up to 5% to 8% of the pediatric population [3–5]. Allergies to milk, egg, wheat, and soy in infants are usually outgrown by 3 years of age, but allergies to fish, crustaceans, peanuts, and tree nuts are usually permanent and sometimes life-threatening [6]. Approximately 100 people per year in the United States die due to IgE-mediated food hypersensitivity [5]. Many of these deaths could be prevented by proper administration of epinephrine in a timely manner. Published series of fatal and near-fatal food reactions show that fatal outcomes are more likely to be associated with a delay in the administration of epinephrine and with eating away from home [7•,8•]. However, most perceived adverse reactions to food are not IgE-mediated, are not immune-mediated, and are not reproducible.

EVALUATION OF ADVERSE REACTIONS TO FOODS

Accepted methods for the diagnosis and management of adverse reactions to food start with a detailed history and physical examination of the patient. If a non–IgE-mediated hypersensitivity reaction involving the intestinal tract is suspected, the patient should be referred to a gastroenterologist. If an IgE-mediated reaction is possible, prick skin tests or in vitro specific IgE assays to specific foods are indicated. Skin test results must be interpreted with caution due to the incidence of false positives; however, one of the most useful applications of skin tests is that the negative predictive value of a negative test is very high (over 95%) in ruling out an IgE-mediated reaction [9]. In vitro specific IgE assays are also useful but appear to be less sensitive. If a patient presents with a definite IgE-mediated reaction and a blood test or skin test for a clearly-implicated food is positive, a diagnosis can usually be confidently established. However, in other cases, food diaries, an elimination diet, and single-blind or double-blind, placebo-controlled food challenges (DBPCFC) are the next steps, especially if an elimination diet (or elemental diet) of 2 weeks has resolved the symptom(s). Published guidelines for the evaluation of adverse food reactions and performing such challenges are available [6,10,11••].

If a patient has a serious adverse reaction to food (asthma, angioedema, laryngoedema, anaphylaxis), they should be referred to an allergy subspecialist if food challenges are needed. However, if the reaction consists of itching, rhinitis, nausea, headache, fatigue, myalgia, or other non–life-threatening symptoms, food challenges—in particular, single-blind challenges of the suspected food hidden in a liquid carrier—could be incorporated into a busy internist's practice. The challenges could provide helpful answers for patients if the results are negative. Ideally, double-blind protocols should be followed if a patient believes they have multiple intolerances, and are absolutely indicated when a single-blind challenge is positive for subjective symptoms. When food hypersensitivity or intolerance is found, no treatment is usually available except avoidance. In trials using DBPCFC, patients with food hypersensitivity or intolerance rarely react to more than one food (*eg*, patients with soy allergy usually tolerate the other legumes) [14], which makes subsequent dietary restriction much easier.

Many patients have read claims about reactions to food and various purported treatments in the press. They may seek support for their views from an internist and, when not forthcoming, may seek help from someone who holds their view. Common symptoms attributed to food allergies are headache, fatigue, difficulty concentrating, myalgia, arthralgia, bloating, stomachache, and loose stools. When such symptoms are carefully evaluated by a DBPCFC, usually no relationship is found. Of course, there are exceptions. For example, in a 1990 study, Parker *et al*. [15] studied 21 people with negative prick-skin tests to an implicated food and three people who claimed sensitivity to white sugar (skin testing was not done in these three). The reactions reported by the subjects included migraines, abdominal pain, swelling, nausea, itching, confusion,

TABLE 5-1. TYPES OF FOOD HYPERSENSITIVITY REACTIONS

IgE-mediated
Immediate (can include any of the following)
 Urticaria, angioedema
 Rhinoconjunctivitis
 Laryngoedema
 Asthma
 Nausea/vomiting, abdominal cramps, diarrhea
 Hypotension
Immediate and late phase
 Atopic dermatitis
 Allergic eosinophilic gastroenteritis
Other IgE-mediated
 Food-dependent exercise induced anaphylaxis
 Food-dependent exercise induced urticaria/angioedema
 Infantile colic (some)

Other immune mechanisms (not clearly delineated)
 Gluten sensitive enteropathy (celiac disease)
 Food protein-induced enterocolitis
 Food protein-induced colitis
 Heiner's syndrome
 Milk-induced thrombocytopenia (rare) [12]
 Dermatitis herpetiformis
 Arthritis (rare) [13]

Adapted from Sampson [10]; with permission.

TABLE 5-2. EXAMPLES OF ETIOLOGY OF FOOD INTOLERANCE REACTIONS

Metabolic
 Lactase deficiency
 Pancreatic insufficiency
Toxins/additives
 Bacterial toxins
 Fungal toxins
 Endogenous toxins
  Uncooked lectins
  Solanine in green potato skin
  Saxitoxin in seafood
  Ciguatera poisoning
  Scombroid poisoning (histamine)
 Infectious
  Bacterial
  Viral
  Parasitic
 Flavoring
  Monosodium glutamate
 Preservatives
  Nitrates/nitrites
  Sulfites
 Antibiotics
 Dyes
Endogenous chemicals with pharmacologic activity
 Caffeine
 Histamine
 Tyramine
 Theobromine
 Tryptamine
 Alcohol
 Phenylethylamine
Psychologic
 Food aversion
 Eating disorder
Unknown

Data from James and Sampson [6], Sampson [10], and Sampson [16••].

fatigue, bloating, and weakness. Only one DBPCFC out of 24 was positive—the elicitation of a migraine headache in a subject with soy intolerance. If evaluated by some of the following methods, however, a patient's beliefs about a food may be incorrectly validated and a cycle of obsession around food avoidance can be started.

UNPROVEN METHODS IN DIAGNOSIS OR THERAPY

Provocation/Neutralization Testing

Provocation/neutralization testing to foods is an unproven technique that involves intracutaneous "provocation" by a test antigen, followed by an observation period of 10 to 20 minutes after each injection, at which time the wheal response is measured and any subjective symptoms are reported. Alternatively, a drop of the antigen can be applied sublingually. Subjective symptoms, such as drowsiness or headache are considered a positive challenge, meaning that the person is "allergic" to the food. The patient then receives a different dose of the antigen as either a sublingual drop or another injection until the "reaction" is "neutralized." This "neutralization" dose would then be taken before an anticipated exposure on a daily or weekly basis, as deemed best by the practitioner [17–19]. It has been touted in the otolaryngology and clinical ecology literature as a safe, effective therapy [19, 20].

Provocation/neutralization testing for adverse food reactions has been shown to be ineffective in a double-blind, placebo-controlled challenge study [20]. This type of procedure relies on a placebo response for effectiveness [21]. The American Academy of Allergy, Asthma, and Immunology (AAAAI) [22, 23•] does not approve of these procedures for the diagnosis and treatment of adverse reactions to foods.

Cytotoxic Food Testing

Cytotoxic food testing hinges on the belief that the morphology or viability of peripheral blood mononuclear cells is affected by contact with foods to which a patient is "allergic" [24]. Typically, a panel of slides will have a dried film of food extract to which a drop of whole blood is added, and the slide viewed. Any morphologic change (crenation or lysis) can be considered positive. There are no valid controls, and investigators have shown that there is no relationship between such changes and clinical symptoms in the case of IgE-mediated food hypersensitivity or when subjective symptoms are attributed to foods [25, 26].

The 4-Day Rotation Diet or Rotary Diversified Diet

The 4-day rotation diet is based on the belief that foods are tolerated better if food groups are rotated completely so that an individual only eats food from one dietary group every 4 to 5 days and not in between [27]. There is no scientific evidence to substantiate this claim, and this diet is burdensome to follow. It may have clinical use as an elimination diet but this has not been evaluated.

Specific IgG (IgG ras-t) Testing

Some laboratories offer in vitro determination of specific IgG- or IgG4-mediated reactions to foods. However, it is normal to produce some IgG (but especially IgA) to the foods we eat the most [28,29]. When subclasses of IgG began to be investigated, there was much interest in IgG4 as a surrogate marker for IgE-mediated allergy, or in its own right as a mediator of inflammation, but it has been shown that normal people produce IgG4 to foods without manifesting symptoms [30–32]. Extremely high levels of IgG to food antigens, which can be visualized by a precipitin assay, are associated and possibly involved in the pathogenesis of food-induced pulmonary hemosiderosis (Heiner's syndrome), which has been seen with cow's milk ingestion [33], and in case reports with egg and pork [34]. There is no proof of IgG antibody involvement in other types of reactions to foods as yet, so such testing is not recommended.

Food Immune Complex Assay Testing

As with circulating food-specific IgG, normal individuals are found to have circulating immune complexes containing food antigens [35–38]. The intestinal mucosa is not impermeable; small amounts of antigen are absorbed and may become part of an immune complex, which is a normal event in the immune response and leads to elimination of the antigen. It has not yet been shown that any clinical disease involves circulating immune complexes to foods. This assay should be considered experimental only [39•].

Applied Kinesiology Testing

In applied kinesiology testing, muscle strength is measured subjectively by a technician using one of the patient's arms while vials containing various foods are held in the patient's opposite hand. A drop in strength indicates "allergy" to a food. No controlled studies validate the claims, nor is there a theoretical scientific explanation. A blinded study of 20 patients showed that results were random and not reproducible [40].

Electrodermal Testing

Electrodermal testing involves the patient being attached to a sometimes elaborate-appearing machine that uses a galvanometer to measure skin conductance. The patient holds the negative electrode in one hand and the positive electrode is applied to various acupuncture points in the lower extremities believed to be related to food allergy. A glass vial of food allergen is put in contact with an aluminum plate within the circuit. If there is a drop in electrical skin conductance, "allergy" is diagnosed [41]. There are no controlled studies and there is no scientific rationale to substantiate these claims.

CONCLUSIONS

Many subjective symptoms are associated with the ingestion of food. This is not surprising, considering that much of our daily life revolves around the procurement, preparation, and ingestion of foodstuffs. Adverse reactions to foods can be immune-mediated, in which case a paradigm of descriptions under the term *food hypersensitivity* may help facilitate communication among physicians and patients, or nonimmune-mediated *food intolerance*, which is far more common. In many cases, it is acceptable to simply acknowledge that we truly do not know all the effects of various phytochemicals, lectins, lipids, proteins, and fibers on humans and that the possibility of various unexplained adverse reactions (including immune) to specific foods is real. However, if a patient is pursuing significant or just plain difficult dietary restrictions (*eg*, no corn products, including all corn syrup, sweeteners, and sugars), and especially if a patient is the recipient of restrictions at the hand of someone else (*eg*, the infirm, elderly, and young) then, by all means, blinded food challenges should be pursued to determine if there is a definite link between a specific symptom and diet (and in the most common scenario, to prove a lack of association). This may be facilitated by referral to a subspecialist.

The broad range of IgE-mediated food hypersensitivity, varying from minor mouth itching to anaphylaxis, should be remembered. All patients with potentially life-threatening reactions should be prescribed epinephrine. During recruitment for our ongoing studies, we spoke with individuals who responded to a local Sacramento press release asking for volunteers with anaphylactic sensitivity to tree nuts, peanuts, or seeds. Out of 31 patients who were treated in the emergency room with epinephrine for life-threatening reactions, only 21 had ever been advised to carry epinephrine for self-administration by any physician (emergency room, primary care, or allergist). In addition, many volunteers told us that they had never discussed their food hypersensitivity with their primary care physician. Thus, there are significant numbers of patients with potentially life-threatening IgE-mediated food hypersensitivity who would benefit from evaluation, counseling, and prescription of epinephrine, in addition to many more who have food beliefs and intolerances causing lifestyle hindrances (and possibly malnutrition) that may benefit from evaluation. Some of the latter may hold such strong beliefs about foods that they are not interested in further evaluation of their "allergies."

REFERENCES AND RECOMMENDED READING

Recently published papers of particular interest have been highlighted as:
- Of interest
- Of outstanding interest

1. Sloan AE: A perspective on popular perceptions of adverse reactions to foods. *J Allergy Clin Immunol* 1986, 78:127–132.
2. American Academy of Allergy and Immunology/NIAID: *Adverse Reactions to Foods*. Edited by Anderson JA, Sogn DD. Washington, DC: NIH Publication no. 84-2442; 1984:1–6.
3. Kayosaari M: Food allergy in Finnish children aged 1 to 6 years. *Acta Paediatric Scand* 1982, 71:815–819.
4. Bock SA: Prospective appraisal of complaints of adverse reactions to foods in children during the first 3 years of life. *Pediatr* 1987, 79:683–688.
5. Sampson HA, Metcalfe DD: Food allergies. *JAMA* 1992, 268:2840–2844.
6. James JM, Sampson HA: An overview of food hypersensitivity. *Pediatr Allergy Immunol* 1992, 3:67–78.
7.• Sampson HA, Mendelson L, Rosen JP: Fatal and near-fatal anaphylactic reactions to food in children and adolescents. *N Engl J Med* 1992, 327:380–384.
   This case series helped identify risk factors for fatal reactions to foods.
8.• Yunginger JW, Sweeney KG, Sturner WQ, *et al.*: Fatal food-induced anaphylaxis. *JAMA* 1988, 260:1450–1452.
   This case series also helped identify risk factors for fatal reactions to foods.
9. Sampson HA: In vitro diagnosis and mediator assays for food allergies. *Allergy Proc* 1993, 14:259–261.
10. Sampson HA: Adverse Reactions to Foods. In *Allergy Principles and Practice*, edn 4. Edited by Middleton E, Reed CE, Ellis EF, *et al*. St. Louis: Mosby; 1993:1661–1686.
11.•• Bock SA, Sampson HA, Atkins FM, *et al.*: Double-blind placebo-controlled food challenge as an office procedure: A manual. *J Allergy Clin Immunol* 1988, 82:986–997.
   This is a step-by-step outline of how to stringently conduct DBPCFCs.
12. Caffrey EA, Sladen GE, Isaacs PET, *et al.*: Thrombocytopenia caused by cow's milk. *Lancet* 1981, 2:316.
13. Panush RS, Stroud RM, Webster E: Food-induced (allergic) arthritis: inflammatory arthritis exacerbated by milk. *Arthritis Rheum* 1986, 29:220–226.
14. Bernhisel-Broadbent J, Sampson HA: Cross-allergenicity in the legume botanical family in children with food hypersensitivity. *J Allergy Clin Immunol* 1989, 83:435–440.
15. Parker SL, Leznoff A, Sussman GL, *et al.*: Characteristics of patients with food-related complaints. *J Allergy Clin Immunol* 1990, 86:503–511.
16.•• Sampson HA: Immediate reactions to foods in infants and children. In *Food Allergy: Adverse Reactions to Food and Food Additives*, edn 2. Edited by Metcalfe DD, Sampson HA, Simon RA. Cambridge, MA: Blackwell Science; 1997:169–182.
   This chapter is an excellent review of the different types of hypersensitivity responses to foods. The entire text is highly recommended as the most comprehensive reference available on the subject of adverse reactions to food.
17. Willoughby JW: Provocative food test technique. *Ann Allergy* 1965, 23:543–553.
18. King WP, Rubin WA, Fadal RG, *et al.*: Provocation-neutralization: a two-part study. Part I. The intracutaneous provocative food test: a multi-center comparison study. *Otolaryngol Head Neck Surg* 1988, 99:263–271.
19. King WP, Rubin WA, Fadal RG, *et al.*: Provocation-neutralization: a two-part study. Part II. Subcutaneous neutralization therapy: a multi-center study. *Otolaryngol Head Neck Surg* 1988, 99:272–277.
20. Jewett DL, Fein G, Greenberg MH: A double-blind study of symptom provocation to determine food sensitivity. *N Engl J Med* 1990, 323:429–433.
21. Ferguson A: Food sensitivity or self-deception? *N Engl J Med* 1990, 323:476–478.
22. American Academy of Allergy, Asthma, and Immunology: Position statements: controversial techniques. *J Allergy Clin Immunol* 1981, 67:333–338.
23.• American Academy of Allergy, Asthma, and Immunology: Position statements: clinical ecology. *J Allergy Clin Immunol* 1986, 78:269–277.
   This and all position statements by the AAAAI can be viewed on the World Wide Web at http://www.aaaai.org.
24. Bryan WTK, Bryan MP: Cytotoxic reactions in the diagnosis of food allergy. *Otolaryngol Clin North Am* 1971, 4:523–534.
25. Lieberman P, Crawford L, Bjelland J, *et al.*: Controlled study of the cytotoxic food text. *JAMA* 1974, 231:728–730.
26. Benson TE, Arkins JA: Cytotoxic testing for food allergy: evaluations of reproducibility and correlation. *J Allergy Clin Immunol* 1976, 58:471–476.
27. Randolph TG: An ecologic orientation in medicine: comprehensive environment control in diagnosis and therapy. *Ann Allergy* 1965, 23:7–22.

28. Korenblatt RE, Rothberg RM, Minden P, Farr RS: Immune response of human adults after oral and parenteral exposure to bovine serum albumin. *J Allergy* 1968, 41:226–236.
29. Rothberg RM, Farr RS: Anti-bovine serum albumin and anti-alpha lactalbumin in the serum of children and adults. *Pediatrics* 1965, 35:571–588.
30. Merrett J, Burr MI, Merrett TG: A community survey of IgG4 antibody levels. *Clin Allergy* 1983, 13:397–407.
31. Layton GT, Stanworth DR: The quantitation of IgG4 antibodies to three common food allergens by ELISA with monoclonal anti-IgG4. *J Immunol Methods* 1984, 73:347–356.
32. Halpern GM, Scott JR, Sun J, et al.: IgG4 antibody levels in normal healthy adults: a follow-up study. *J Allergy Clin Immunol* 1986, 77:124.
33. Heiner DC, Sears JW: Chronic respiratory disease associated with multiple circulating precipitins to cow's milk. *Am J Dis Child* 1960, 100:500–502.
34. Lee SK, Kniker WT, Cook CD, et al.: Cow's milk-induced pulmonary disease in children. *Adv Pediatr* 1978, 25:39–57.
35. Paganelli R, Levinsky RJ, Brostoff J, et al.: Immune complexes containing food proteins in normal and atopic subjects after oral challenge and effect of sodium cromoglycate on antigen absorption. *Lancet* 1979, 1:1270–1272.
36. Haddad ZH, Vetter M, Friedman J, et al.: Detection and kinetics of antigen-specific IgE and IgG immune complexes in food allergy. *Ann Allergy* 1983, 51:255.
37. Leary HL, Halsey JF: An assay to measure antigen-specific immune complexes in food allergy patients. *J Allergy Clin Immunol* 1984, 74:190–195.
38. Paganelli R, Quinti I, D'Offizi GP, et al.: Immune-complexes in food allergy: a critical reappraisal. *Ann Allergy* 1987, 59:157–161.
39.• Terr AI: Unconventional theories and unproven methods in allergy. In *Allergy Principles and Practice*, edn 5. Edited by Middleton E, Reed CE, Ellis EF, et al. St. Louis: Mosby; 1998:1767–1793.

This is a thorough review of all unproven methods of diagnosis and treatment of food allergy or other allergies.

40. Garrow JS: Kinesiology and food allergy. *Br Med J* 1988, 296:1573–1578.
41. Tsuei JJ, Lehman CW, Lam FMK, Zhu DAH: A food allergy study utilizing the EAV acupuncture technique. *Am J Acupuncture* 1984, 12:105.

Integrative Treatment of Fibromyalgia and Chronic Fatigue/Immune Dysfunction Syndrome

Keith Berndtson

The terms *alternative medicine*, *complementary medicine*, and *integrative medicine* are often used interchangeably. The phrase *complementary and alternative medicine* (CAM) is also frequently used. Not all authors agree about how these terms are defined. For the sake of clarity, I have assigned working definitions for these terms. *Alternative medicine*, perhaps the most widely used and recognized term, refers to all healing methods and traditions not routinely taught in the education and training programs of conventional medicine, including the more controversial alternative healing methods. *Complementary medicine* is a less divisive term that presumes that some alternative approaches are safe and work reasonably well, and that we will call them complementary to conventional medical approaches until such time as they can themselves be considered conventional. *Integrative medicine* refers to a clinical approach that seeks to combine the strengths of conventional and alternative medicine, with a bias toward options that are considered safe and that will, on review of the available evidence, offer reasonable expectations of benefit to the patient. This chapter summarizes current thinking on the treatment of fibromyalgia and chronic fatigue/immune dysfunction syndrome (CFIDS) from an integrative perspective.

CONVENTIONAL VERSUS INTEGRATIVE MEDICINE

Significant differences are present in the core philosophies from which conventional and integrative methods approach the clinical care of patients. Three of the most important differences are considered briefly here.

Reductionism versus Holism

By reducing our understanding of the human body to terms of molecular biology, conventional biomedicine has achieved major breakthroughs in the diagnosis and treatment of many diseases, especially those of an acute or critical nature. A reductionistic model favors the concept of upward causation, in which molecular activities determine a person's cellular and organ system functions, and, by extension, his or her relative state of health or disease. Less emphasis is placed on matters that are more difficult to understand in molecular terms, such as psychosocial phenomena, or the role of emotions in determining health, simply because it is hard to describe mental or emotional phenomena in precise molecular terms (notwithstanding fascinating treatments of the subject that have appeared)[1•]. Reductionist theorists also have trouble with the idea of downward causation, which holds that thoughts and emotions can drive molecular function and, by extension, the relative state of health or disease. Integrative medicine embraces both upward and downward causation within a general systems model of multilevel, multidirectional causes and effects.

Clinical Implications of Complex Biologic Systems

Molecular biology has elaborated impressive models for understanding cell function and the interrelationships of homeostatic systems. From receptor dynamics and the movement of intracellular messengers, to genetic expression and the control of cell proliferation and energy production, to the mediating processes of digestion, elimination, inflammation, and repair, reductionistic biomedicine has penetrated the invisible workings of the body to an awesome degree. Even so, good reasons exist for us to remain humble before the mysterious subtlety and complexity of the human body. For instance, credible speculation supports the idea that meaningful information is communicated within homeostatic systems at the level of weak electromagnetic fields [2•]. If this is true, it will take years of dedicated effort to support the concept with solid scientific evidence. If true, however, complementary interventions, such as homeopathy or acupuncture, that may operate at such subtle homeostatic levels deserve careful consideration as clinical options today.

From a philosophic perspective, integrative medicine, as opposed to conventional medicine, is willing to believe that CAM therapies work at some level within complex biologic systems, and shares this perspective with patients, who are ultimately in the business of collecting information, weighing options, and going forward with a strategy for health care. An integrative medical approach acknowledges the limits to our scientific understanding of complex biologic systems and maintains its focus on the patient rather than on the disease.

Disease-Centered versus Patient-Centered Medicine

Disease-centered practitioners are often accused of getting so caught up in the pathophysiology of an illness that they lose sight of the many other facets of illness that factor into the clinical care of human beings. A patient-centered approach must be based on empathetic listening, understanding, and a willingness to explain and consider the antecedents and triggers of illness peculiar to the life a given patient has lived [3•]. A patient-centered approach recognizes the healing potential of simply being heard, and it uses the power of positive meaning to foster healing.

A patient-centered approach looks beyond disease pathophysiology to consider how biography influences biology. For patients with complex forms of chronic illness, if an alternative path is considered safe and offers reasonable expectations of benefit, and the patient wants to explore it, an integrative clinician is willing to serve as trail guide. Patient and clinician together agree to proceed, responding and adapting to the patient's course of treatment as partners. As evidenced by the high rate at which they seek CAM therapies [4,5], few patients are more in need of guidance concerning CAM options than those with fibromyalgia or CFIDS.

Diagnosing Fibromyalgia and Chronic Fatigue/Immune Dysfunction Syndrome

The classic diagnostic criteria for fibromyalgia were proposed by the American College of Rheumatology in 1990 (Table 6-1)[6]. The diagnostic criteria for CFIDS were proposed by the Centers for Disease Control and Prevention in 1994 (Table 6-2)[7]. Various modifications of the diagnostic criteria for both fibromyalgia and CFIDS have been proposed. Some have suggested that fibromyalgia and CFIDS are the same illness, but they should be distinguished. Fibromyalgia patients, for example, tend not to experience recurrent, low-grade fevers. CFIDS patients do not typically present with a chronic, widespread pain syndrome. Many patients, however, meet the criteria for both. What impresses most clinicians who work with these patients is the quantity of nonspecific abnormalities that have been documented, and the range of credible hypotheses about causes and pathogenesis that have stemmed from these observations.

One of these hypotheses states that a substantial subgroup of CFIDS patients may suffer from an aberrant RNase-L enzyme, which, in turn, hampers antiviral defenses and may cause other homeostatic insults as well [8]. Several investigative leads point to a form of brain injury, the consequences of which include impaired processing of information in areas that may include the thalamus, limbic system, prefrontal cortex, hypothalamus, or other centers. The pattern of injury may vary from patient to patient. In this view, a molecular regulatory system somehow gets deranged, and the result is as though "microbullets" were sprayed at neural networks connecting these brain centers. These patients have multiple symptoms, and yet no known pathognomonic markers in the periphery. Pain signal processing, communication along various endocrine axes, sleep cycling, and autonomic function could all be affected.

Remember that the name is not the thing itself, and that in fibromyalgia and CFIDS, the thing itself is better described as a nonspecific, psycho-neuro-immuno-endocrinologic illness

TABLE 6-1. AMERICAN COLLEGE OF RHEUMATOLOGY CRITERIA FOR THE CLASSIFICATION OF FIBROMYALGIA*

History of widespread pain†
  Pain is considered widespread when all of the following are present:
   Pain in the left side of the body
   Pain in the right side of the body
   Pain above the waist
   Pain below the waist
   Axial skeletal pain (cervical, anterior chest, thoracic, or lumbosacral)
  Pain in 11 of 18 tender points on digital palpation†
   Bilateral, suboccipital muscle insertions
   Bilateral, intertransverse spaces, C5–C7
   Bilateral, trapezius, midpoints on upper border
   Bilateral, supraspinatus, medial border of scapular spine
   Bilateral, above and lateral to second costochondral junctions
   Bilateral, 2 cm distal to lateral epicondyles
   Bilateral, gluteal (upper, outer quadrants)
   Bilateral, greater trochanter (posterior to prominence)
   Knees, bilateral, medial fat pads proximal to joint line

*1990
†Widespread pain present for at least 3 months; palpation force of approximately 4 kg produces pain.

TABLE 6-2. CENTERS FOR DISEASE CONTROL AND PREVENTION CRITERIA FOR CHRONIC FATIGUE SYNDROME

A case of chronic fatigue syndrome is defined by the presence of the following:
Clinically evaluated, unexplained, persistent, or relapsing chronic fatigue of new or definite onset (not lifelong), not the result of ongoing exertion, and not substantially alleviated by rest. Results in substantial reduction in previous levels of occupational, educational, social, or personal activities.
Concurrent occurrence of four or more of the following symptoms, all of which must have persisted or recurred during 6 or more consecutive months of illness and must not have predated the fatigue:
Self-reported impairment in short-term memory or concentration severe enough to cause substantial reduction in previous levels of occupational, educational, social, or personal activities
Sore throat
Tender cervical or axillary lymph nodes
Muscle pain
Multijoint pain without joint swelling or redness
Headaches of a new type, pattern, or severity
Unrefreshing sleep
Postexertional malaise lasting more than 24 hours

resulting in a range of debilitating conditions that, in addition to pain, fatigue, and nonrestorative sleep, can include a range of "allied health problems." These problems include, but are not limited to, migraine headaches, allergies, interstitial cystitis, impaired cognition, irritable bowel syndrome, dizziness and vertigo, regional abnormalities in cerebral blood flow, temporomandibular joint syndrome, mitochondrial dysfunction, Raynaud's phenomenon, multiple chemical sensitivity, decreased natural killer cell function, and non-specific, low-grade autoimmunity (Table 6-3 lists examples of health conditions allied with fibromyalgia and CFIDS).

A few patients meeting the criteria for fibromyalgia or CFIDS have another diagnosable condition that accounts for their symptoms. Some of these conditions are listed in Table 6-4. Still at issue is whether a significant percentage of patients diagnosed with fibromyalgia or CFIDS actually suffer from some form of major depression. Family history studies support the possibility of depression [9], but medical history studies support the notion that, in most fibromyalgia/CFIDS patients, depression follows the onset of their multisystem problems, and it is thus reactive rather than primary [10]. In these patients, primary depression may be a comorbid condition.

Rarely, a patient with a supportable but suspect diagnosis of fibromyalgia or CFIDS is stuck in a pattern of illness behavior with perhaps too much at risk in getting well. Malingering for the purpose of receiving disability payments has been reported [11], but the insurance industry and governmental agencies confronted with the dilemma of judging disability on cases of fibromyalgia or CFIDS are recognizing that many claims are valid and so they are calling for research aimed at better discriminating types of fibromyalgia- or CFIDS-related disabilities [12].

Although much uncertainty remains about the causes and pathophysiology of fibromyalgia and CFIDS, the body of positive information on therapeutic strategies is increasing. When approached from an integrative medical perspective, the prognosis for fibromyalgia and CFIDS is optimistic.

TABLE 6-3. "ALLIED" HEALTH PROBLEMS ASSOCIATED WITH FIBROMYALGIA AND CHRONIC FATIGUE/IMMUNE DYSFUNCTION SYNDROME

Allergies
Chronic indigestion
Chronic sinusitis
Cognitive impairment
Dizziness and vertigo
Eczema
Hashimoto's thyroiditis
Interstitial cystitis
Idiopathic neuropathies
Irritable bowel syndrome
Low-grade, non-specific autoimmunity
Migraine headaches
Mitochondrial dysfunction
Multiple chemical sensitivity
Raynaud's phenomenon
Regional blood flow abnormalities
Temporomandibular joint syndrome

INTEGRATIVE TREATMENT ISSUES
Interviewing the Patient

Treatment of fibromyalgia and CFIDS begins with listening to the patient. The experience of being listened to and validated is new to many of these patients, some of whom have been to several physicians before consulting an empathetic practitioner. The act of listening builds rapport and begins the healing process. The past medical and social histories of these patients are often lengthy and complicated. Given the time constraints placed on most practices, however, it may be necessary to divide the intake interview into two or even three sessions.

TABLE 6-4. DIFFERENTIAL DIAGNOSIS OF FIBROMYALGIA AND CHRONIC FATIGUE/IMMUNE DYSFUNCTION SYNDROME

Adverse drug reactions
Anemia
Anorexia nervosa
Autoimmune disease
    Inflammatory bowel disease
    Myasthenia gravis
    Rheumatoid arthritis
    Scleroderma
    Sjögren's syndrome
    Vasculitides
Chronic myofascial pain
    (regional rather than widespread pain)
Chronic renal failure
Cirrhosis
Depression
Diabetes mellitus
Drug or alcohol abuse
Hyponatremia
Hypopituitarism
Hypothyroidism
Infectious disease
    Fungal infections
    Chronic hepatitis B or C
    HIV
    Lyme disease
    Parasitic infections
Malingering/secondary gain
Multiple sclerosis
Occult malignancy
Sarcoidosis
Sleep apnea

A patient-centered approach to history-taking works to gain a sense of the person's unique biography. A useful way to begin is to ask, "When was the last time you felt perfectly well?" The patient may pinpoint the start of his or her troubles to a specific flulike illness, accident, or other trauma, saying he or she has never been the same since. In these cases, evidence suggests that chemical or mechanical insults to central nervous system function triggered a cascade of imbalances from which the patient has been unable to recover [13,14]. In other cases, the patient may indicate that the start of his or her troubles was a period of time, lasting several months to years, associated with an insidious, steady decline in health and the appearance of new symptoms. In these cases, it is useful to question the patient about what occurred in his or her life over the year or two preceding this decline. It is common to learn that the patient was experiencing chronic physical, mental, or emotional strain punctuated by acutely stressful events. Some patients will ponder the question for a few moments, then look away, tears welling, and say, "I can't remember ever feeling well." These patients may be suffering from reactive or primary depression, which needs to be treated accordingly. They also may simply be reflecting with sadness on the negative meaning of feeling so poorly and being so misunderstood for so long.

Studies estimate the prevalence of victimization experience (*eg,* physical, emotional, or sexual abuse) preceding the onset of fibromyalgia and CFIDS to be somewhere between 50% and 65%, although little evidence to date has validated any causal association [15]. It may be that patients who have been victims of abuse in the past are primed to feel violated anew by their fibromyalgia or CFIDS.

It is not uncommon for these patients to present with the infamous "positive review of systems," in which almost every organ system is involved in one way or another. This is the fate of those suffering from a condition whose downstream consequences are increasingly traced to abnormalities in signal processing at multiple levels within the central nervous system [16].

The Healing Path

The interview, when approached with sensitivity, empathy, and patience, will elicit critical information about the person's biography, precedents of illness stemming from his or her life, triggers associated with illness onset, allied health conditions present, predominant symptom patterns, and which therapies have already been tried and with what results. When history, physical examination, and laboratory investigation lead to a supportable diagnosis of fibromyalgia, CFIDS, or both, it becomes time to map out a treatment plan. From an integrative medical perspective, the treatment plan is frequently referred to as a *healing path*, because this term better conveys the idea of treatment as a journey with its ups and downs, in which patient and physician together clear the way to an improved quality of life for the patient.

The healing path should specify the main problems and the treatment goals, and then determine which endpoints will be used to gauge progress toward those goals. It should also specify which additional diagnostic evaluations are warranted and why, which kinds of patient education and empowerment tools are recommended, which medications and nutritional or botanical supplements will aid recovery, and which forms of conventional or CAM therapies should be used to support the healing process. Movement along the path is a dynamic process aimed at restoring balance at multiple system levels. It needs to be revisited and revised at regular intervals.

When designing an integrative healing path for patients with fibromyalgia or CFIDS, the following areas should be addressed: pain, energy, sleep, hormone balance, autonomic function, digestion and elimination, nutritional status, allergies, immune system function, mood, exercise, and coping and support. Treatments focused in one area will often yield dividends in another. The goal (and the challenge) of an integrative healing path for patients with fibromyalgia or CFIDS is to identify a critical mass of imbalances in homeostasis and to restore balance to these systems more or less simultaneously over a period of 6 to 12 months.

Pain

It is not clear whether the chronic, widespread pain phenomena observed in patients with fibromyalgia or CFIDS are primarily central, autonomic, or peripheral in nature. It may prove to be some combination, the pathophysiology of which differs from subgroup to subgroup. Narcotic pain relievers are rarely justified, and patients who present while receiving this therapy should accept a tapering schedule as part of the healing path. The same is true for chronic, long-term use of nonsteroidal anti-inflammatory drugs, because the risk of gastritis or nephropathy may exceed the drug's analgesic benefits. Moreover, the drugs' mechanism of action does little to address the neuroendocrine pain-related factors in these patients. Various pharmacologic agents have been reported by Goldstein [17] to provide significant relief, but results are hard to predict and are based primarily on case studies.

Acupuncture treatment is routinely helpful in the management of chronic pain [18]. According to experienced practitioners, acupuncture also has the potential to help restore homeostatic balance at other levels in these patients [19]. It is not clear whether significant differences exist between different acupuncture styles (*ie*, traditional Chinese, Japanese, Korean, French classical) or methods (dry needling with or without electrical stimulation, ear, scalp, moxibustion). Perhaps the various styles and methods have equivalent healing potential. The overall effectiveness of acupuncture in the treatment of fibromyalgia and CFIDS probably lies in the skill with which a practitioner applies his or her techniques not simply toward pain management, but toward general health promotion and the "unblocking" of the patient's chi, or essential life force.

Massage therapy, the systematic manipulation of the soft tissues of the body, is also favored by many of these patients, suggesting that at least some peripheral component to the widespread pain is amenable to manual medicine [20]. Techniques can affect musculoskeletal, circulatory, lymphatic, and nervous system tissues. In addition to help with pain management, massage techniques can also trigger emotional release and contribute to the relief of psychologic distress [21]. Trigger point therapy, including injections, can be used to help break the cycle of spasm and pain [22]. Chiropractic interventions, in addition to treating pain and related biomechanical issues, can offer much to these patients as part of an integrative approach to therapy. In the same way that acupuncture works to promote general health, chiropractic manipulation, by decreasing the "noise" through which nervous system information must flow, may work to unblock innate healing intelligence [23].

Oral supplementation with a combination of magnesium and malic acid has been reported to be useful in managing the pain of fibromyalgia [24]. An intravenous combination of magnesium citrate, calcium gluconate, vitamin C, and B vitamins administered by slow push through an antecubital vein has also been reported useful in patients with fibromyalgia [25••]. Whether the benefits are due to the spasmolytic effects of magnesium, antioxidant support, enzyme support, or other properties is not known, but the slow intravenous push of this "nutritional cocktail" is able to create a large concentration gradient between extracellular and intracellular spaces, speeding up tissue repletion of these micronutrients.

Energy

Supplementation with magnesium and malic acid and other nutrients may help boost energy in addition to diminishing pain. Of particular help are the "mitochondrial resuscitant factors": coenzyme-Q-10, acetyl-L-carnitine, and reduced nicotinamide-adenine dinucleotide (NADH)[26]. These nutrients are co-factors in oxidative phosphorylation and in the conversion of oxygen into chemical energy.

Restoring balanced homeostatic function in any of the psychophysiologic systems discussed in this chapter can be expected to improve energy by decreasing metabolic drain or increasing metabolic efficiency.

Sleep

Improving sleep with pharmaceuticals can improve energy, decrease pain, and enhance self-reported quality of life in patients with fibromyalgia or CFIDS [27–30]. In practice, clinicians typically have a choice of therapeutic options, and, based on the patient's clinical profile and personal preferences, they will cycle through them one or more at a time until the patient reports some degree of improvement. Medications worth trying include amitriptyline, nortriptyline, cyclobenzaprine, and zolpidem. Natural medicines with reported uses include St. John's Wort [31], valerian, and melatonin [32,33]. In general, these patients have less trouble with falling asleep than with sleeping well through the night. Remedies that help patients cycle through their sleep stages better will provide the most benefit. Patient education concerning behaviors that promote good sleep hygiene, including the use of relaxation tapes, may offer additional help.

Hormone Balance

The thyroid gland produces two major versions of thyroid hormone: T4 and T3. Of the total amount of T3 in the body, only about 20% comes from the thyroid gland itself. The other 80% is made when the enzyme 5-deiodinase in cells throughout the body converts T4 into T3 [34]. Inside these cells, where most metabolism takes place, T3 is a more active "thyroid messenger" than T4. People who suffer decreased conversion of T4 into T3 by this enzyme have fewer "thyroid messages" getting through at the cellular level, despite normal routine thyroid blood test results. Other mechanisms (*eg*, central, genetic) by which low thyroid status may exist despite normal blood test results have been proposed as well [35••,36••,37,38]. Whatever the mechanism, these people have a condition that could be called chronic "sick euthyroid" syndrome, or *subtle hypothyroidism*.

In most cases of subtle hypothyroidism, basal body temperature will be low. Reverse T3 levels may be elevated in the blood. Therefore, if a patient has symptoms consistent with hypothyroidism (*eg*, the reverse T3 is high or the basal body temperature is low), even if routine thyroid blood test results are normal, it is appropriate to consider an empiric trial of thyroid hormone supplementation. If, as hypothesized, the amount of available T3 inside the cells of this group of patients is too low, then empiric treatment should begin with either thyroid extract or pure T3. Thyroid extract is a form of thyroid supplement that contains T4, T3, and diiodotyrosine.

Synthetic L-thyroxine preparations are not typically used because they contain only T4, despite the fact that batch-to-batch variability is lower with synthetic forms of T4. With either the thyroid extract or pure T3, treatment begins at physiologic doses, that is, a fraction (say, one sixth to one third) of what a normal thyroid produces in a day.

Before treatment, patient and doctor decide which symptoms will be used to gauge the short-term effects of the thyroid supplement. Common examples include energy, mood, ability to concentrate, fluid retention, cold intolerance, and ability to get up in the morning (other symptoms, such as weight, susceptibility to infection, menstrual cycle abnormalities, body temperature, and cholesterol levels can take several months to change). Within 2 to 3 weeks of monitoring, one of three things tends to occur. The patient may develop symptoms of too much thyroid hormone (jitteriness, racing pulse, irritability, difficulty sleeping, or chest pain). The risk of these side effects is less than 10%; if they occur, halt the trial. On the other hand, the patient may feel mildly, moderately, or much better (*eg*, more energy, improved concentration, elevated mood). If this happens, maintain that dosage for a period of 3 to 18 months. During this time, other therapies should be working to restore homeostatic balance, which supports the ability to taper off of thyroid supplementation without relapse. Finally, the patient may experience no change at all. If this happens, adjust the dosage or type of thyroid supplement and continue the trial.

Overall, this empirical trial process can take anywhere from 2 to 12 weeks before a clear conclusion about whether a case of subtle hypothyroidism exists and how best to treat it can be reached. When patients are closely monitored, the biggest risk is waiting up to 12 weeks before learning that thyroid is not the cause. For many patients, the bigger risk is having a subtle form of hypothyroidism go undetected and untreated.

These patients may also suffer from patterns of glucocorticoid resistance. Low levels of adrenal function may further aggravate low levels of thyroid function, as well as interfere with a successful response to thyroid treatment [39]. For this reason, it helps to evaluate adrenal cortical status when considering an empiric trial of thyroid supplementation. This can be done in several ways, including an adrenocorticotropin stimulation test to evaluate adrenal cortisol production capacity, morning and evening salivary measures of cortisol, or serum levels of dehydroepiandrosterone (DHEA). The safety and application of physiologic and low pharmacologic doses of cortisol have been extensively reviewed by Jeffries [40]. Cortisol supplementation alone, however, is not likely to suffice as a method of treatment.

Fibromyalgia and CFIDS patients may also have difficulty processing estrogen and progesterone signals in the body [25••]. Monitoring and balancing thyroid, adrenal, and reproductive hormones as a group are often required for an empiric trial to succeed in controlling symptoms and restoring homeostatic balance. The tonic herbs chasteberry and angelica can be used to help restore reproductive hormone balance in women [41]. Natural hormone supplementation should be based on documented levels of estradiol or progesterone in a known phase of the cycle. Use of oral contraceptives to correct menstrual cycle imbalances should be considered a last resort.

DHEA is the most ubiquitous corticosteroid hormone in the human body, with multiple anabolic effects and a low toxicologic profile [42]. Patients with systemic lupus erythematosus (with or without exogenous adrenal suppression) are often low in DHEA levels and experience symptomatic improvement with DHEA supplementation [43]. Patients with HIV experience faster deterioration if their DHEA levels are low [44]. These observations are used by some clinicians to support the use of low doses of DHEA in patients with fibromyalgia or CFIDS whose baseline levels are low or low-to-normal.

If the subtle neuroendocrine abnormalities found in patients with fibromyalgia or CFIDS are related to chemically-induced injuries to the neural networks connecting limbic, hypothalamic, thalamic, prefrontal, hypophyseal, and other areas of the brain, these abnormalities may easily involve hormones beyond those already mentioned. Thus, it is not surprising to see reports involving vasopressin, aldosterone, oxytocin, somatomedin-C, or growth hormone in the fibromyalgia/CFIDS literature [Fleschas J, unpublished data, Hendersonville, NC].

Autonomic Function

The autonomic nervous system may be directly or indirectly involved in the pathogenesis of fibromyalgia and CFIDS [45,46]. Autonomic involvement may play roles in producing pain, fatigue, nonrestorative sleep, headaches, palpitations, irritable bowel syndrome, postexertional malaise, cold hands and feet, or other symptoms commonly seen in these patients. Neurally mediated hypotension, a form of dysautonomia, is associated with insufficient aldosterone levels [47]. Aldosterone helps mediate sodium retention by the kidneys. As circulating sodium levels drop, third-spacing of the fluid component of the blood results in hypovolemia and symptoms of hypovolemia (*eg*, low resting blood pressure, postexertional malaise, orthostatic symptoms, and difficulty concentrating) in the circulation compartment. These symptoms can respond dramatically to administration of fludrocortisone, a synthetic aldosterone analogue. Because many symptoms experienced by patients with fibromyalgia or CFIDS may result from central or peripheral forms of dysautonomia, pharmacologic agents must be considered. Goldstein [17] has reported case-specific, symptom-reducing results from agents including acetazolamide, baclofen, ergoloid mesylates, gabapentin, histamine-2 receptor antagonists, hydralazine, hydrochlorothiazide, lidocaine, mexiletine, nimodipine, oxytocin, pindolol, risperidone, spironolactone, sumatriptan, tacrine, and venlafaxine, although controlled data are not available at this time.

Of considerable interest in the management of autonomic manifestations of fibromyalgia or CFIDS is the use of voluntary self-regulation methods. These methods include guided imagery, self-hypnosis, biofeedback-assisted relaxation techniques, progressive muscle relaxation, autogenic training, mindfulness practice, yoga, meditation, and tai chi. The ability of these methods to grant patients control over aspects of autonomic function is well established [48].

Digestion and Elimination

Little in the conventional literature associates issues of digestion and elimination with fibromyalgia or CFIDS. For this connection we must turn to the naturopathic and functional medicine literature [34,35••]. Here we find an unconventional but clinically practical framework linking gut, liver, and immune system function to such phenomena as irritable bowel syndrome, food allergies, intestinal candidiasis, and, by extension, chronic sinusitis, arthralgias, and a host of other symptoms commonly found in patients with fibromyalgia or CFIDS.

Teeth, saliva, stomach, pancreas, and gall bladder cooperate to digest what is eaten into micronutrient building blocks, which are absorbed across the small intestinal surface. Fats enter the circulation through lacteals, and the balance of what is absorbed enters the portal vein circulation and is carried to the liver, which screens out that which must be metabolized and eliminated through urine or bile. About 40% of the body's immune system exists in and around the gut, which makes sense, because the antigen load passing through the gut wall is considerable. If, for whatever reason, the small intestine becomes hyperpermeable to macromolecules, the immune system must expend increased energy to keep up with antigen processing, a concept well established in the conventional medical literature [49]. The liver functions to "mop up" after whatever the immune system cannot handle. In these simple terms, then, maldigestion of food promotes an imbalanced ecology of microflora in the gut (what naturopaths call "intestinal dysbiosis"), resulting in toxic chemical stresses that compromise gut wall transport functions ("leaky gut"). This, in turn, can cause increased production of immune complexes and low-grade inflammatory responses to antigen ("toxin overload"). Over time, the liver enzyme-mediated detoxification pathways cannot keep up ("sluggish liver"). What develops is a picture of increased sensitization to food antigens, high levels of circulating immune complexes composed of various antigens, and accumulation of low molecular weight toxins, all of which increase the body's burden of oxidative stress. By adding more "noise" to the body's homeostatic and regulatory systems, energy is drained, cell-to-cell communication is compromised, balance is lost, and multiple symptoms result.

Diagnostic tests that help the practicing clinician investigate these conditions include the intestinal hyperpermeability test (mannitol and lactulose are ingested and urinalysis assesses intestinal permeability to these low- versus high-molecular-weight substances), and a comprehensive digestive and stool analysis (looking at protein and starch digestion, fat absorption, bowel floral ecology, and various metabolic markers of gut chemical balance). Treatment consists of using digestive enzymes, betaine hydrochloride, probiotics (*eg*, acidophilus and bifidobacter), anti-infective agents (pharmaceutic or botanical), antioxidants, liver detoxification protocols, elimination diets, and nutritional supplements targeted at restoring normal permeability to the gut wall. Readers are referred to the works of Golan [35••] and Pizzorno [36••] for a more detailed discussion of treatment strategies.

Nutritional Deficiencies

With the aforementioned problems related to digestion and elimination, nutritional deficiencies of various types may result from decreased assimilation. Protein maldigestion may be accompanied by amino acid, vitamin, and mineral deficiencies. These deficiencies may be associated with decreased synthesis or activity of neurotransmitters, cytokines, enzymes, or other important regulatory molecules. For example, a recent study has documented elevated homocysteine and decreased vitamin B_{12} levels in the cerebrospinal fluid of patients with CFIDS [50].

Of additional concern is the likelihood that upregulation of certain metabolic pathways will cause increased use and early depletion of critical nutrients and cofactors involved in minimizing oxidative stress, maintaining intracellular redox balance, cell-to-cell communication, and intracellular communication. When confident that nutrients are being assimilated, the clinician places patients on a high-potency multiple vitamin to provide fundamental nutritional support, which can be built on with targeted nutritional supplementation as indicated.

Allergies

Conventional allergy specialists find little credible evidence to support the claim that delayed sensitization to food antigens occurs, much less that acceptably sensitive and specific laboratory testing exists to detect the problem [51], although a study suggesting clinical uses for in vitro testing for food allergens has been published. The holistic medicine community itself is divided about the use of in vivo allergy testing [52]. Evidence clearly suggests, however, that elimination diets can relieve chronic symptoms [53]. There is also evidence that food-supplemented detoxification programs can aid in the management of chronic health problems [54].

To examine the food allergy hypothesis empirically, without testing, ask the patient to eliminate all dairy, eggs, wheat, corn, citrus, refined sugar, caffeine, alcohol, and processed or additive-rich food from his or her diet for a minimum of 3 weeks. Although up to 6 months may be required for some patients to become fully desensitized, 3 weeks is usually long enough to produce symptomatic improvement. After 3 weeks, foods from each class can be reintroduced, one at a time, 3 days apart, while the patient monitors for symptom recurrence. Cheney [55] has observed that treating food allergies through dietary elimination occasionally provides substantial benefit for patients with fibromyalgia or CFIDS. Sensitivities to inhaled allergens certainly can add to the burden of suffering of these patients. Conventional and alternative options for managing the respiratory manifestations of allergy and infection have been thoroughly reviewed by Ivker [56•].

Immune System Function

Some patients with CFIDS experience upregulation of RNase-L, which may impede antiviral defenses as well as interfere with intracellular protein metabolism with hard to predict but considerable downstream consequences. No specific treatment for this defect has yet been proposed. Decreased natural killer cell function has also been observed in patients with CFIDS. Natural killer cells are important to antiviral and antifungal defenses. Thus, a defect in this aspect of immune defense can partially account for the problems CFIDS patients have preventing reactivation of Epstein-Barr virus, human herpesvirus 6, and other chronic viruses [57,58]. This finding may also account for the frequency with which intestinal candidiasis and elevated *Candida* immune complexes are seen in these patients [25••].

Immune system boosting agents, including acyclovir and related antivirals, have produced benefits to these patients. The herb astragalus has been shown to enhance natural killer cell function, with clinical improvement in treated patients [59]. Relaxation techniques also have been shown to enhance natural killer cell activity [60].

Intestinal candidiasis is a poorly studied but recognized condition that appears to occur in many patients with fibromyalgia or CFIDS [25••,34,61]. Management of candidiasis in these patients rests on a three-pronged strategy. First, patients should eliminate refined sugar, baker's yeast, brewer's yeast, and foods containing mold. Second, they should reimplant their guts with probiotics, because these organisms compete with *Candida* species for cell-binding sites. Finally, antifungal agents should be used. Choices include antifungal botanical combinations, nystatin, fluconazole, or itraconazole. Virtually no available data establish effective dosage or durations of treatment with these agents.

Mood

Anxiety can be treated in the short-term with benzodiazepines, but long-term use should be avoided. Kava may help and is not thought to be addictive, but it should be avoided in patients receiving benzodiazepine therapy and used with caution in patients who will not avoid alcohol [62]. Depression, if severe, should be treated with antidepressant medications, such as serotonin reuptake inhibitors (fluoxetine, nefazodone, paroxetine, sertraline), tricyclics (amitriptyline, doxepin, imipramine, nortriptyline), tetracyclics (mirtazipine), mixed neurotransmitter reuptake inhibitors (venlafaxine), trazodone, or bupropion. These patients should be monitored closely for adverse effects, with dosage adjustment, medication switches, or psychiatric referral as needed.

Counseling is an essential healing path component for most of these patients. Cognitive therapy, voluntary self-regulation training, psychodynamic counseling, behavioral counseling, or an eclectic approach can all be helpful. From an alternative, mind–body–medicine perspective, considerations include the use of flower essences [63]. Homeopathic remedies can have many applications along the healing path [64], including treatment of fibromyalgia [65], and can be of particular use in addressing emotional issues, anxiety, and depression.

Mood and emotion-related problems can also be addressed through body work. Reiki, therapeutic touch, and various types of massage therapy can be especially useful. They can trigger emotional releases, which need to be properly supported and integrated into the counseling relationship. Through the laying on of hands, these alternative modalities have a unique ability to build hope and optimism about the future, as well as trust and confidence in the healing partnership.

Exercise

Clinicians disagree whether aerobic exercise is a bonanza or bane for patients with fibromyalgia or CFIDS. If fatigue is due in part to deconditioning of muscles and circulation, very gradual increases in aerobic activity are capable of reducing pain and adding energy. If the patient has difficulty converting oxygen into chemical energy, aerobic exercise simply increases oxidative stress on the system. In this case, brief episodes of weight resistance and stretching exercise will be better tolerated. The key to energy management is knowing one's activity limits, and staying within them, despite the temptation to use a good day to make up for a month's worth of lost time. Many of these patients benefit from work with a teacher of the Feldenkrais method (a method of movement and neuromuscular re-education), with whom they will learn how to use their muscles and joints with maximum efficiency and to expand their limits safely, without setbacks from overuse or poor mechanics.

Coping and Support

Patients should be encouraged to participate in support groups or to become involved in the fibromyalgia and CFIDS patient communities through newsletters, meetings, and conferences. Of course, they should participate in outside activities within their individual stamina limits. Many published sources of information exist on coping with fibromyalgia and CFIDS that offer useful information to patients and their families [66,67]. Many patients report that their ability to cope was helped best by educating their spouse or other loved ones in a way that validated how real and complex their illness is. It is truly unfortunate that many clinicians, let alone family members, feel that fibromyalgia and CFIDS are purely psychologic conditions at best, fictional at worst.

CONCLUSIONS

Fibromyalgia and CFIDS are poorly understood, chronic, multisymptom illnesses. Layer after layer of homeostatic imbalance has been found in patients meeting diagnostic criteria for these conditions. These imbalances exist at biochemical, biomechanical, psychosocial, and spiritual levels, and should be addressed using a patient-centered approach. By identifying and treating a critical mass of problems in simultaneous fashion over 6 to 12 months, patients with fibromyalgia or CFIDS can expect moderate-to-major improvement in symptoms and quality of life [68,69].

Healing paths should address pain, energy, sleep, hormone balance, autonomic function, digestion and elimination, nutritional deficiencies, allergies, immune system function, mood, exercise, and coping and support issues (Table 6-5). The integrative team can include allopathic physicians, osteopathic physicians, chiropractic physicians, nurses, acupuncturists, homeopaths, nutritionists, bodyworkers of various types, and counselors trained in psychotherapy and mind-body interventions. The treatment plan constitutes a partnership that includes the patient, the physician, and the integrative medical team. This healing path should be revisited periodically to monitor progress and troubleshoot along the way. With so many tools, an integrative approach, by combining the strengths of conventional and alternative medicine, seems best suited to the treatment of fibromyalgia and CFIDS.

Table 6-5. Integrative Treatment of Fibromyalgia and Chronic Fatigue/Immune Dysfunction Syndrome

FM/CFIDS	Applicable Interventions
Pain	Pharmaceuticals, hormones; nutriceuticals; botanicals; chiropractic; acupuncture; massage/bodywork; mind–body counseling; exercise; therapeutic touch; homeopathy, flower essences; group support
Energy	Pharmaceuticals, hormones; nutriceuticals; botanicals; chiropractic; acupuncture; nutritional counseling; exercise
Sleep	Pharmaceuticals, hormones; nutriceuticals; mind–body counseling; exercise; homeopathy, flower essences
Hormone function	Pharmaceuticals, hormones; nutriceuticals; botanicals; chiropractic; nutritional counseling
Autonomic function	Chiropractic; acupuncture; massage/bodywork; mind–body counseling
Digestion/elimination	Pharmaceuticals, hormones; nutriceuticals; botanicals; chiropractic; acupuncture; nutritional counseling, homeopathy, flower essences
Nutritional deficiencies	Nutriceuticals; nutritional counseling
Allergies	Pharmaceuticals, hormones; nutriceuticals; botanicals; acupuncture; nutritional counseling; exercise; homeopathy, flower essences
Immune function	Pharmaceuticals, hormones; nutriceuticals; botanicals; chiropractic; acupuncture; mind–body counseling; nutritional couseling; exercise; therapeutic touch
Mood	Pharmaceuticals, hormones; nutriceuticals; botanicals; chiropractic; acupuncture; massage/bodywork; mind–body counseling; therapeutic touch; homeopathy, flower essences; group support
Coping/support	Mind–body counseling; nutritional counseling; therapeutic touch; homeopathy, flower essences; group support

References and Recommended Reading

Recently published papers of particular interest have been highlighted as:
- Of interest
- •• Of outstanding interest

1.• Pert C: *Molecules of Emotion*. New York: Scribner; 1997.
Pert links consciousness to ligand-receptor dynamics, creating a framework for understanding the molecular basis of thought and emotion.

2.• Bellavite P, Signorini A: *Homeopathy: A Frontier in Medical Science*. Berkeley: North Atlantic; 1995.
This book is notable for its articulate and insightful discussion of the ways in which information may be communicated within complex biologic systems. This work opens the door to refereed discussions of the physical mechanisms underlying homeopathy, acupuncture, and other subtle interventions.

3.• Galland L: *The Four Pillars of Healing*. New York: Random House; 1997.
This book is a cogently written introduction to integrative, functional medicine perspectives about health, illness, and patient-centered care.

4. Pioro-Boisset M, Esdaile JM, Fitzcharles MA: Alternative medicine use in fibromyalgia. *Arthritis Care Res* 1996, 9:13–17.

5. Dimmock S, Troughton PR, Bird HA: Factors predisposing to the resort of complementary therapies in patients with fibromyalgia. *Clin Rheumatol* 1996, 15:478–482.

6. Wolfe F, Smythe HA, Yunus MB, *et al.*: The American College of Rheumatology 1990 criteria for the classification of fibromyalgia: report of the multicenter criteria committee. *Arthritis Rheum* 1990, 33:160–172.

7. Fukuda K, Straus SE, Hickie I, *et al.*: The chronic fatigue syndrome: a comprehensive approach to its definition and study. *Ann Intern Med* 1994, 121:953–959.

8. Suhadolnik RJ, Peterson DL, O'Brien K, *et al.*: Biochemical evidence for a novel low molecular weight 2-5A-dependent RNase L in chronic fatigue syndrome. *J Interferon Cytokine Res* 1997, 17:377–385.

9. Katz RS, Kravitz HM: Fibromyalgia, depression and alcoholism: a family history study. *J Rheumatol* 1996, 23:149–154.

10. Kreusi MJP, Dale J, Straus S: Psychiatric diagnoses in patients who have chronic fatigue. *J Clin Psych* 1989, 50:53–56.

11. Capen K: The courts, expert witnesses and fibromyalgia. *Can Med Assoc J* 1995, 153:206–208.

12. Wolfe F, Aarflot T, Bruusgaard D, *et al.*: Fibromyalgia and disability: report of the Moss International Working Group on medico-legal aspects of chronic widespread musculoskeletal pain complaints and fibromyalgia. *Scand J Rheumatol* 1995, 24:395–396.

13. Cheney PR: Proposed pathophysiologic mechanism of CFIDS. *CFIDS Chronicle* 1994:1–6.

14. Buskila D, Neumann L, Vaisberg G, *et al.*: Increased rates of fibromyalgia following cervical spine injury: a controlled study of 161 cases of traumatic injury. *Arthritis Rheum* 1997, 40:446–452.

15. Boisset-Pioro MH, Esdaile JM, Fitzcharles MA: Sexual and physical abuse in women with fibromyalgia. *Arthritis Rheum* 1995, 38:235–241.

16. Olin R: Fibromyalgia: a neuro-immuno-endocrinologic syndrome? [Swedish]. *Lakartidningen* 1995, 92:755–758.

17. Goldstein J: *Betrayal by the Brain: the Neurologic Basis of Chronic Fatigue Syndrome, Fibromyalgia Syndrome, and Related Neural Network Disorders*. New York: Haworth Press; 1996.

18. Patel M, Gutzwiller F, Paccaud F, Marazzi A: A meta-analysis of acupuncture for chronic pain. *Int J Epidemiol* 1989, 18:900–906.

19. Berndtson K, Moulton K, Uretz A: Clinical uses of acupuncture. *Chicago Med* 1996, 100:10–13.

20. Kaarda B, Tosteinbo O: Increase of plasma beta-endorphins in connective tissue massage. *Gen Pharmacol* 1989, 20:487–489.
21. Joachim G: The effects of two stress management techniques on feelings of well-being in patients with inflammatory bowel disease. *Nursing Papers* 1983, 15:5–18.
22. Jayson MI: Fibromyalgia and trigger point injections. *Bull Hosp Joint Dis* 1996, 55:176–177.
23. Hasselberg PD: *Chiropractic in New Zealand: Report of the Commission of Inquiry.* New Zealand: Government Printer; 1979.
24. Russell IJ, Michalek JE, Flechas JD, Abraham GE: Treatment of fibromyalgia syndrome with Super Malic: a randomized, double-blind, placebo-controlled, crossover pilot study. *J Rheumatol* 1995, 22:953–958.
25.•• Teitelbaum J: *From Fatigued to Fantastic!* edn 2. Garden City Park, NY: Avery Press; 1996.

Dr. Teitelbaum's popular book has become a classic among patients and clinicians interested in an integrative approach to fibromyalgia and CFIDS. It is a good source of specific information regarding diagnostic and treatment protocols.

26. Bland J: Fibromyalgia and chronic myofascial pain. In *Applying New Essentials in Nutritional Medicine.* Gig Harbor, WA: HealthComm Seminars, 1995:1–22.
27. Goldenberg D, Mayskiy M, Mossey C, *et al.*: A randomized, double blind crossover trial of fluoxetine and amitriptyline in the treatment of fibromyalagia. *Arthritis Rheum* 1996, 39(suppl):1852–1859.
28. Bennett RM, Gatter RA, Campbell SM, *et al.*: A comparison of cyclobenzaprine and placebo in the management of fibrositis: a double-blind controlled study. *Arthritis Rheum* 1988, 31:1535–1542.
29. Carette S, Bell MJ, Reynolds WJ, *et al.*: Comparison of amitriptyline, cyclobenzaprine, and placebo in the treatment of fibromyalgia: a randomized, double blind clinical trial. *Arthritis Rheum* 1994, 37:32–40.
30. Moldofsky H, Lue FA, Mously C, *et al.*: The effect of zolpidem in patients with fibromyalgia: a dose ranging, double-blind, placebo-controlled, modified crossover study. *J Rheumatol* 1996, 23:529–533.
31. Murray M: Common questions about St. John's wort extract. *Am J Nat Med* 1997:14–19.
32. Dressing T: Insomnia: are valerian/melissa combinations of equal value to benzodiazepine? *Therapiewoche* 1992, 42:726–736.
33. Zhdanova IV, Wurtman RJ, Lynch HJ, *et al.*: Sleep-inducing effects of low doses of melatonin ingested in the evening. *Clin Pharmacol Ther* 1995, 57:552–558.
34. Schimmel M, Utiger RD: Thyroidal and peripheral production of thyroid hormones. *Ann Intern Med* 1977, 87:760–768.
35.• Golan R: *Optimal Wellness.* New York: Ballantine Books; 1995:381–385.

Golan offers a unique synthesis of conventional and alternative medicine in this encyclopedic collection of information that draws on naturopathic and holistic perspectives. Written for the lay public, Golan includes excellent self-care advice for patients.

36.•• Pizzorno J: *Total Wellness.* Rocklin, CA: Prima Publishing; 1996.
Pizzorno is the president of Bastyr University, a leading naturopathic school, and is an articulate spokesman for naturopathic clinical perspective. The book is meticulously referenced and covers the foundations of functional medicine perspective in depth.

37. Bode HH, Danon M, Weintraub BD, *et al.*: Partial target organ resistance to thyroid hormone. *J Clin Invest* 1973, 52:776–782.
38. Lowe JC, Cullum ME, Graf LH Jr, Yellin J: Mutations in the c-erbA beta I gene: do they underlie euthyroid fibromyalgia? *Med Hypotheses* 1997, 48:125–135.
39. Hill SR Jr, Reiss RS, Forsham PH, *et al.*: The effect of adrenocorticotropin and cortisone on thyroid function: thyroid-adrenocortical interrelationships. *J Clin Endocrinol* 1950, 10:1375–1400.
40. Jeffries WM: *Safe Uses of Cortisol* edn 2. Springfield, IL: Thomas CC; 1996.
41. Murray M: A comprehensive evaluation of premenstrual syndrome. *Am J Nat Med* 1997:6–22.
42. Gordon GB, Shantz IM, Talalay P: Modulation of growth, differentiation, and carcinogenesis by dehydroepiandrosterone. *Adv Enzyme Reg* 1987, 26:355–383.
43. Van Vollenhoven RF, Engleman EG, McGuire JL: Dehydroepiandrosterone in systemic lupus erythematosus. *Arthritis Rheum* 1995, 38:1826–1831.
44. Jacobson MA, Fusaro RE, Galmarini M, Lang W: Decreased serum dehydroepiandrosterone is associated with increased progression of human immunodeficiency virus in men with CD4 cell counts of 200–499. *J Infect Dis* 1991, 64:864–868.
45. Vaeroy H, Qiao ZG, Morkrid L, Forre O: Altered sympathetic nervous system response in patients with fibromyalgia (fibrositis syndrome). *J Rheumatol* 1989, 16:1460–1465.
46. Van Denderen JC, Boersma JW, Zeinstra P, *et al.*: Physiologic effects of exhaustive physical exercise in primary fibromyalgia syndrome (PFS): is PFS a disorder of neuroendocrine reactivity? *Scand J Rheumatol* 1992, 21:35–37.
47. Rowe PC, Bou-Holaigah I, Kan JS, *et al.*: Improvement in symptoms of chronic fatigue syndrome is associated with reversal of neurally mediated hypotension [abstract]. *Pediatr Res* 1995, 37:33A.
48. Achterberg J: Mind-body interventions. In *Alternative Medicine: Expanding Medical Horizons: a Report to the National Institutes of Health on Alternative Medical Systems and Practices in the United States.* Washington, DC: U.S. Government Printing Office; 1992:3–43.
49. Sanderson IR, Walker WA: Uptake and transport of macromolecules by the intestine: possible role in clinical disorders. *Gastroenterology* 1993, 104:622–639.
50. Regland B, Andersson M, Abrahamsson L, *et al.*: Increased concentrations of homocysteine in the cerebrospinal fluid in patients with fibromyalgia and chronic fatigue syndrome. *Scand J Rheumatol* 1997, 26:301–307.
51. American Academy of Allergy and Immunology: Position statement: measurement of specific and nonspecific IgG4 levels as diagnostic and prognostic tests for clinical allergy. *J Allergy Clin Immunol* 1995, 95:652–654.
52. el Rafei A, Peters SM, Harris N, Bellanti JA: Diagnostic value of IgG4 measurements in patients with food allergy. *Ann Allergy* 1989, 62:94–99.
53. Grant ECG: Food allergies and migraine. *Lancet* 1979, 1:966–969.
54. Bland JS, Barrager E, Bland K: A medical food supplemented detoxification program in the management of chronic health problems. *Altern Ther* 1995, 1:62–71.
55. Cheney P: Treatment at the Cheney Clinic. *CFIDS Chronicle* 1998:13–14.
56.• Ivker R: *Sinus Survival: the Holistic Medical Treatment for Allergies, Asthma, Bronchitis, Colds, and Sinusitis* edn 3. New York: Jeremy Tarcher/Putnam; 1995.

This book summarizes the conventional full court press for a range of chronic respiratory disorders, as well as a comprehensive summary of alternative thinking and treatment strategies.

57. Buchwald D, Cheney PR, Peterson DL, *et al.*: A chronic illness characterized by fatigue, neurologic and immunologic disorders, and active human herpesvirus 6 infection. *Ann Intern Med* 1992, 116:103–113.
58. Galbraith DN, Clements GB, Nairn C: Evidence for enteroviral persistence in humans. *J Gen Virol* 1997, 78:307–312.
59. Yang YZ, Jin PY, Guo Q, *et al.*: Effect of astragalus membranaceus on natural killer cell activity and induction with coxsackie B viral myocarditis. *Chin Med J* 1990, 103:304–307.
60. Kiecolt-Glaser JK, Glaser R, Williger D, *et al.*: Psychosocial enhancement of immunocompetence in a geriatric population. *Health Psych* 1985, 4:25–41.

61. Bodey P, Sobel JD: Lower intestinal candidiasis. In *Candidiasis: Pathogenesis, Diagnosis, and Treatment*. New York: Raven Press; 1993.
62. Brown DJ: *Herbal Prescriptions for Better Health*. Rocklin, CA: Prima Publishing; 1996:145–150.
63. Scheffer M: *Bach Flower Therapy: Theory and Practice*. Rochester, VT: Healing Arts Press, 1988.
64. Kleinjen J, Knipschild P, Riet G: Clinical trials of homeopathy. *Br Med J* 1991, 302:316–323.
65. Fisher P, Greenwood A, Huskisson EC, *et al*.: Effect of homeopathic treatment on fibrositis. *Br Med J* 1989, 299:365–366.
66. Fibromyalgia Network: *A Newsletter for People with Fibromyalgia Syndrome/Chronic Fatigue Syndrome*. Edited by Thorson K. Tucson, AZ: Health Information Network; 1998.
67. Hoh D: *The CFIDS Chronicle: The Bimonthly Publication of the Chronic Fatigue and Immune Dysfunction Syndrome Association of America*. Charlotte, NC: Chronic Fatigue and Immune Dysfunction Syndrome Association of America; 1998.
68. Teitelbaum J, Bird B: Effective treatment of severe chronic fatigue: a report of a series of 64 patients. *J Musculoskel Pain* 1995, 3:91–110.
69. Hoh D: Effective treatment: an unusual study tests entire protocol. *CFIDS Chronicle* 1998:16–17.

Acupuncture

Mary Ellen Scheckenbach

The practice of acupuncture is a an intricate and delicate art, one part of the vast world of Oriental medicine—a medicine that describes a very different movement of life in nature from that which forms the usual Western conception. The fundamental premise of acupuncture presupposes the existence of a complex network of pathways of *qi* (energy), which is the life force that animates all living matter. Early Chinese texts describing the theory and application of acupuncture provide few clues to the discovery and development of the principles of the *qi* movement. The use of these ancient principles in clinical practice, however, has given rise to a coherent practice of the art.

Because Western medical science is founded on a different body of knowledge (*eg*, biology, chemistry, and physics), no easy translation of theory exists between the two medicines. In particular, the search for scientific verification of the existence of *qi* remains elusive. In the same way that we cannot see wind but we feel it and know it exists, so in acupuncture we cannot know the ultimate reality of *qi* but can witness and study its effects in living systems. The task of establishing the reality of acupuncture has therefore given way to ascertaining a demonstrated efficacy of acupuncture. This task, taking place in the second half of the 20th century, relies largely on the use of modern, randomized, controlled, and blinded clinical studies. Using this method of investigation, derived from a very different paradigm of causality in nature, we may have the good fortune to learn more about the two systems of medicine reciprocally.

Although acupuncture has been practiced in China for over 2000 years, its introduction in the West came only in the 16th century, when reports were brought back to Europe by Jesuit missionaries traveling in Asia. Trade relations and empire building brought Europeans in contact with many aspects of Oriental medicine, such as acupuncture, herbal medicine, and the principles of living in accordance with natural laws to preserve health and achieve longevity. Translations of Chinese texts and original medical works by Dutch and German physicians began to appear in the 17th centuries, mostly in association with travels to trading posts for the Dutch East India Company. Later, 19th-century French physicians brought acupuncture to France from colonies in Indochina [1].

Documented use of acupuncture in the United States dates to 1826, when Franklin Bache, a grandson of Benjamin Franklin, translated the French text *Memoir on Acupuncturation* by Morand. Bache, a physician and chemist, later wrote an account of his experimentation on prisoners at the Pennsylvania state penitentiary, where they received acupuncture treatment for the pain of rheumatism and neuralgia [1]. Acupuncture is cited in the Civil War field surgeon's manual, *An Epitome of Practical Surgery* [2]. In 1892, Sir William Osler devoted attention to the success of acupuncture treatment for lumbago and sciatica in his *The Principles and Practice of Medicine* [3].

Little is known of the extent of practice of acupuncture and Oriental medicine among Chinese and Japanese immigrants to the United States since the late 19th and early 20th centuries. Certainly many of the modalities of Oriental medicine were practiced, given the availability of materials at hand (*ie*, needles and herbs). It must also be remembered that certain effects sought through acupuncture needles could be achieved through the manual arts of acupressure and *shiatsu*.

Despite this long worldwide history, the legal practice of acupuncture in the United States dates only to 1973 and the passage of laws in Nevada, Oregon, and Maryland regulating its use for the purpose of research. Since that time, laws in 36 states and the District of Columbia have been passed to regulate the practice of acupuncture for both physicians and nonphysicians. Approximately 30 colleges have been established and accredited by the Accreditation Commission for Acupuncture and Oriental Medicine. Most acupuncturist physicians in the United States are trained through the American Academy of Medical Acupuncture. Educational standards and legal requirements continue to evolve to ensure accessibility to practitioners and the highest quality of care.

In the past few years, significant changes to the legal and scientific status of acupuncture have been accomplished at the federal level. These changes have broad implications for the use of acupuncture by all Americans and for the institutions, both medical and economic, that deliver health care in our society.

Since 1972, acupuncture needles and some ancillary devices had been labeled as "investigational devices" by the U.S. Food and Drug Administration (FDA). Recognizing the need for trained practitioners to have access to specialized needles and electroacupuncture devices and citing the lack of proven effectiveness, the FDA made acupuncture tools available for "investigational" use. The issue of safety was addressed in 1980, at which time it was determined that no significant risks existed. On March 29, 1996, the FDA reclassified acupuncture needles into the Class II category (safe and effective, but requiring restrictions) [4].

NATIONAL INSTITUTES OF HEALTH CONSENSUS REPORT

Between November 3 and November 5, 1997, nearly 25 years after the first legalization of acupuncture, the National Institutes of Health (NIH) sponsored a consensus conference to explore the efficacy of acupuncture, its risks, and its place in our current health-care system [5•]. The panel was an independent, nonfederal body that evaluated the data and presented discussions to create a consensus statement. The members reviewed scientific and medical data from national and international sources. They sorted through the array of clinical studies performed with varying approximation to the preferred model of a randomized, placebo-controlled, double-blind study and explored issues of basic science with regard to mechanisms of action in acupuncture. The NIH panel also sought to explore public policy issues governing the use and distribution of acupuncture in the United States, its accessibility, and matters of regulations, standards, and safety.

Organized by the NIH Office of Alternative Medicine and the NIH Office of Medical Applications of Research, the conference was cosponsored by the National Cancer Institute, the National Heart, Lung, and Blood Institute, the National Institute of Allergy and Infectious Diseases, the National Institute of Arthritis and Musculoskeletal and Skin Diseases, the National Institute of Dental Research, the National Institute of Drug Abuse, and the NIH Office of Research on Women's Health. During the 3 days of presentations, this forum gathered together national and international experts in the fields of acupuncture, pain, psychology, psychiatry, physical medicine and rehabilitation, drug abuse, family practice, internal medicine, health policy, epidemiology, statistics, physiology, and biophysics as well as members of the public. Supporting scientific and medical data were drawn from national and international databases with some 2300 citations indexed from January 1970 to September 1997. Controlled trials have been conducted in the areas of acute and chronic pain and many areas of internal medicine including allergy, immunology, gastroenterology, cardiology, reproductive health, and addictions. There have also been studies in biochemistry, physiology, veterinary medicine, and research methodology. Particular attention was paid to research methods and the difficulty that researchers face in carrying out a standard, placebo-controlled, double-blind trial of acupuncture [5•].

In addition to reviewing medical data, the NIH panel invited presenters to describe and explain the theoretic underpinnings of acupuncture as understood in Asia, and particularly China, over the past 2500 years. The model used by the Chinese and described in *The Yellow Emperor's Classic of Internal Medicine*, which dates from about 200 BC, presupposes the existence of *qi*, or energy, that circulates through the body in an organized fashion along pathways called meridians [6]. Each meridian governs the function of a particular organ and other aspects of physiologic, mental, and emotional effect assigned to that organ. Interruption in this flow or a decrease in the amount of energy transmitted accounts for pathologic changes in physiologic and emotional health.

In the NIH consensus statement [5•], acupuncture was found to be effective for certain limited conditions based on the best clinical data then available. These included adult postoperative and chemotherapy-induced nausea and vomiting, postoperative pain, and dental pain. Acupuncture was found an acceptable alternative or adjunct treatment in cases of addiction, stroke rehabilitation, headache, menstrual cramps, tennis elbow, fibromyalgia, myofascial pain, osteoarthritis, low back pain, carpal tunnel syndrome, and asthma. The panel added that "further research is likely to uncover additional areas where acupuncture interventions will be useful" [5•].

The NIH consensus conference statement [5•] addressed the following questions in its discussions:

What is the efficacy of acupuncture, compared with that of placebo or sham acupuncture, in those conditions for which sufficient data are available for evaluation?

What is acupuncture's place in the treatment of various conditions for which sufficient data are available, in comparison or in combination with other interventions (including no intervention)?

What is known about the biologic effects of acupuncture that may help us understand how it works?

What issues need to be addressed so that acupuncture can be incorporated appropriately into today's health-care system?

What are the directions for future research?

In this chapter, we examine each of these questions and review in detail the supporting presentations that were used to arrive at the panel's statement.

EFFICACY OF ACUPUNCTURE COMPARED WITH PLACEBO ACUPUNCTURE AND STANDARD CARE

Despite acupuncture's reputation as primarily a treatment for pain, its use in postoperative and postchemotherapeutic emesis has been an area of significant research. Several studies were performed by Dundee *et al.* [7–10] over a period of 5 years on approximately 500 women. These clinical trials evaluated the effect of manual and electroacupuncture at *Pericardium 6* on emesis as a sequela to minor gynecologic surgery and cancer chemotherapy treatment. *Pericardium 6* is located on the wrist between the tendons *palmaris longus* and *flexor carpi radialis* about 2 inches proximal to the wrist crease. Findings from the studies showed a consistent significant reduction in postoperative emesis and an effect equivalent to the use of antiemetic medication (*eg,* cyclizine). In trials evaluating the effectiveness of acupuncture stimulation of *Pericardium 6* in combination with chemical antiemetic agents after chemotherapy treatment, 80% of women reported no emesis during 24 hours following treatment. Sustained suppression of emesis was achieved through acupressure applied with wrist bands containing a button placed over *Pericardium 6* that was pressed for 5 minutes every 2 hours after the initial treatment [10].

The second area of significant research ("significant" being determined by a higher quality of research methodology) demonstrated the efficacy of acupuncture in the treatment of postoperative pain. Three randomized clinical studies of postoperative pain comparing acupuncture's effects with those of analgesic medication were evaluated. Types of surgeries included gynecologic (especially hysterectomy), abdominal, rectal, and lumbar. Measures of acupuncture's efficacy were obtained using control groups that received either no acupuncture, transcutaneous electrical nerve stimulation (TENS), or analgesic medication, or who received treatment under general anesthesia so that patients were unaware of who had been treated and not treated. Results of the studies demonstrated that acupuncture is equivalent or superior to pain medication or is effective in significantly lowering pain medication use compared with controls who received no acupuncture [11–13].

Postoperative dental pain was assessed in three trials that compared acupuncture's effects with those of analgesic medication and placebo acupuncture. Forty patients, mostly undergoing wisdom tooth extraction, reported less pain with acupuncture and pain medication than with either acupuncture, medication, or placebo alone, both immediately after surgery and several hours later [14]. This study demonstrated a more sophisticated design, comparing randomly assigned groups that received acupuncture and codeine, acupuncture and placebo medication, control needling (also known as *placebo acupuncture* or *sham acupuncture* with needling at a short distance from the true acupuncture point) and codeine, or control needling and placebo medication. Lao *et al.* [15] studied postoperative dental pain by comparing acupuncture treatment with placebo acupuncture. Patients receiving true acupuncture reported less intense pain and significantly longer time without pain than the placebo group. When acupuncture was compared with medication by Lapeer *et al.* [16], no difference in pain reduction immediately postoperatively was observed, but significantly less pain was reported in the acupuncture group during the 10 days following surgery. Uncontrolled studies of dental pain relief that showed acupuncture to be effective in inducing both immediate and lasting analgesia in over 80% of patients were based on clinical observation findings [17–19].

Interesting studies of increased dental pain threshold following electroacupuncture were performed on human and monkey subjects [20–23]. These findings suggested a significant increase in pain threshold in both groups when electroacupuncture was applied for 30 minutes on the point of *Large Intestine 4*, or *hegu*, located between the first and second metacarpals of the hand.

Numerous studies on the most common pain syndromes for which individuals seek acupuncture therapy were presented to the NIH panel. These syndromes included headache, neck and low back pain, myofascial and joint pain, and osteoarthritis. Although many reported findings show the efficacy of acupuncture treatment for these conditions, serious design flaws in methodology limited the acceptance of some results and conclusions [24••]. In addition, much research continues to take the form of clinical observation. For example, of physician-acupuncturists surveyed, 96% found acupuncture to be effective for these conditions [25].

What might seem like very limited areas of clear efficacy shown for acupuncture, such as relief in nausea and vomiting, postoperative surgical pain, and dental pain, show most vividly the constraints that inadequate research has placed on answering the question of efficacy. Interestingly, a common aspect of these conditions is that they were all similarly induced in each subject. This is crucial because the effectiveness of using a standardized acupuncture protocol relies largely on each study subject having the same diagnosis from an Oriental medical perspective. In the cases noted, these induced conditions might all have received the same Oriental medical diagnosis. Consequently, in these instances, one might be able to perform a standardized treatment with more success. In the case of many other sorts of conditions, such as back pain, tennis elbow, or migraines, the causes are likely to be much more multifactorial from the perspective of Oriental medicine. Treating complex and differing Oriental medical diagnoses with standardized protocols would, therefore, not necessarily produce clear and consistent results.

Assessing the efficacy of such a complex modality used for so many conditions and diseases is akin to asking whether pharmaceutical agents in general are as effective as another type of health-care tool. The answer is complex, has been reached through billions of dollars of research over many years, and is rooted in decades of clinical experience.

Role of Acupuncture in the Treatment of Various Conditions in Comparison or Combination with Other Interventions

The choice of treatment strategies by a medical practitioner is informed by several factors, and sometimes efficacy proven by controlled trials is not one of them. There are many instances in Western clinical practice in which techniques or protocols are not supported by substantial research data and yet are clearly useful in clinical experience. Decision-making factors include recent findings of clinical observation in the medical literature, related anecdotal experiences of colleagues, and assessment of risk or potential side effects among various choices. Sometimes the particularities of a patient's history or presentation will warrant the choice of one strategy over another. Treatments selected for their overall appropriateness may indeed be effective despite a lack of confirming data. In the case of acupuncture, the NIH panel noted that "the data in support of acupuncture are as strong as those for many accepted Western medical therapies" [5•].

In cases of pain due to musculoskeletal conditions, such as fibromyalgia, epicondylitis, myofascial pain, some kinds of headaches, and osteoarthritis, a large body of literature exists citing positive clinical outcomes in the use of acupuncture to treat these conditions. When compared with conventional medical practice for the treatment of pain, such as steroidal and nonsteroidal anti-inflammatory drugs or steroid injections, acupuncture often fares well in producing relief [15,26–31]. Acupuncture treatment has the advantage of producing far fewer adverse effects than standard drug therapies. In fact, the American Medical Association (AMA) stated in a 1981 assessment that the practice of acupuncture has very few complications [32].

Other data from controlled trials suggest that acupuncture could also be useful in conditions of low back pain, addiction, stroke rehabilitation, carpal tunnel syndrome, and asthma [33–39]. The NIH panel [5•] also noted that the World Health Organization indicates more than 40 conditions for which acupuncture may be of benefit. The conclusion of the consensus statement regarding the place of acupuncture in treatment for the various conditions listed clearly suggests that, given the relative safety of acupuncture and its relative effectiveness compared with conventional medical treatment, acupuncture treatment "may be a reasonable option" and "should be a part of a comprehensive management program" for those conditions.

Biological Effects of Acupuncture

Deciphering the physiologic mechanisms of acupuncture-related phenomena is a recent endeavor in the history of acupuncture. Oriental medical theory presents a vast and complex theoretical basis of action for acupuncture. Unfortunately, this system presupposes the existence of an extensive network of interaction among energetic phenomena that has never been validated from a Western scientific perspective. The system is internally consistent for clinical use, but so far it remains impenetrable to our modern understanding of natural laws (ie, physics, biology, and chemistry). Oriental medicine is often poetic and metaphoric in its descriptions of natural events, which further eludes our conceptual grasp.

Early studies focused on acupuncture-related analgesia using mostly rabbit and rat models and measuring objective reactions to acute and chronic pain stimuli through observation of escape behavior or vocalization. More recent research reveals that acupuncture apparently activates the endogenous opioid system to produce analgesia. With the discovery of opioid receptors by Pert and Snyder in 1973 [40] and further advances in opioid identification and cloning in the 1990s, various interactions between acupuncture and the opioid system have been studied. Early work confirmed the existence of this interaction with the inhibition of an acupuncture analgesic effect in the presence of the opioid antagonist naloxone [41,42].

Although acupuncture stimulation traditionally is executed through complex manual needle manipulation, electroacupuncture has often been used in studies. This change has led to several interesting findings. Different electrical frequencies of stimulation were found to be associated with the release of different opioid peptides in both animal and human models [43,44]. Selected or combined release of the peptides, enkephalin, β-endorphin, and dynorphin was achieved by the manipulation of frequencies between 2 Hz and 100 Hz with a potent analgesia obtained by the synergistic activation of the three peptides [45,46]. In addition, central nervous system monoamines are found to have various effects on acupuncture analgesia, with serotonin mediating the effect in the brain and spinal cord and the catecholamines, dopamine and noradrenaline, antagonizing acupuncture analgesia in the brain and increasing it in the spinal cord [47–49].

Antiopioid peptides, cholecystokinin, and orphanin FQ were found to be released with prolonged electroacupuncture stimulation, creating "acupuncture tolerance" and inhibiting analgesia, thus mimicking morphine tolerance after repeated injections [50–52]. Tolerance was reversed with intracerebroventricular injection of cholecystokinin antiserum [53]. Interestingly, about one third of animals are "low responders" to acupuncture, and these were found to have low levels of opioid peptides and high levels of cholecystokinin on electroacupuncture stimulation [43]. Furthermore, when the cholecystokinin gene is suppressed by the antisense technology, a low responder can be converted to a high responder and can thereby benefit from acupuncture treatment [54].

Clearly, acupuncture involves more than opioid-mediated analgesia. There are many biologic responses involving complex physiologic changes that are only beginning to be examined. Stimulation at a given point involves local and distal pathway activation affecting aspects of the central nervous system and other physiologic systems, mediating alterations between the brain and the periphery. Many studies have demonstrated changes in blood pressure, blood flow, secretions of neurotransmitters and neurohormones, and immunologic functions, among other factors. As important as these findings are, few associations can yet be established between these changes and the various clinical effects observed. The pathways of analgesia, however, have afforded a singular opportunity to understand at least one dimension of the effect of acupuncture.

Advanced imaging techniques, specifically single-photon emission computed tomography (SPECT), have been employed to further elucidate fundamental mechanisms. In the paper by Alavi *et al.* [55], five study subjects who suffered from chronic pain and on whom acupuncture was an effective treatment were given SPECT scans before and after acupuncture treatment on the same day. Baseline scans showed a marked asymmetry in the cerebral blood flow in the thalami in all five study subjects as compared those of with controls. After acupuncture treatment, all patients exhibited a lateral shift in the opposite direction, with four of the five achieving an equilibration of thalamic activity.

The search for these mechanisms is only complicated by referring to Oriental medical physiology. The assumption of a vast network of *qi* or energy activation creating a complex reaction and evoking response from many organ systems simultaneously does not further inform Western physiology at present. No validation by instrumentation of this *qi* network has yet been achieved and the "anatomy and physiology of the acupuncture points...remain controversial" [5•].

One final word on biologic mechanisms must take into account the "nonspecific" effects of treatment that many therapeutic modalities share. Acupuncture treatment produces biologic alterations (*eg*, changes in blood pressure, blood flow) that are similar to those of such activities as relaxation training and vigorous exercise. Although these effects may not be specific to acupuncture, they certainly can enhance or limit its clinical effect and compound the placebo effect. The NIH panel [5•] summarized a number of factors that affect treatment outcome: the clinician–patient relationship; the level of trust between clinician and patient; the patient's expectations; and whether the beliefs and backgrounds of the clinician and patient are compatible. The panel also listed a number of factors "that together define the therapeutic milieu" [5•]. For many acupuncturists, the quality of their relationship with the patient is central to the therapeutic phenomenon, the balancing of *qi* within the body, mind, and spirit of the patient [56]. Eliminating this aspect for the sake of clinical standardization may reduce the effectiveness of treatment.

Issues to Address Before Acupuncture is Incorporated into the Current Health-Care System

The NIH panel [5•] indicated several domains in which certain advancements must be made for acupuncture to be integrated further into the current Western health-care system. These domains included communication among professionals, patient education, uniformity of licensure and standards, and economic access. "It has been reported that more than 1 million Americans currently receive acupuncture each year. Continued access to qualified acupuncture professionals for appropriate conditions should be ensured" [5•].

Communication Among Professionals

Communication between acupuncturists (physician and nonphysician) and conventional physicians should be encouraged and fostered despite the difficulties of communicating from different models—one based on a model of Oriental medical physiology and energy balancing and the other a disease-oriented diagnostic and treatment model. If treatment is sought from both groups of professionals, information and communication should be facilitated by all parties in the interest of complete care for the patient.

Patient Education

The panel saw increased patient education, preferably prior to treatment, as an important goal due to the public's general unfamiliarity with acupuncture needles and practices. "Linguistically and culturally appropriate" information should be provided to patients that outlines the scope of acupuncture practice, the expectations of prognosis, the relative risks, and the safety measures used [5•].

Uniformity of Licensure and Standards

Although acupuncture licensure or registration exists in 36 states and the District of Columbia, considerable variation exists among credentialing requirements, titles, scopes of practice, and access to non–English-language examinations and credentialing. Although states may exercise this prerogative, most acupuncture education for nonphysicians in the United States is governed by the standards of the Accreditation Commission for Acupuncture and Oriental Medicine, a credentialing body recognized by the U.S. Department of Education. These standards for accredited schools require 1725 didactic hours in acupuncture and Western anatomy, physiology, and pathology, and require 660 hours of clinical internship. A national examination used by many states for licensure or registration is administered by the National Certification Commission for Acupuncture and Oriental Medicine (NCCAOM), conferring a Diplomate of Acupuncture that indicates entry-level competency in the field.

Educational and credentialing standards for physicians also vary from state to state. Some require no specialized training in acupuncture, whereas others require a passing grade on the NCCAOM examination. Most physicians trained in the United States have completed a minimum 200-hour program at the American Academy of Medical Acupuncture. As the profession evolves, more uniformity will develop; the panel identified progress toward uniformity as one means by which greater public confidence would be created.

Economic Access

Access to acupuncture care is a function of health insurance coverage for many Americans. Although many insurers provide or are considering providing coverage for this service, lack of coverage can present an obstacle to treatment. Health insurance plans and Medicaid plans vary from state to state. Medicare does not provide coverage for acupuncture services. The NIH panel [5•] concluded that expanded coverage by private, state, and federal insurers would "help remove financial barriers to access." Given the relatively small number of acupuncturists in the United States and the concentration of their practices on the east and west coasts, more universal coverage would presumably create a demand that could not be easily met.

DIRECTIONS FOR FUTURE RESEARCH

The NIH panel highlighted several areas for future research in acupuncture, with particular focus directed toward how to demonstrate, if possible, the efficacy of acupuncture for various conditions. The acceptance of any new therapeutic tool into modern, evidence-based medical practice requires more rigorous research than ever before. Few high-quality, randomized, controlled trials assessing the efficacy of acupuncture exist in the literature. When designing a study, special attention must be paid in the future to control selection, placebo effects, sample size, and designing a study that reflects the actual practice of acupuncture in a clinical setting. For example, as useful as it is to demonstrate the efficacy of *Pericardium 6* in the treatment of postoperative nausea, it is highly unlikely that an acupuncturist would select only one point for a given condition or use the same point on every patient every time for therapy of a given condition. Finally, the panel recommended the use of outcomes research and clinical epidemiologic studies to clarify further the conditions for which acupuncture may be an appropriate treatment choice.

To further complicate the design dilemma, many different styles of acupuncture are practiced in the United States and worldwide. The three most common styles in the United States come from China, Japan, and France, although some Korean and Vietnamese styles are common in areas of the country. Each style emphasizes different aspects of the huge body of knowledge of Oriental medicine. Moreover, practitioners trained in multiple styles may use all of them depending on the particulars of the patient's case. Centuries of clinical observation also suggest that the quality of the practitioner's *qi* has an influence on therapeutic outcomes. This is why practitioners are encouraged to pursue personal development of the internal arts, such as meditation, *tai ji*, or *qi gong*.

If the considerations mentioned are taken into account and the efficacy of acupuncture is demonstrated more broadly, this may beg the question about the validity of the Oriental model of an organized energy system. The NIH panel [5•] posed this question for future research and suggested that exploration of this model might also yield "new insights into medical research." In addition, the Western biochemical and physiologic effects of acupuncture should be studied further.

Finally, research into areas of public policy that would have an impact on the use and access of acupuncture deserves attention. Issues of cost effectiveness, reimbursement by private and public third-party payers, and standards and creation of uniformity in education, licensing, and accreditation should be "founded on quality demographic data and effectiveness research" [5•].

CONCLUSIONS

The impact of the NIH panel's consensus statement was immediate and widespread. Front page coverage in major American newspapers announced the conclusions of the consensus report following its release. This historic event has accelerated the creation of a place for acupuncture treatment to be performed within conventional Western medical settings. Numerous complementary and alternative medicine clinics and medical academic programs are being established around the United States. Although acupuncture is only one modality practiced in these clinics and programs, it would seem the consensus statement has helped to spur the acceptance of complementary medicine in general.

NEW RESEARCH

Since the consensus panel convened in November of 1997, studies have been published in referenced literature covering many of the same research topics as have been studied in the past two decades. Two areas continue to dominate the literature—clinical studies and studies of the biologic mechanisms of acupuncture.

Clinical Studies

Two studies demonstrated acupuncture's efficacy in ameliorating the postoperative sequelae of pain and nausea. In one study, 81 patients underwent gynecologic laparoscopic surgery and received acupuncture stimulation at *Pericardium 6* for nausea and vomiting in a randomized, controlled study [57]. The incidence of nausea and vomiting was reduced from 65% to 35% in the hospital and from 69% to 31% after discharge on the same day as compared with placebo. In a more sophisticated design, 100 women were randomly assigned to four study groups after lower abdominal surgery [58]. The four groups received patient-controlled anesthesia (PCA) of hydromorphone, transcutaneous acupoint electrical stimulation (TAES), or both, in the following configurations: PCA alone, PCA and sham-TAES (with no electrical stimulation), PCA and low-TAES, or PCA and high-TAES. Outcomes were recorded for PCA requirement, pain scores, opioid-related side effects, and the need for antiemetic and antipruritic medications. Results showed a 65% and 35% decrease in PCA for high and low TAES, respectively. Reduced nausea, dizziness, and pruritus were also marked. Sham-TAES produced only a 23% reduction in pain medication requirements.

In England, a 1-year follow-up study was performed on stroke patients treated with acupuncture an average of 40 days poststroke. Patients were randomly assigned to a treatment or control group accounting for gender and the side of hemispheral localization of the lesion. Initial acupuncture treatment was added to individually designed, multidisciplinary treatment regimens in a rehabilitation-hospital setting. Acupuncture treatments were also designed and administered according to the principles of classical acupuncture and carried out over a 6-week period. Outcomes were measured by the Motor Assessment Scale (MAS), the Sunnaas Index of Activity of Daily Living (ADL), and the Nottingham Health Profile (NHP). The group that received the acupuncture treatments showed significant improvement both during the treatment phase and even more in the following year than the controls, leading to the possibility of long-term beneficial effects of acupuncture treatment at certain stages poststroke [59].

Although acupuncture in the United States is probably most often used for pain relief, acupuncture in Asia is used also as a primary or adjunct treatment in internal medicine.

Two studies looked at the effect of acupuncture on the symptoms of irritable bowel syndrome (IBS) and Raynaud's syndrome. In the first, a pilot study, seven patients recorded self-assessments of their condition on a diary card while receiving acupuncture treatment for IBS. Significant improvements in symptoms of bloating and general well-being were noted and a recommendation for further study was made [60]. In the study on Raynaud's syndrome, of 33 patients (including 16 controls), 17 were treated during the middle 2-week period of a 23-week study that occurred during the winter months [61]. In addition to daily patient diaries, which recorded vasospastic attacks, nailfold capillaroscopy was performed at weeks 1, 12, and 23. According to patient reports, attacks were reduced by 63%. The mean duration of capillary flow-stop reactions was significantly reduced, with the control group noting no changes, which was a significant finding.

One area of acupuncture applications that has received little research attention is pediatric medicine. In one study, 22 children with childhood-onset migraine were divided into a treatment group and placebo acupuncture group, with 10 healthy children acting as controls. In addition to changes in frequency and intensity of headaches, opioid levels were also monitored, specifically panopioid activity and β-endorphin–like immunoreactivity. At the outset, the control group displayed significantly greater total opioid activity in plasma than the children with migraines. After the tenth treatment, these differences were nearly eliminated in the treatment group, with no significant changes measured in the placebo group. Elevations in panopioid activity and β-endorphin levels rose concurrently with a decrease in migraine frequency and intensity [62].

STUDIES OF BIOLOGIC MECHANISMS

As we have seen in the study of childhood migraines, some clinical studies are beginning to measure biologic markers of physiologic change before, during, and after acupuncture treatment to begin to identify mechanisms of action. A few recent studies of the biologic mechanisms of action of acupuncture also blend into the realm of clinical applicability. Unraveling acupuncture's seemingly elusive clinical logic may elucidate some physiologic relationships.

In the past year, studies have chiefly examined markers in the areas of cardiology, gastroenterology, and neurology. In a Japanese study, heart rate was measured after acupuncture stimulation of *Pericardium 4* on the anterior forearm. Either a reduced heart rate or no change was noted. Any heart rate decrease thus achieved was inhibited by administration of atropine or propranolol, which led researchers to conclude that this effect was the result of simultaneous increased vagal activity and decreased cardiac sympathetic activity [63]. Hypertension is frequently treated with acupuncture in Asia and in the West, assuming an endocrine mechanism at work. In an uncontrolled study, 50 patients with untreated essential hypertension were treated with acupuncture for 30 minutes. Blood pressure and heart rate decreased significantly, whereas no significant change in plasma vasopressin or cortisol levels occurred. A significant decline in plasma renin activity, however, suggested a mechanism that warrants further investigation [64].

Proceeding from the studies of postsurgical nausea and vomiting alleviation by acupuncture therapy, researchers recorded gastric motility in nine healthy people. Electrogastrography recorded myoelectrical activity in a fasting state during which continuous electroacupuncture was applied. The percentage of slow waves (2 to 4 cycles per minute) significantly increased following normalization of arrhythmia during acupuncture [65]. In another study, stimulated and unstimulated salivary responses were affected by manual acupuncture and electroacupuncture in eight healthy people. Some neuropeptides affect salivary secretion; acupuncture may activate these [66].

Neurologic research has produced results suggesting specific brain and nervous system activity pursuant to acupuncture treatment. Cerebral oxygen saturation was measured before, during, and after acupuncture stimulation in 12 healthy people. Measurements obtained with the cerebral oximeter and robotic transcranial Doppler sonography revealed small increases in saturation and significant increases in blood-flow velocity within the right middle cerebral artery [67].

Treatment of eye disorders with acupuncture is common in Oriental medicine. One study correlated the stimulation of a vision-related acupuncture point with the corresponding brain localization for vision [68]. Activation in the occipital lobes was measured by functional magnetic resonance imaging (MRI) during stimulation of an acupuncture point on the lateral aspect of the foot and during direct stimulation of the eye using a light source. Monitoring 12 volunteers, close correlation was seen between visual and acupuncture stimulation. Stimulation to a nonacupuncture point 2 to 5 cm from the study point produced no activation of the occipital lobes [68].

In an ongoing pain investigation, researchers measured pain thresholds in a controlled study using electrical tooth-pain stimulation [69]. Electroacupuncture was performed at *Large Intestine 4* and *Large Intestine 11* (between the first and second metacarpals and at the lateral end of the elbow crease) to inhibit pain. Multiunit efferent postganglionic sympathetic nerve activity was recorded in a muscle fascicle of the peroneal nerve along with mean arterial pressure, heart rate, and skin blood flow, measured during and after treatment. Researchers found that electroacupuncture increased the pain threshold, which was concurrent with a transient increase in muscle sympathetic nerve activity [69].

Finally, in an effort to assess the actual clinical efficacy of acupuncture as experienced by real patients in the United States, a study survey was conducted by a medical anthropologist among 575 patients at eight clinics throughout the country [70,71]. The respondents completed a quantitative and qualitative questionnaire reporting on their experience of care. Of respondents, 91.5% reported their symptoms or conditions had improved or disappeared, with concurrent reductions in the use of prescription medications, office visits to medical doctors, and avoidance of surgery in many instances. The study showed high satisfaction with acupuncture medical care, most of which was paid for by the patients [70,71].

DISCUSSION OF RESEARCH ISSUES

Methodologic considerations are crucial in the evaluation of any study. One source of difficulty in evaluating the efficacy of acupuncture lies in the problems of research design. The standard of randomized, double-blind clinical trials is virtually impossible to achieve in an acupuncture study. Complicating factors, not present in pharmaceutical trials, plague nearly every aspect of study design. Assumptions are made to create shortcuts that ultimately degrade outcome results [72].

One of the most significant areas of complication in current research lies in selecting appropriate control groups. Comparing the effects of acupuncture treatment with those of no treatment does not control for placebo effects or for the nonspecific effects of acupuncture treatment, or any treatment, which can be considerable [73]. Creating an actual placebo treatment has typically fallen into two categories: 1) bogus treatment, *eg*, applying mock TENS units, and 2) sham acupuncture. The third common comparison is to standard Western health care, usually in the form of pharmacotherapy [74,75].

Accounting and controlling for placebo and nonspecific effects include careful handling of many factors unique to an acupuncture trial. An obvious influence on outcomes derives from the beliefs, expectations, and conceptions of acupuncture treatment held by the patient. The complex communication interactions involved in any skilled physical treatment, verbal and nonverbal, can unwittingly suggest all sorts of expectations to the patient. Even minor variations in a consent form stating whether a subject will receive "true" or "sham" treatment versus "treatment A (true)" or treatment B "(sham)" can create bias [74,76,77].

In addition to the nonspecific effects shared by many other modalities already discussed, there exists in acupuncture trials a phenomenon called the "intermediate effect." The problem of intermediate effect occurs between the effect of no acupuncture treatment and the effect of true acupuncture treatment and is frequently encountered when sham acupuncture, or "minimal needling," is used as a control. Some analgesic effect has been noted with mere needle insertion and produces intermediate effects that are neurally mediated responses to noxious stimuli, probably manifest through diffuse noxious inhibitory control (DNIC) [78–80].

Comparison with no treatment, besides being ineffectual for placebo control, raises the ethical problem of no "intent to treat" [73,81,82]. Placebo treatment with a nonfunctioning TENS unit or needles that are merely taped to the skin can sometimes only control for placebo effects in subjects who have little familiarity with actual acupuncture treatment. More recently, mock needling has taken the form of pressing on the skin with the blunt end of the needle handle [83], using an empty guide tube with no needle inside [15], and a using blunted cocktail stirrer inside a guide tube [84]. Assessing patient knowledge of whether true treatment is being administered has been part of some studies to evaluate the particular method as a credible control. A modified version of the credibility scale, originally created by Borkovec and Nau [85], has been used to determine that acupuncture and mock TENS are equally credible in treating neck pain according to the opinion of study subjects [86].

Sham acupuncture has varied in use over the years and as yet no consensus has formed within the research community as to its best application. Sham acupuncture includes such practices as inserting the needle to a shallow insertion depth, needling with no needle manipulation in an area within centimeters of the "true" point, needling of less "active" points, and proper needling of a point not commonly used for the condition being studied. Each of these methods has presented its own complications.

Needling shallowly (*ie*, not to the depth of the acupuncture point below the skin) will probably not produce the *de qi* sensation of brief tingling and aching classically described as a hallmark of a successful needle insertion for treatment [87]. (It should be stressed, however, that some traditions, especially in Japan, employ painless needling techniques.) The absence of sensation in shallow or nearby needling is apparent. Participants in a study who have received acupuncture in the past would presumably notice this lack of sensation and thereby suspect they had not been given true acupuncture; this suspicion would erode their "being blind," in study terms. Even in acupuncture-näive populations, comparison of the experience between the acupuncture group and control group reveals the difference in needle sensation.

Nearby needling has been problematic as a result of variability in the size of acupuncture points and their locations [88]. Because the size of an acupuncture point is classically described as the space into which "a half of a grain of rice" would fit, exact locations of both the acupuncture point and the sham point are critical. Furthermore, we have no absolute certainty that a "nonpoint" area will produce no physiologic effect when stimulated. Needling points that are not primarily indicated for the study condition but that may produce effects raise ethical questions of improper treatment.

The use of sham acupuncture treatment, with superficial and minimal needling being currently preferred, provides the most control for placebo effect and nonspecific effects. In fact, superficial and minimal needling does trigger most of the nonspecific effects of acupuncture needling [89]. This fact also hampers analysis of research study conclusions, however, because sham acupuncture needling that produces intermediate effects between no acupuncture and acupuncture dilutes some of true acupuncture's apparent effect.

A recent innovation from Germany has produced the first "placebo needle," which can visually disguise whether a needle has actually been inserted into the skin. A tiny plastic sheet covers the insertion area and the needle handle moves down over the shaft of the needle, which produces the illusion of needle insertion. This movement is accompanied by a slight pricking sensation and no penetration. None of the 60 volunteers in the study suspected that the needle did not penetrate the skin [90].

Comparison with standard biomedical care also offers many unique advantages. First, the ethical "intent to treat" is satisfied because all study participants receive some form of treatment. Furthermore, it is possible to eliminate the use of controls because there is an adequate comparison group. The presence of a control group, however, may be additionally useful in controlling for the effect of the difference in the experience of receiving a pill versus undergoing a treatment with complex interpersonal interaction involving more time and attention [73]. Other variables that could be compared with conventional care include degree and duration of effect, cost effectiveness, occurrence of side effects, rate of return to activities of daily living and work, and overall well-being. When compared with conventional care, acupuncture efficacy need only match that degree of efficacy.

A review of 52 clinical trials comparing acupuncture with conventional care revealed many difficulties in study design or reporting of study conditions [75]. These ubiquitous problems throw into question both positive and negative study outcomes. Positive outcomes may be confounded, for example, by a treatment assessor who was not blinded, thus leading to a bias toward effectiveness. Negative outcomes throw suspicion on inadequate treatment design or delivery, neither of which is usually described in detail [73].

This last consideration brings to bear an issue of ultimate importance in evaluating the efficacy of acupuncture—treatment design and execution. For the sake of standardization, acupuncture is performed in research settings in ways never conducted in clinical practice in the United States or in Asian countries. The fundamental concept in acupuncture is treatment of the individual and the individual's condition according to the diagnostic principles of Oriental medicine. This means that each person who presents with low back pain, tennis elbow, migraines, or asthma is treated in a unique fashion. No uniform protocols exist for acupuncture treatment according to Western biomedical diagnoses. The exact pathologic condition, according to Oriental medical diagnostic principles, must exist in order to use the same treatment on all study subjects. Standardization of treatment protocols, easily accomplished in drug trials, creates a procrustean bed in which acupuncture research designs have attempted to fit. Eliminating a practitioner's ability to do the "appropriate" treatment certainly undermines the efficacy of treatment. It would be similar to requiring researchers to treat all infections (of viral and various bacterial pathogens) with penicillin. In contrast, a few studies have used the traditional Oriental medical model to diagnose and treat, but the extrapolation of these clinical results, from a Western scientific viewpoint, is obviously hampered by nonstandardization of the treatment.

Understanding the basis for diagnosis in acupuncture clarifies why such difficulties exist in clinical trial study design. Using the same acupuncture points for lateral epicondylitis in 25 patients yields poorer results than performing individual diagnoses and selecting points based on those diagnoses. For example, a difference of 1 inch between patients in the exact location of the pain, variability of exacerbation of pain by movement, or changes in the weather can necessitate choosing different points. Some acupuncture points that effectively treat tennis elbow are found near the elbow, whereas others are found on the lateral aspect of the leg, distal to the patella. Uniformity of treatment protocols required by most clinical trials is anathema to the fundamental principles of Oriental medicine, whereas the lack thereof bedevils any rational Western medical investigation.

A more complex difficulty arises when choosing which acupuncture tradition or style to use when deciding on a treatment protocol. For example, when treating pain, some styles suggest points at or near the site of pain, whereas others may suggest points at the opposite end of the body from where the pain is experienced. A practitioner in clinical practice may choose from several styles when treating a condition as common as low back pain.

In many research settings, an assumption is frequently made that acupuncture is a simple technique that is easily learned. Many studies have employed inadequately trained personnel to perform acupuncture [24••]. Although this seems advantageous to achieve blinding, the reality of introducing an acupuncture needle into the qi and nature of a human being is a highly complex and delicate art. Clinical results are certainly compromised by inadequately trained and inexperienced practitioners.

The final major issue complicating research design involves blinding. The double-blind trial that works so well to assess the efficacy of pharmaceuticals presents enormous difficulties for acupuncture research trials (assuming one uses a trained acupuncturist). Although pharmaceutical and placebo pills can be created to look identical and thereby blind the physician to the distinction, it is not possible to completely blind the acupuncturist administering a treatment protocol. After all, knowing whether or not one is on an acupuncture point is fundamental to the training of an acupuncturist. One suggested compromise is a modified double-blind scheme in which the person administering the treatment is not blinded but the patient and the assessor are [73]. Strict uniformity of interaction and treatment technique would obviously be required of the acupuncturists performing the treatment to reduce bias (perceived by the subject) as much as possible.

Other more minor difficulties with research conducted in the past have included poor or no randomization, too few treatments performed to achieve an effect, unidentified antecedent or intervening variables, subject groups that were too small, and little accounting for internal and external validity, among others [72,76].

Conclusions

Acupuncture medical theory presupposes the existence of energy as a dynamic substrate for the functioning of the physical, mental, and spiritual levels of a human being. The treatment experience encompasses much more than the action of needle insertion. Traditionally, acupuncture practice has required the practitioner to have great command of one's internal qi so as to be compassionately present to the body, mind, and spirit of the patient in order to diagnose and treat energetic imbalances at each of these levels. This internal mastery also allows one to effect greater command of the qi through the needle. These are highly developed concepts of the reality of healing in acupuncture—some of which occur in the ordinary reality of healing we experience throughout life.

We all know the healing effect of being in the presence of a truly caring physician when we are sick. Being truly and compassionately heard can restore hope, clear the mind to solve problems, and renew a deeper commitment to self care. As children, we understood how our pains were healed by the loving presence and tender care of an adult, in concert with nature. Nature heals best in the presence of love and understanding.

We remember many traumas and illnesses as fully physical and emotional experiences. We often associate these times with the image of someone who either cared for us or neglected to do so. This presence or lack thereof affects the healing at many levels of our being. As adults, we frequently lack ready arms into which we can nestle for comfort when we are ill. As a result, we tend to ignore the emotional dimension of our physical maladies because it is too painful to experience those feelings fully when alone. Conversely, we may minimize the impact of emotional stress that could be contributing to physical illness.

At a deeper level of our beings, some instances of sickness and healing leave indelible marks on our spirit that we recognize as we grow older. These experiences render us more open to the wonder of being alive or more closed and protected against all that might further harm us.

Oriental medical theory attempts to embrace these commonly experienced dimensions of the impacts of disease on our emotional health and on our spirit, as well as on our bodies. The differential diagnosis of acupuncture theory incorporates evaluation at the level of the body, mind, and spirit of our being. The internal balance of one's feelings and spirit is not merely interesting but clinically important both in diagnosis and treatment. To treat only the body in crisis is considered, by Oriental medical tradition, an inferior level of care and sometimes dangerous.

The refinement of the practitioner's internal *qi*, which allows for the deeply compassionate experience and assessment of another human being, also lends greater command to the movement of *qi* through the instrument of the needle. As one can master the flexion and extension of one's arm, one can also master the manipulation of *qi* through the needle. This concept, fundamental to acupuncture theory for 2000 years, is rarely raised in the West because little cultural context is in place to understand it. Its importance begins to be apparent when, for example, the same acupuncture point can be needled to achieve opposite effects depending on how the practitioner directs the *qi*.

The manipulation of *qi* through the needle activates the person's own resources to stimulate self-healing and seek a return to equilibrium. All change happens more easily and swiftly when unopposed. Creating a setting in which the *qi* can move with ease and in fundamentally altering ways is essential to the outcome of treatment. More than any other single factor, the relationship between patient and practitioner creates the milieu of healing. This serves as a foundation on which the treatment rests.

This complex phenomenon is clinical reality for most acupuncture as performed in the United States today, but it is a far cry from the drug-testing model of current research. Although a drug trial can approximate clinical reality because a pharmaceutical product can be given by anyone to anyone with the appropriate diagnosis, acupuncture trials do not approximate clinical reality. Acupuncture never treats back pain; acupuncture treats a person who, through living life, experiences back pain. The task of the medicine is to achieve an understanding of the functioning of a human being at the level of the body and the mind and the spirit under the conditions of navigating a life. The complex degree of understanding of a human being engendered by a traditional Oriental medical diagnosis that leads to an energetic assessment and treatment plan cannot be approximated during the sort of clinical trials in current use.

Despite these difficulties, acupuncture research goes on, continually refining methodology that can honor both the scientific method of medical investigation and the principles of Oriental medicine. Given the many individualized components in an acupuncture treatment, a new paradigm of research is needed. It is essential to create research methods that conform to clinical reality, rather than reduce clinical reality to the confines of a research methodology designed for other purposes. The thousands of attempts to do the latter have created a paucity of data, despite the expenditure of enormous resources over decades. Amid a vast number of these imperfect studies, the NIH consensus panel [5•] has attempted to arrive at a supportable, substantiated preliminary conclusion as to the efficacy of acupuncture. The number of such studies reinforces both the promise of acupuncture as an effective treatment modality and the need for more research.

REFERENCES AND RECOMMENDED READING

Recently published papers of particular interest have been highlighted as:
- Of interest
- •• Of outstanding interest

1. Helms JM: *Acupuncture Energetics: A Clinical Approach for Physicians*. Berkeley, CA: Medical Acupuncture Publishers; 1995.
2. Warren E: *An Epitome of Practical Surgery*. Richmond, VA: West and Johnson; 1863.
3. Osler W: *The Principles and Practices of Medicine*. New York: Appleton; 1892.
4. Medical devices: reclassification of acupuncture needles for the practice of acupuncture. *Federal Register* 1996, 61:64616–64617.
5.• National Institutes of Health: *Consensus Development Conference Statement on Acupuncture, November 3–5, 1997*. Rockville, MD: National Institutes of Health, 1997.
   This is the full text of the NIH panel statement.
6. Unschuld PU: *Medicine in China*. Berkeley, CA: University of California Press; 1985.
7. Dundee JW, Ghaly RG, Bill KM, *et al.*: Effect of stimulation of the P6 antiemetic point on postoperative nausea and vomiting. *Brit J Anaesth* 1989, 63:612–618.
8. Ghaly RG, Fitzpatrick KTJ, Dundee JW: Antiemetic studies with traditional Chinese acupuncture: a comparison of manual needling with electrical stimulation and commonly used antiemetics. *Anesthesia* 1987, 42:1108–1110.
9. Dundee JW, Ghaly RG, Fitzpatrick KTJ, *et al.*: Acupuncture prophylaxis of cancer chemotherapy-induced sickness. *J Roy Soc Med* 1989, 82:268–271.
10. Dundee JW, Yang J: Prolongation of the antiemetic effect of P6 acupuncture by acupressure in patients having cancer chemotherapy. *J Roy Soc Med* 1990, 83:360–362.
11. Christensen PA, Noreng M, Anderson PE, *et al.*: Electroacupuncture and postoperative pain. *Br J Anaesth* 1989, 62:258–262.

12. Facco E, Manani G, Angel A, et al.: Comparison study between acupuncture and pentazocine analgesic and respiratory post-operative effects. *Am J Chin Med* 1981, 9:225–235.
13. Martelete M, Fiori AMC: Comparative study of the analgesic effect of transcutaneous nerve stimulation (TNS), electro-acupuncture (EA), and meperidine in the treatment of post-operative pain. *Acupunct Electrother Res* 1985, 10:183–193.
14. Sung YF, Kutner MH, Cerine FC, et al.: Comparison of the effects of acupuncture and codeine on postoperative dental pain. *Anesth Analg* 1977, 56:473–478.
15. Lao L, Bergman S, Langenberg P, et al.: Efficacy of Chinese acupuncture on postoperative oral surgery pain. *Oral Surg Oral Med Oral Path* 1995, 79:423–428.
16. Lapeer GL, Biedermann HJ, Hernsted JJ: Acupuncture analgesia for postoperative dental pain. *J Can Dent Assoc* 1987, 53:479–480.
17. Selden HS: Pain and perception modification with acupuncture: a clinical study. *J Endod* 1978, 4:356–361.
18. Silva SA: Acupuncture for the relief of pain of facial and dental origin. *Anesth Prog* 1989, 36:242–248.
19. Wong T: Use of electrostimulation of acupuncture points in general dental practice. *Anesth Prog* 1989, 36:243–244.
20. Ha H, Tan EC: Effect of acupuncture on pain threshold measurement of tooth pulp in the monkey. *Am J Chin Med* 1982, 14:68–72.
21. Ha H, Wu RS, Contreras RA, et al.: Measurement of pain threshold by electrical stimulation of tooth pulp afferent in the monkey. *Exp Neurol* 1978, 61:260–269.
22. Chapman RC, Sato R, Martin RW, et al.: Comparative effects of acupuncture in Japan and the United States on dental pain perception. *Pain* 1982, 12:312–328.
23. Ernst M, Lee MH: Influence of naloxone on electro-acupuncture analgesia using an experimental dental pain test: review of possible mechanisms of action. *Acupunct Electrother Res* 1987 12:5–22.
24.•• Birch S, Hammerschlag R: *Acupuncture Efficacy: A Compendium of Controlled Clinical Trials*. Tarrytown, NY: National Academy of Acupuncture and Oriental Medicine; 1996.
This is a concise review of some of the better trials performed in acupuncture.
25. Diehl D, Kaplan G, Coulter I, et al.: Use of acupuncture by American physicians. *J Altern Complement Med* 1997, 3:119–126.
26. DeLuze C, Bosia L, Zirbs A, et al.: Electroacupuncture in fibromyalgia: results of a controlled trial. *Br Med J* 1992, 305:1249–1252.
27. Hesse J, Mogelvang B, Simonsen H: Acupuncture versus metoprolol in migraine prophylaxis: a randomized trial of trigger point inactivation. *J Intern Med* 1994, 235:451–456.
28. Lenhard L, Waite PME: Acupuncture in the prophylactic treatment of migraine headaches: pilot study. *N Z Med J* 1983, 96:663–666.
29. Molsberger A, Hille E: The analgesic effect of acupuncture in chronic tennis elbow pain. *Br J Rheumatol* 1994, 33:1162–1165.
30. Takeda W, Wessel J: Acupuncture for the treatment of pain of osteoarthritic knees. *Arthritis Care Res* 1994, 7:118–122.
31. Vincent CA: A controlled trial of the treatment of migraine by acupuncture. *Clin J Pain* 1989, 5:305–312.
32. American Medical Association: Proceedings of the House of Delegates at the 130th Annual Convention. June 7–11, 1981.
33. Kleijnen J, ter Riet G, Knipschild P: Acupuncture and asthma: a review of controlled trials. *Thorax* 1991, 46:799–802.
34. Konefal J, Duncan R, Clemence C: The impact of the addition of an acupuncture treatment program to an existing Metro-Dade County outpatient substance abuse treatment facility. *J Addict Dis* 1994, 13:71–99.
35. Lewith GT, Watkins AD: Unconventional therapies in asthma: an overview. *Allergy* 1996, 51:761–769.
36. MacDonald AJ, Macrae KD, Master BR, et al.: Superficial acupuncture in the relief of chronic low back pain. *Ann R Coll Surg Engl* 1983, 65:44–46.
37. Naeser MA, Alexander MP, Stiassny-Eder D, et al.: Real vs. sham acupuncture in the treatment of paralysis in acute stroke patients: a CT scan lesion site study. *J Neuro Rehab* 1992, 6:163–173.
38. Naeser MA, Alexander MP, Stiassny-Eder D, et al.: Acupuncture in the treatment of hand paresis in chronic and acute stroke patients: improvement observed in all cases. *Clin Rehab* 1994, 8:127–141
39. Naeser MA, Hahn KK, Lieberman B: Real vs. sham laser acupuncture and microamps TENS to treat carpal tunnel syndrome and worksite wrist pain: pilot study. *Lasers Surg Med* 1996, 8(suppl):7.
40. Pert CB, Snyder SH: Opiate receptor: demonstration in nervous tissue. *Science* 1973, 179:1011–1014.
41. Mayer JD, Price DD, Rafii A: Antagonism of acupuncture analgesia in man by the narcotic antagonist naloxone. *Brain Res* 1977, 21:368–372.
42. Pomeranz B, Chiu D: Naloxone blocks acupuncture analgesia and causes hyperalgesia: endorphin is implicated. *Life Sci* 1976, 19:1757–1762.
43. Fei H, Xie GX, Han JS, et al.: Low and high frequency electroacupuncture stimulation releases enkephalin and dynorphin A and B in rat spinal cord. *Chin Sci Bull* 1987, 32:1496–1501.
44. Han JS, Chen XH, Sun SL et al.: Effect of low- and high-frequency TENS on metenkephalin-Arg-Phe and dynorphin A immunoreactivity in human lumbar CFS. *Pain* 1991, 47:295–298.
45. Chen XH, Guo SF, Chang CG, et al.: Optimal conditions for eliciting maximal electroacupuncture analgesia with dense-and-disperse mode of stimulation. *Am J Acupunct* 1994, 22:47–53.
46. Huang L, Ren MF, Lu JH, et al.: Mutual potentiation of the analgesic effect of [met superscript 5] enkephalin, dynorphin A-(1-13) and morphine in the spinal cord of the rat. *Acta Physiol Sin* 1987, 9:454–461.
47. Han JS, Chou PH, Lu CC, et al.: The role of central 5-HT in acupuncture analgesia. *Sci Sin* 1979, 22:91–104.
48. Xu W, Qi XC, Han JS: Serotonin receptor subtypes in spinal antinociception in the rat. *J Pharmacol Exp Ther* 1994, 269:186–189.
49. Xie CW, Tang J, Han JS: Central norepinephrine in acupuncture analgesia: differential effects in brain and spinal cord. *Advances in Endogenous and Exogenous Opioids*. Tokyo: Kodansha; 1981:288–290.
50. Han JS, Li SJ, Tang J: Tolerance to acupuncture and its cross tolerance to morphine. *Neuropharmacology* 1981, 20:593–596.
51. Tian JH, Xu W, Fang Y, et al.: Bidirectional modulatory effect of orphanin FQ on morphine induced analgesia: antagonism in brain and potentiation in spinal cord of the rat. *Br J Pharmacol* 1997, 120 676–680.
52. Tian JH, Xu W, Zhang Y, et al.: Involvement of endogenous orphanin FQ in electroacupuncture induced analgesia. *Neuroreport* 1997, 8:497–500.
53. Han JS, Ding XZ, Fan SG: CCK-8: antagonism on electroacupuncture analgesia and a possible role in electroacupuncture tolerance. *Pain* 1986, 27:101–115.
54. Tang NM, Dong HW, Wang XM, et al.: Cholecystokinin antisense RNA increases the analgesic effect induced by EA or low dose morphine: conversion of low responder rats into high responders. *Pain* 1997, 71:71–80.
55. Alavi A, LaRiccia PJ, Sadek AH, et al.: Neuroimaging of acupuncture in patients with chronic pain. *J Altern Complement Med* 1997, 3(suppl):47–53.
56. Worsley JR: *Traditional Acupuncture, Volume II: Traditional Diagnosis*. Royal Leamington Spa, UK: The College of Traditional Acupuncture; 1990.
57. al-Sadi M, Newman B, Julious SA: Acupuncture in the prevention of postoperative nausea and vomiting. *Anaesthesia* 1997, 52:658–661.
58. Wang B, Tang J, White PF, et al.: Effect of the intensity of transcutaneous acupoint electrical stimulation on the postoperative analgesic requirement. *Anesth Analg* 1997, 85:406–413.

59. Kjendahl A, Sallstrom S, Osten PE, et al.: A one year follow-up study on the effects of acupuncture in the treatment of stroke patients in the subacute stage: a randomized, controlled study. *Clin Rehab* 1997, 11:192–200.
60. Chan J, Carr I, Mayberry JF: The role of acupuncture in the treatment of irritable bowel syndrome: a pilot study. *Hepato-Gastroenterology* 1997, 44:1328–1330.
61. Appiah R, Hiller S, Caspary L, et al.: Treatment of primary Raynaud's syndrome with traditional Chinese acupuncture. *J Int Med* 1997, 241:119–124.
62. Pintov S, Lahat E, Alstein M, et al.: Acupuncture and the opioid system: implications in management of migraine. *Pediatr Neurol* 1997, 17:129–133.
63. Nishijo K, Mori H, Yosikawa K, et al.: Decreased heart rate by acupuncture stimulation in humans via facilitation of cardiac vagal activity and suppression of cardiac sympathetic nerve. *Neurosci Lett* 1997, 227:165–168.
64. Chiu YJ, Chi A, Reid IA: Cardiovascular and endocrine effects of acupuncture in hypertensive patients. *Clin Exp Hypertens* 1997, 19:1047–1063.
65. Lin X, Liang J, Ren J, et al.: Electrical stimulation of acupuncture points enhances gastric myoelectrical activity in humans. *Am J Gastroenterol* 1997, 92:1527–1530.
66. Dawidson I, Blom M, Lundeberg T, et al.: The influence of acupuncture on salivary flow rates in healthy subjects. *J Oral Rehab* 1997, 24:204–208.
67. Litscher G, Schwarz G, Sandner-Kiesling A, et al. Effects of acupuncture on the oxygenation of cerebral tissue. *Neurol Res* 1998, 20(suppl):S28–S32.
68. Cho ZH, Chung SC, Jones JP, et al.: New findings of the correlation between acupoints and corresponding brain cortices using functional MRI. *Proc Natl Acad Sci U S A* 1998, 95:2670–2673.
69. Knardahl S, Elam M, Olausson B, et al.: Sympathetic nerve activity after acupuncture in humans. *Pain* 1998, 75:19–25.
70. Cassidy CM: Chinese medicine users in the United States, part I: utilization, satisfaction, medical plurality. *J Altern Complement Med* 1998, 4:17–27.
71. Cassidy CM: Chinese medicine users in the United States, part II: preferred aspects of care. *J Altern Complement Med* 1998, 4:189–202.
72. Singh BB, Berman BM: Research issues for clinical designs. *Complement Ther Med* 1997, 5:3–7.
73. Hammershlag R: Methodological and ethical issues in clinical trials of acupuncture. *J Altern Complement Med* 1998, 4:159–171.
74. Vincent C, Lewith G: Placebo controls for acupuncture studies. *J Roy Soc Med* 1995, 88:199–202.
75. Hammershlag R, Morris MM: Clinical trials comparing acupuncture with biomedical standard care: a criteria-based evaluation of research design and reporting. *Complement Ther Med* 1997, 5:133–140.
76. Vincent CA, Richardson PH: The evaluation of therapeutic acupuncture: concepts and methods. *Pain* 1986, 24:1–13.
77. Birch S: Credibility of treatment in controlled trials of acupuncture. *J Altern Complement Med* 1997, 3:315–321.
78. Le Bars D, Willer JC, De Broucker T, et al.: *Neurophysiological Mechanisms Involved in the Pain Relieving Effects of Counterirritation and Related Techniques Including Acupuncture.* Heidelberg, Berlin: Springer; 1989.
79. Le Bars D, Villaneuva L, Willer JC, et al.: Diffuse noxious inhibitory control (DNIC) in animals and man. *Acup Med* 1991, 9:47–57.
80. Liu X, Zhu B, Zhang SX: Relationship between electroacupuncture analgesia and descending pain inhibitory mechanism of nucleus raphe magnus. *Pain* 1986, 24:383–396.
81. Stanley B: An integration of ethical and clinical considerations in the use of placebos. *Psychopharmacol Bull* 1988, 24:18–20.
82. Rothman KJ, Michels KB: The continuing unethical use of placebo controls. *N Engl J Med* 1994, 331:394–398.
83. Hesse J, Mogelvang B, Simonsen H: Acupuncture versus metoprolol in migraine prophylaxis: a randomized trial of trigger point activation. *J Intern Med* 1994, 235:451–456.
84. White AR, Eddleston C, Hardie R, et al.: A pilot study of acupuncture for tension headache, using a novel placebo. *Acup Med* 1996, 14:11–15.
85. Borkovec TD, Nau SD: Credibility of analogue therapy rationales. *J Beh Ther Exp Psychiatr* 1972, 3:257–260.
86. Petrie JP, Hazelman BL: A controlled study of acupuncture in neck pain. *Br J Rheumatol* 1986, 25:271–275.
87. Bensky D, O'Connor J: *Acupuncture: A Comprehensive Text. Shanghai College of Traditional Medicine.* Seattle: Eastland Press; 1981.
88. Zhang K, Dang R, Guan L, et al.: A morphological study on the receptors of acupuncture points. *J Tradit Chin Med* 1982, 2:251–260.
89. Birch S: Testing the clinical specificity of needle sites in controlled clinical trials of acupuncture. *Proc Soc Acup Res* 1995, 2:274–294.
90. Streitberger K, Kleinhenz J: Introducing a placebo needle into acupuncture research. *Lancet* 1998, 352:364–365.

Spinal Adjustment for Low Back Pain

Daniel Redwood

In recent years, spinal manual therapy (SMT), also known as spinal adjustment or manipulation, has moved from the fringes to center stage among treatment options for low back pain (LBP), an extremely common yet challenging condition. When the Agency for Health Care Policy and Research (AHCPR) released its landmark 1994 practice guideline, *Acute Low Back Pain in Adults* [1], only two methods out of dozens evaluated were judged to have convincing documentation in the scientific literature—SMT and nonsteroidal anti-inflammatory drugs (NSAIDs). The AHCPR panel, chaired by an orthopedic surgeon and primarily composed of conventionally trained medical physicians, concluded that of these two methods, only SMT both relieved pain and restored function. SMT, 94% of which is provided by chiropractors [2], was not only the sole "alternative" treatment to pass muster, but it also surpassed a whole gamut of conventional techniques, rising straight to the top of the list. Recognition of this procedure's unique effectiveness for LBP and its promise in treating other ailments [3,4] has led to increased efforts to integrate chiropractic care more fully into conventional health delivery.

In 1998, the National Institutes of Health (NIH) inaugurated the Consortial Center for Chiropractic Research (CCCR) under the auspices of the NIH Office of Alternative Medicine and the National Institute of Arthritis and Musculoskeletal and Skin Diseases. Based at the Palmer Center for Chiropractic Research in Davenport, Iowa, the CCCR is a joint venture by five chiropractic schools, a medical school, and a school of veterinary medicine. CCCR's mission is to support a multidisciplinary group of researchers and clinicians to perform basic, preclinical, clinical, epidemiologic, and health-care services research on chiropractic. Among its key goals are developing an environment for training future scientists and encouraging collaboration between basic and clinical scientists and between the chiropractic and conventional medical communities.

CONTEMPORARY CHIROPRACTIC

Chiropractic is now the third largest independent health-care profession, after conventional medicine and dentistry. America's 55,000 chiropractors are portal-of-entry providers, educated and licensed in both diagnosis and treatment. Approximately 22 million Americans receive chiropractic care annually. Chiropractic scope of practice is limited not by anatomic region but by procedure. It excludes surgery and pharmaceuticals, focusing on SMT and related therapies. Chiropractors are licensed in the United States, Canada, and in a growing number of other nations. Educational standards are supervised by government-recognized accrediting agencies, including the Council on Chiropractic Education (CCE) in the United States. After fulfilling prechiropractic college science prerequisites, chiropractic students complete a 4-year chiropractic school program that includes a wide range of courses in anatomy, physiology, pathology, and diagnosis as well as spinal adjustment, nutrition, physical therapy, and rehabilitation. Basic science faculty hold masters' and doctoral degrees in their academic areas of expertise. Most clinical faculty are themselves chiropractors.

Chiropractic care has been covered by Medicare and worker's compensation insurance since the 1970s and is included in most private sector health insurance policies. At present, a small majority of health maintenance organization (HMO) policies cover chiropractic, as do a larger majority of preferred provider organization (PPO) policies. The advent of managed care has proved to be a challenge for chiropractors as it has for many medical practitioners, because in many cases referral from a primary care physician (PCP) is required before patients can receive reimbursable chiropractic care. Most PCPs are relatively unfamiliar with chiropractic, thus seriously impeding patients who need access to chiropractic services. This chapter is written for PCPs interested in current developments in chiropractic, with a special focus on LBP.

PRIMARY CARE PHYSICIANS, CHIROPRACTORS, AND LOW BACK PAIN

Primary care physicians serve as portal-of-entry providers for about one third of patients seeking treatment for LBP [5]. In managed-care settings, PCPs often occupy the crucial gatekeeper role. Studies show, however, that PCPs are frustrated with their ability to offer effective care for LBP patients [6]. Moreover, most patients are dissatisfied with this care [7]. Cherkin et al. [8], whose work uncovered these disturbing patterns, sought to remedy the situation by developing an educational program to provide family physicians with specific information, tools, and techniques associated with more satisfying and cost-effective care for LBP. Implementation of this program resulted in significant increases in the proportion of providers who felt confident that they knew how to manage LBP, and who believed their patients were satisfied. When the patients themselves were evaluated, however, outcomes had not improved and the patients remained dissatisfied, even those whose physicians had perceived the greatest benefit.

Cherkin et al. [8] and others [9,10] have found significantly higher rates of patient satisfaction among chiropractic patients, the majority of whom seek care for LBP. It is likely that the explanation lies in the efficacy of chiropractic treatment and in the nature of the chiropractor–patient relationship. Robert Mootz, the Associate Medical Director of the Chiropractic Department of the Washington Department of Labor and Industries, describes the chiropractor–patient encounter as "characterized by extensive hands-on evaluation, clear and concrete explanations, hands-on treatment that often feels good and is sometimes associated with an immediate improvement in symptoms, and repeated follow-up with the doctor" [11,12].

Given the body of evidence supporting the efficacy of SMT for LBP [1,13,14] and the fact that patients are highly satisfied with chiropractic care, PCP referral of many LBP patients to chiropractors appears at first glance to be a winning situation. When these referrals occur, PCPs are relieved of some of their most frustrating cases, chiropractors have the chance to do what they do best, and patients achieve desirable clinical outcomes that leave them satisfied with both the chiropractor and the PCP. Still, PCP attitudes toward spinal manipulation and chiropractors lag far behind conclusions contained in evidence-based practice guidelines, such as the AHCPR [1]

document. In 1995, Cherkin et al. [15] reported that only 35% of physicians considered SMT "effective for some patients," compared with 93% who considered physical therapy effective, even though the literature offers greater support for SMT than for physical therapy, as clearly noted by the AHCPR panel [1].

A substantial history underlies this pattern. Until the 1980s, American Medical Association policies declared it unethical for medical doctors to refer to chiropractors or accept referrals from them, a practice eventually found to be illegal by the Supreme Court in *Wilk versus AMA et al.* From the founding of the chiropractic profession in 1895 through the 1960s, chiropractic education left much to be desired and research on SMT was minimal. In the past 3 decades, however, these troublesome trends have been dramatically reversed. Interprofessional cooperation has increased in the academic and clinical arenas [16], and chiropractic education in the past few decades has undergone a period of sustained positive change no less profound than that which followed Abraham Flexner's landmark 1910 report on medical education [17].

The time is ripe for healing old rifts and changing outdated beliefs to reflect current realities. In my lectures to fourth-year medical students, I have found a welcome openness to chiropractic that bodes well for future interprofessional relations. To best serve our patients, communication and understanding must be improved between PCPs and chiropractors. PCPs, most of whom graduated from medical school when the curriculum either included nothing about manual therapies or dismissed them in disparaging terms, need a working knowledge of spinal joint dysfunction, along with an understanding of what chiropractic is, when it is likely to be helpful, how safe it is, and to whom they can confidently refer their LBP patients.

Subluxation

In significant ways, structure determines function. A fundamental tenet of chiropractic is that proper physiologic function requires balance among the bony structures of the body. When this balance is lost, whether from trauma or gradual compensatory shifting, stress accumulates. Structurally, much of this stress focuses at the weight-bearing joints of the axial skeleton. Because spinal joints function as mechanical fulcrums and also lie adjacent to nerve roots that branch out from the spinal cord, spinal joint dysfunction (also called *subluxation*, which in chiropractic use refers to a joint malfunction with neural involvement) is a complex entity. Contemporary models of the subluxation complex, drawing on recent advances in basic science and clinical research, incorporate the components shown in Table 8-1 [18].

Depending on the specifics of the injury or cumulative stress pattern, one or more of these components may predominate in a particular case. For example, some LBP is primarily myologic (due to muscle strain) with secondary kinesiologic or inflammatory aspects. Other cases are largely kinesiologic, with minimal muscular involvement. In each individual circumstance, appropriate treatment depends on proper evaluation.

Compensation

When considering joint dysfunction, it is important to bear in mind that the spine functions as a unit. Dysfunction at one

Table 8-1. Components of the Subluxation Complex

Type	Symptom
Kinesiologic	Motion segment hypomobility or hypermobility
Neurophysiologic	Irritation of nerve receptors or nerve tissue, compression of neural elements, decreased axoplasmic transport
Myologic	Spasm or hypertonicity of muscles
Connective tissue	Immobilization leading over time to fibrofatty consolidation, fibrous deposition, and deposition of bone salts; shrinkage of articular cartilage from loss of proteoglycans; adhesions between adjacent connective tissues
Inflammatory	Inflammatory response elicited by joint immobilization

From Cleveland [18]; with permission.

level can trigger compensatory changes at other spinal levels, or in other musculoskeletal areas (*eg*, hip, knee, or ankle). In describing these relations, McAndrews [*quoted in* 16] has used the artful metaphor of a mobile hanging over a child's crib to illustrate the concept of dynamic equilibrium. When one of the mobile's strings is cut, all of its suspended ornaments start to bounce and shift erratically until a new equilibrium is achieved. In this new state of equilibrium, the ornaments have shifted, both in relation to the central axis and in relation to each other. The body's musculoskeletal system works in much the same way. When equilibrium is disrupted (by injury, chronic postural stress, or other causes) structural patterns are altered to a greater or lesser degree, depending on the nature and intensity of the forces that threw off the old pattern of balance. Over time, compensatory imbalances can embed themselves deeply, as muscles, ligaments, cartilage, and even bone undergo changes in structure and function. The result is chronic musculoskeletal imbalance and pain.

A key corollary of the principle of compensation is that the site of pain may not be the site of the pain's cause. Some cases of knee pain, for instance, result from structural injury to the knee, but others are compensations for mechanical joint dysfunction in the lumbar spine or sacroiliac joints. Similarly, a case of LBP might include a fixated sacroiliac, but this could in turn be a compensation for a problem elsewhere in the spine. From the chiropractor's point of view, palpating for areas of significant joint restriction is relevant not only where symptoms are present, but throughout the spine and related areas of the musculoskeletal system.

Screening the Patient

In evaluating patients to determine whether spinal adjustments are indicated, the crucial first step is to rule out "red flag" situations, most of which require immediate referral to other specialists. SMT is absolutely contraindicated in anatomic areas where the following occur: malignancies; bone and joint infection; acute myelopathy or acute cauda equina syndrome; acute fractures and dislocations, or healed fractures and dislocations with signs of ligamentous rupture or instability; acute rheumatoid, rheumatoid-like, or nonspecific arthropathies including ankylosing spondylitis characterized by episodes of acute inflammation, demineralization, or ligamentous laxity with anatomical subluxation or dislocation; active juvenile avascular necrosis; or unstable os odontoideum [19].

After screening for these "red flags" has ruled out contraindications to manual adjustment, the next step is to ascertain whether spinal joint dysfunction is present. Restriction of joint motion, or "fixation," is the key sign of spinal joint dysfunctions likely to benefit from SMT. Leach [20] describes a triad of diagnostic signs indicating segmental dysfunction. These are 1) point tenderness or altered pain threshold to pressure in the adjacent paraspinal musculature or over the spinous process; 2) abnormal contraction or tension within the adjacent paraspinal musculature; and 3) loss of normal motion in one or more planes. Highly refined psychomotor skills are necessary to diagnose spinal joint dysfunction and to perform the manual maneuvers best suited to its correction.

Some joint dysfunctions involve hypermobility, characterized by ligamentous laxity frequently of traumatic etiology. Hypermobility may be clinically diagnosed by eliciting a repeated click when a joint is moved through its normal range of motion. Forceful manipulation of hypermobility should be avoided (because this can further increase the hypermobility), but nearby joints that have become fixated to compensate for the hypermobile joint should be adjusted. Muscles in the area should be strengthened and toned to minimize stress on the hypermobile joint.

Unless the PCP possesses the well-honed motion palpation skills necessary to determine that such spinal joint dysfunction is absent, moderate to severe back pain that does not appear to be moving toward resolution within a few to several days should be evaluated by a specialist who can competently make such a determination. Chiropractors and osteopaths who use spinal manipulation on a regular basis (only a minority of osteopaths does) are the professionals best trained to do so. In practical terms, given the numbers and geographic distribution of practitioners in each of these specialties, this will most often mean referral to a chiropractor.

When a chiropractor determines that spinal joint dysfunction is not present, he or she may proceed with other appropriate therapy, such as exercise recommendations or the use of physical therapy modalities. Where joint dysfunction is noted, he or she will manually adjust the problematic joint(s) to restore proper biomechanic function. Lengthy immobilization can cause serious compromise of musculoskeletal structures including muscle, tendon, ligament, cartilage, disk, and bone [21]. By imparting motion into dysfunctionally fixated vertebral joints, manipulation alters the environment of the motion segment. As noted, this may evoke positive change not only in kinesiologic function, but in the neurophysiologic, inflammatory, connective tissue, and myologic aspects of the subluxation complex as well.

RESEARCH ON MANUAL ADJUSTMENT FOR LOW BACK PAIN

A substantial body of research has addressed the efficacy of SMT in the treatment of LBP. Consensus panels evaluating the data have consistently placed SMT on the short list of recommended procedures for acute, uncomplicated LBP [1,2,22]. These reports are based on controlled clinical trials; approximately 40 such papers have been published as of this writing.

Among the most influential trials were those conducted by Meade [23,24••] with over 700 patients. Meade compared chiropractic manipulation with standard hospital outpatient treatment for LBP, which consisted of physical therapy and wearing a corset. He concluded that, "for patients with low-back pain in whom manipulation is not contraindicated, chiropractic almost certainly confers worthwhile, long-term benefit in comparison to hospital outpatient management." Describing the applicability of these findings for PCPs, he stated, "Our trial showed that chiropractic is a very effective treatment, more effective than conventional hospital out-patient treatment for low-back pain, particularly in patients who had back pain in the past and who [developed] severe problems. One of the unexpected findings was that the treatment difference–the benefit of chiropractic over hospital treatment–actually persists for the whole of that 3-year period" [25].

Meade's studies [23,24••] were the first large randomized clinical trial to demonstrate substantial short-term and long-term benefits from chiropractic care. Because it dealt with both acute and chronic LBP patients, Meade's data supports the use of SMT for both populations.

ACUTE VERSUS CHRONIC LOW BACK PAIN

A crucial issue not yet resolved by consensus panels and meta-analyses is whether chiropractic adjustments should be recommended for patients with both chronic and acute LBP (Tables 8-2 and 8-3). Strong agreement exists that SMT is appropriate for many acute LBP cases, but the jury is still out regarding chronic LBP (a minority view can be found in the work of van Tulder et al. [26], who conclude that evidence supports SMT for chronic but not acute cases of LBP). The current perceived insufficiency of data favoring SMT for chronic LBP has led some analysts to rate it as inappropriate for chronic LBP. When Shekelle et al. [27••] rated the "appropriateness" of decisions to initiate manipulative therapy, they deemed manipulation inappropriate for all cases of chronic LBP. Although this perception lowered the percentage of cases in which chiropractic was considered appropriate, both Shekelle's group and an accompanying editorial by Micozzi [28] aptly noted that the study offers convincing reasons for PCPs to refer many more of their LBP patients to chiropractors.

EVIDENCE FOR MANUAL METHODS IN CHRONIC CASES

Physicians reading that manipulation is considered "inappropriate" for chronic LBP may conclude that, until further convincing evidence emerges, referral of patients with chronic LBP to chiropractors would be an error. Physicians frequently refer chronic LBP patients to physical therapists, however, based on perceptions of its effectiveness and appropriateness that vastly exceed that found in research documentation [15]. Because a PCP's decision about whether and where to refer patients with LBP hinges on which treatments are expected to yield the most satisfactory outcomes, a summary of studies on SMT for chronic LBP may aid the decision-making process.

Aside from Meade's work [23,24••], perhaps the most impressive of these is a prospective study performed at the University of Saskatchewan hospital orthopedics department

TABLE 8-2. ACUTE LOWER BACK PAIN

Patient	Male, 26 years of age, electrician
Chief complaint	LBP with intermittent tingling in left inguinal region
Duration	10 days
Intensity	Moderate, occasionally severe
Original cause	Work-related lifting injury
History	Patient was lifting boxes and a teletypewriter from a high shelf and placing them on the floor. While doing this, he felt sharp pain, centrally located in the lower lumbar area.
Exam findings	Motor, sensory and reflex function normal. Bilateral spasm of lumbar paraspinal muscles, with pain on palpation. Restricted joint mobility at L5-S1 and both sacroiliac joints.
Diagnosis	Lumbar strain with L5-S1 segmental dysfunction
Treatment	Eight spinal adjustments in 3-week period. Electronic muscle stimulation used during early acute phase.
Response	Gradual decrease in symptoms, with no pain after 2 weeks of treatment.
Comments	No further episodes at 2-year follow-up

by Kirkaldy-Willis and Cassidy [29]. The approximately 300 subjects in this study were "totally disabled" by LBP, with pain present for an average of 7 years. All had gone through extensive, unsuccessful medical treatment before participating as research subjects. After 2 to 3 weeks of daily chiropractic adjustments, over 80% of these patients without spinal stenosis had good to excellent results, reporting substantially decreased pain and increased mobility. After chiropractic treatment, over 70% improved to the point of having no work restrictions. Follow-up 1 year later demonstrated that the changes were long-lasting. Even those with a narrowed spinal canal, who represented a particularly difficult subset, showed a notable response. More than half improved, and about one in five had no pain and were working 7 months after treatment.

In a randomized trial of 209 patients, Triano et al. [30••] compared SMT to education programs for chronic LBP, which they defined as pain lasting 7 weeks or longer or representing more than 6 episodes in 12 months. These investigators found greater improvement in pain and activity tolerance in the SMT group and noted that "immediate benefit from pain relief continued to accrue after manipulation, even for the last encounter at the end of the 2-week treatment interval." They concluded that "there appears to be clinical value to treatment according to a defined plan using manipulation even in LBP exceeding 7 weeks duration."

Koes et al. [31] compared manipulation with physiotherapy and treatment by a general practitioner (GP) in a randomized trial of 256 chronic cases that included back and neck pain. Physiotherapy included exercises, massage, heat, electrotherapy, ultrasound, and short-wave diathermy. GP care included medication (analgesics, NSAIDs) and advice about posture, rest, and activity, among other things. Data compiled by these workers indicated that both manipulation and physiotherapy were far more effective than GP treatment, with SMT surpassing physiotherapy. This advantage was sustained at 12-month follow-up.

Another randomized trial by Bronfort et al. [32••] compared the effects of SMT and NSAID treatments, each combined with supervised trunk exercise for 174 patients with chronic LBP (Table 8-3). Both therapeutic regimens were found to produce similar and clinically important improvement over time that was considered superior to the expected natural history of long-standing chronic LBP. The SMT/trunk-strengthening exercise group showed a sustained reduction in medication use at 1-year follow-up. In addition, continuation of exercise during the follow-up year was associated with better outcomes, regardless of experimental group.

PREVENTING ACUTE CASES FROM BECOMING CHRONIC

High priority must be accorded to acute LBP patients to prevent them from becoming chronic because the prognosis is better for acute than for chronic patients. A key factor that leads physicians to minimize this concern, however, is the conventional wisdom that 90% of LBP cases resolve on their own within a short time. Recent findings published in the *British Medical Journal* call for urgent rethinking of the assumption that most LBP patients seen by PCPs attain resolution of their complaints [33••]. Contrary to prevailing assumptions, the research done by Croft

TABLE 8-3. CHRONIC LOW BACK PAIN WITH COMPLICATIONS

Patient	Male, 40 years of age, carpet salesperson and installer
Chief complaint	LBP
Duration	18 years
Intensity	Moderate, gradually worsening
Original cause	Motor vehicle accident
History	In the collision, the patient's van was hit by a truck and spun around, catapulting him onto the pavement. Referred by PCP to chiropractor after 2 weeks of poor response to medication and rest. Pain resolved with several weeks of chiropractic care. Injured at work 1 year later lifting a 75-pound box. Pain again resolved with manual therapy. Periodic LBP episodes during next 16 years. Patient hospitalized for transverse myelitis 1 year before seeking chiropractic treatment at my office. His recovery from transverse myelitis was complete except for residual "half-numbness" in the groin.
Exam findings	Motor and reflex function normal. Decreased sensation at L1 dermatome, with remainder of sensory exam normal. Multiple trigger points throughout lumbar and gluteal regions. Restricted mobility of both sacroiliac joints, L5-S1, and C2-3.
Diagnosis	Chronic lumbosacral strain with sacroiliac, lumbar, and cervical subluxations.
Treatment	Spinal adjustments of the affected areas, starting at three per week for 3 weeks, gradually decreasing frequency over next few months.
Response	Gradual decrease in pain. After 3 months, patient seen once per month for next year. After that, seen on as-needed basis, averaging twice per year. After several months, all sensation returned to patient's groin area.
Comments	This case indicates the usefulness of spinal manipulation in a complicated chronic case of LBP. Both the low back pain and the groin numbness resolved. At 6-year follow-up, patient has occasional brief episodes of LBP, generally requiring one chiropractic session per episode.

et al. [33••] found that at 3- and 12-month follow-ups, only 21% and 25% percent of patients, respectively, had completely recovered in terms of pain and disability. However, only 8% of patients continued to consult their physicians for longer than 3 months. In other words, most patients continued to have LBP but stopped seeing their physicians about it. Their dissatisfaction with PCP care was also reminiscent of conclusions given in earlier works by Cherkin *et al.* [7,8].

Croft *et al.* [33••] concluded that LBP should be viewed as a chronic problem with a "pattern of grumbling symptoms" and pain- and disability-free periods with recurring acute episodes. This is based on two observations about LBP that appear consistently in research: 1) a history of LBP is the "strongest risk factor for a new episode," and 2) nearly half the population will experience LBP by age 30. This data contradicts claims that complete recovery occurs in 90% of patients with LBP.

The patients in Croft's study [33••] were not referred for manual manipulation and most became chronic. Based on the AHCPR guidelines [1], which emphasize the functionally restorative qualities of SMT, early chiropractic adjustments could possibly have prevented this progression in many cases. Recall that follow-up in both the Meade (1- and 3-year) [23,24••] studies and the Kirkaldy-Willis and Cassidy (1-year) [29] study showed that the beneficial effect of manipulation was sustained for extended time periods. The decision not to refer patients to chiropractors appears to mean that many LBP patients will develop long-term problems that could have been avoided.

LOW BACK PAIN WITH LEG PAIN

For patients with LBP who have pain radiating into the leg (Table 8-4), differential diagnosis is crucial. Specifically, motor, sensory, and reflex testing should be used to screen for signs of radicular syndromes and cauda equina syndrome. A recent British study of PCPs, however, found that most of these physicians do not examine routinely for muscle weakness or sensation, and 27% do not regularly check reflexes [34]. Such factors play a central role in determining which cases should be referred directly for surgical consultation and which should be referred for chiropractic.

According to AHCPR guidelines [1], manipulation is appropriate for acute LBP cases that include pain radiating into the lower extremity. Even in cases in which radicular signs, such as muscle weakness or decreased reflex response, are present, preliminary evidence [35,36•] suggests that chiropractic can yield beneficial results. In a series of 424 consecutive cases, Cox and Feller [35] report that 83% of 331 lumbar disk syndrome patients completing care (13% of whom had previous low back surgeries) had good to excellent results. (Excellent was defined as more than 90% relief of pain and return to work with no further care required. Good was defined as 75% relief of pain and return to work with periodic manipulation or analgesia required). A median of 11 treatments and 27 days to attain maximal improvement was determined.

Ben Eliyahu [36•] observed 27 patients receiving chiropractic care for cervical-disk and lumbar-disk herniations, the majority being lumbar cases. Pre- and post-treatment magnetic resonance imaging (MRI) scans were performed. Of the 27 patients, 80% had a good clinical outcome and 63% of the posttreatment MRIs showed herniations either reduced in size or completely resorbed (Tables 8-5 and 8-6).

Cassidy *et al.* [37] reported that, of 14 patients with lumbar-disk herniation, all but one obtained significant clinical improvement and relief of pain after a 2- to 3-week regimen of daily side posture manipulation of the lumbar spine directed toward improving spinal mobility. All patients were scanned using computed tomography (CT) before and 3 months after treatment. In most cases, the appearance of the disk herniation on CT scan remained unchanged after successful treatment, whereas in five cases a small decrease was noted in the size of the herniation. In one case a large decrease was noted.

OTHER CONSIDERATIONS WHEN REFERRING PATIENTS TO CHIROPRACTORS
Safety

Although no health-care intervention is wholly without side effects, SMT for the low back is an extremely safe procedure by any standard. Cauda equina syndrome is usually considered the most serious possible adverse response to lumbar manipu-

TABLE 8-4. LOW BACK PAIN WITH SEVERE LEG NUMBNESS

Patient	Male, 25 years of age, police officer
Chief complaint	Acute LBP, numbness radiating down left leg to ankle
Duration	1 day
Intensity	Severe and unremitting
Original cause	Weight-lifting
History	Acute LBP after lifting heavier than usual weight from squatting position
Exam findings	Straight leg raising positive on left at 30°. Positive Braggard's on left. Numbness to pinprick throughout lateral aspect of lower left leg. No muscle strength on left great toe extension.
Diagnosis	Prolapsed L5-S1 disk
Treatment	Immediate referral to neurosurgeon, who performed surgery later that day.
Response	Successful surgery, uneventful recovery.
Comments	Example of prompt referral on a case for which chiropractic care was inappropriate.

lation. In a detailed literature review of manipulation for LBP, Shekelle *et al.* [13] estimated the occurrence of cauda equina syndrome from SMT to be less than one case per 100 million manipulations. Terrett and Kleynhans [38] analyzed other disk-related complications from low-back SMT and found only 65 cases reported in the literature between 1911 and 1991. Of these, almost half were from manipulation under anesthesia, a relatively rare procedure.

Concern has sometimes been expressed that chiropractors may endanger patients by missing important diagnostic signs. Chiropractic colleges and regulatory boards are acutely aware of the importance of proper diagnosis and maintain high standards. A study by Taylor *et al.* [39•] helps put this matter into perspective. They compared the interpretations made by students, clinicians, radiology residents, and radiologists from both chiropractic and medicine of abnormal lumbar spine radiographs. Not surprisingly, radiologists and radiology residents from both professions scored highest. No significant difference was found between chiropractic and medical radiologists or between chiropractic and medical clinicians.

Cost Effectiveness

Although the potential health benefit for the patient should always be the primary consideration when considering referral to a chiropractor, cost is also a factor. A widely quoted North Carolina study [9] found that, among doctors treating LBP cases, PCPs were the least expensive and orthopedic surgeons were the most expensive. The cost of chiropractic care in the study was closer to that of the orthopedists. However, this study stands virtually alone among numerous others that have found chiropractic to be the most cost-effective treatment for LBP [40–47]. Manga's comprehensive report [47] on LBP, commissioned by the provincial government of Ontario, concluded that chiropractic was the most effective and cost-

TABLE 8-5. LOW BACK PAIN IN PATIENT WITH PAST SURGERY

Patient	Female, 52 years of age, secretary
Chief complaint	Left-sided LBP radiating into gluteal area
Duration	6 years, with significant worsening of pain in previous 6 weeks
Intensity	Variable. Occasionally severe after major exertion or standing for more than an hour
Original Cause	Unknown
History	L5 laminectomy 4 years earlier.
Exam Findings	Motor, sensory, and reflex function normal. Lumbar musculature tight bilaterally but not in spasm. Tenderness on palpation of left posterior superior iliac spine and left gluteus medius muscle. Markedly restricted mobility of left sacroiliac joint.
Diagnosis	Sacroiliac subluxation
Treatment	Spinal adjustments three per week for 2 weeks, then two per week for 3 weeks, then one per week for 3 weeks.
Response	Significant improvement in sacroiliac mobility; 95% decrease in pain. Improvement sustained on follow-up at 6 and 12 months.
Comments	Chiropractic care can be helpful for some patients with a history of low back surgery.

TABLE 8-6. LOW BACK PAIN RADIATING INTO LEG

Patient	Female, 39 years of age, registered nurse
Chief complaint	LBP. Pain and numbness radiating into left gluteals, hip, and posterior and lateral thigh.
Duration	3 months
Intensity	Moderate to severe, worsening in preceding 2 weeks
Original cause	Unknown
History	Several previous episodes of LBP in past several years, occasionally including sciatica-like symptoms. Seen at emergency room 2 months before presenting at chiropractic office. Flexeril and Darvocet prescribed, along with 5 days off work. Symptoms remitted, but later returned with greater intensity.
Exam findings	Exquisite tenderness on palpation of L4-5 area. Straight leg raising elicits LBP, but only at 70° to 75°. Motor, sensory, and reflex function within normal limits. Substantial restriction of left sacroiliac joint mobility.
Diagnosis	Sacroiliac syndrome (SI motion dysfunction with sciatica-like leg symptoms)
Treatment	Seven spinal adjustments over 3-week period. Ultrasound applied to lumbar paraspinal muscles for muscular relaxation and pain relief. Stretching exercises for sacroiliac/hip/low back prescribed.
Response	After first treatment, patient reported that all numbness was gone, and that she had slept through the night for the first time in 2 weeks. Pain gradually decreased over following 3 weeks. Follow-up at 6 months indicated no recurrence.

effective method of treatment. Stano [48], using an elegant set of calculations on a massive insurance database of over 400,000 patients from which a randomized sample of over 6000 was analyzed in depth, concluded that when all episodes of care are considered, the mean total costs are $1000 for each medical episode and $493 for each chiropractic episode.

The main message here for the PCP considering referral to a chiropractor is that, in general, studies show chiropractic to be either very cost effective or moderately cost effective. Questions of cost should not deter PCPs from making such referrals.

Choosing the Individual Chiropractor

For PCPs, distinguishing among chiropractic practitioners is a necessary part of the referral process. As would be the case with referral to a medical specialist, the key is to find the right blend of professional competence and interpersonal rapport. Curtis and Bove [49], a family physician and a chiropractor, respectively, listed the following guidelines for identifying a competent chiropractor:

- Treats mainly musculoskeletal disorders with manual manipulative techniques
- Does not perform routine radiographs on every patient
- Does not extend duration of treatment unnecessarily
- Writes a response to a referral and outlines evaluation and therapy
- Does not charge "front end" lump sum for whole treatment program
- Is willing to have the physician visit the office to observe treatment
- Provides good feedback from patients on care

I would add that it is important to refer to a chiropractor who is able to clearly distinguish among the proven, the probable, and the speculative [50]. Some of the most pointed criticism of chiropractic has been in reaction to the tendency of some chiropractors to "globalize" [51], making broad claims on the basis of limited evidence. All health-care professions use unproven methods (only 15% to 20% of conventional medicine's methods are proven by rigorous research) [52,53] but it is never acceptable to make inaccurate claims about these methods and techniques.

As research on SMT develops further and the chiropractic profession continues its path toward higher academic and practice standards, many current controversies will likely come to be seen as historical anomalies. By referring LBP patients for chiropractic care, present-day PCPs can serve their patients well and hasten the arrival of truly integrated health care.

References and Recommended Reading

Recently published papers of particular interest are highlighted as:
- Of interest
- •• Of outstanding interest

1. Bigos S, Bowyer O, Braen G, *et al.*: Acute Lower Back Problems in Adults: *Clinical Practice Guideline, Quick Reference Guide Number 14.* Rockville, MD: Agency for Health Care Policy and Research; 1994. US Department of Health and Human Services, Public Health Service, AHCPR Publication no. 95-0643.

2. Shekelle PG, Adams AH, Chassin MR, *et al.*: The Appropriateness of Spinal Manipulation for Low-Back Pain: *Project Overview and Literature Review (R-4025/1-CCR/FCER).* Santa Monica: RAND; 1991.

3. Rosner AL: Musculoskeletal disorders research. *In Contemporary Chiropractic.* Edited by Redwood D. New York: Churchill Livingstone; 1997:163–187.

4. Masarsky C, Weber M: Visceral disorders research. *In Contemporary Chiropractic.* Edited by Redwood D. New York: Churchill Livingstone; 1997:189–204.

5. Shekelle PG, Markovich M, Louie R: Factors associated with choosing a chiropractor for episodes of back pain care. *Med Care* 1995, 33:842–850.

6. Cherkin DC, MacCornack FA, Berg AO: Managing LBP: a comparison of the beliefs and behaviors of family physicians and chiropractors. *West J Med* 1988, 149:475–480.

7. Cherkin DC, MacCornack FA: Patient evaluations of low back care from family physicians and chiropractors. *West J Med* 1989, 150:351–355.

8. Cherkin D, Deyo RA, Berg AO, *et al.*: Evaluation of a physician education intervention to improve primary care for low back pain I: impact on physicians. *Spine* 1991, 16:1168–1172.

9. Carey TS, Garrett J, Jackman A, *et al.*: The outcomes and costs of care for acute low back pain among patients seen by primary care practitioners, chiropractors, and orthopedic surgeons. *N Engl J Med* 1995, 333:913–917.

10. Coulehan JL: Chiropractic and the clinical art. *Soc Sci Med* 1985, 21:383–390.

11. Mootz RD, Coulter ID, Hansen DT: Health services research related to chiropractic: review and recommendations for research prioritization by the chiropractic profession. *J Manipulative Physiol Ther* 1997, 20:201–217.

12. Cherkin DC, Mootz RD: *Chiropractic in the United States: Training, Practice, and Research.* Rockville, MD: Agency for Health Care Policy and Research; 1997. US Department of Health and Human Services, Public Health Service, AHCPR Publication no. 98-N002.

13. Shekelle PG, Adams AH, Chassin MR, *et al.*: Spinal manipulation for low-back pain. *Ann Intern Med* 1992, 117:590–598.

14. Anderson R, Meeker W, Wirick BE, *et al.*: Meta-analysis of randomized clinical trials on manipulation for low-back pain. *J Manipulative Physiol Ther* 1992, 15:181–194.

15. Cherkin DC, Deyo RA, Wheeler K, Ciol MA: Physician views about treating low back pain. *Spine* 1995, 20:1–10.

16. Redwood D: Chiropractic. In: *Fundamentals of Complementary and Alternative Medicine.* Edited by Micozzi M. New York: Churchill Livingstone; 1996:91–110.

17. Vear H: Education and accreditation: a century of progress. In *Contemporary Chiropractic.* Edited by Redwood D. New York: Churchill Livingstone; 1997:15–27.

18. Cleveland CS III: Vertebral subluxation. In *Contemporary Chiropractic.* Edited by Redwood D. New York: Churchill Livingstone; 1997:29–44.

19. Haldeman S, Chapman-Smith D, Peterson DM: *Guidelines for Chiropractic Quality Assurance and Practice Parameters: Proceedings of the Mercy Center Consensus Conference.* Gaithersburg, MD: Aspen Publications; 1993.

20. Leach RA: *The Chiropractic Theories: Principles and Clinical Applications* edn 3. Baltimore: Williams and Wilkins; 1994.

21. Halar EM, Bell KR: Contracture and other deleterious effects of immobility. In *Rehabilitation Medicine: Principles and Practice.* Edited by DeLisa JA. Philadelphia: JB Lippincott; 1993:681–699.

22. Royal College of General Practitioners: *Clinical Guidelines for Management of Acute Low Back Pain.* London: Royal College of General Practitioners; 1997.

23. Meade TW, Dyer S, Browne W, et al.: Low back pain of mechanical origin: randomized comparison of chiropractic and hospital outpatient treatment. *Br Med J* 1990, 300:1431–1437.

24.•• Meade TW, Dyer S, Browne W, et al.: Randomised comparison of chiropractic and hospital outpatient management for low back pain: results from extended follow-up. *Br Med J* 1995, 311:349–350.

This article revisits Meade's landmark 1990 study [23] on LBP. With its large (700+) cohort and long-term follow-up, this study offers strong support for both short- and long-term benefits of chiropractic care for LBP. This was the first major randomized trial directly comparing chiropractic manipulation with conventional medical care for LBP, and it found chiropractic care to be the superior modality.

25. Meade TW: Interview on Canadian Broadcasting Corporation (CBC). Reprinted in *Chiropractic: A Review of Current Research. Foundation for Chiropractic and Research*. Arlington, VA: Foundation for Chiropractic Education and Research; 1992:2.

26. van Tulder MW, Koes BW, Bouter LM: Conservative treatment of acute and chronic nonspecific low back pain: a systematic review of randomized controlled trials of the most common interventions. *Spine* 1997, 22:2128–2156.

27.•• Shekelle PG, Coulter I, Hurwitz EL: Congruence between decisions to initiate chiropractic spinal manipulation for low back pain and appropriateness criteria in North America. *Ann Intern Med* 1998, 129:9–17.

Shekelle's study is noteworthy for subjecting chiropractors' decision-making to rigorous analysis. Despite rating manipulation as inappropriate for all cases of chronic back pain (based on an early 1990s RAND literature review), the study nonetheless concludes that the decision to commence manipulative therapy was appropriate in 46% of cases, uncertain in 25%, and inappropriate in 29%. Noting that these findings are comparable to those for various medical procedures, the authors urge primary care physicians to refer more LBP cases to chiropractors.

28. Micozzi MS: Complementary care: when is it appropriate? Who will provide it? *Ann Intern Med* 1998, 129:65–66.

29. Kirkaldy-Willis W, Cassidy J: Spinal manipulation in the treatment of low back pain. *Can Fam Physicians* 1985, 31:535–540.

30.•• Triano JJ, McGregor M, Hondras MA, Brennan PC: Manipulative therapy versus education programs in chronic low back pain. *Spine* 1995, 20:948–955.

This randomized trial found chiropractic manipulation to be effective for chronic LBP. Pain and activity tolerance improved in the SMT group. Of particular note is the fact that relief continued to accrue after the course of manipulative therapy had been completed.

31. Koes BW, Bouter LM, van Mameren H, et al.: Randomised clinical trial of manipulative therapy and physiotherapy for persistent back and neck complaints: results of one year follow-up. *Br Med J* 1992, 304:601–605.

32.•• Bronfort G, Goldsmith CH, Nelson CF et al.: Trunk exercise combined with spinal manipulative or NSAID therapy for chronic low back pain: a randomized, observer-blinded clinical trial. *J Manipulative Physiol Ther* 1996,19:570–582.

Another of the growing number of post-1994 randomized trials demonstrating effectiveness of chiropractic for chronic LBP. SMT and NSAID treatments were compared, each combined with supervised trunk exercise. Both produced similar improvement beyond the expected natural history of longstanding chronic LBP. The SMT/trunk-strengthening exercise group showed a sustained reduction in medication use at 1-year follow-up.

33.•• Croft PR, Macfarlane GJ, Papageorgiou AC, et al.: Outcome of low back pain in general practice: a prospective study. *Br Med J* 1998, 316:1356–1359.

Testing the conventional wisdom that 90% of LBP cases seen by physicians resolve in a few weeks with or without treatment, this study found that only one fourth of patients were free of pain and disability after 12 months. The 90% figure, they discovered, referred to the percentage of patients that stopped seeing their physicians about their pain.

34. Little P, Smith L, Cantrell T, et al.: General practitioners' management of acute back pain: a survey of reported practice compared with clinical guidelines. *Br Med J* 1996, 312:485–488.

35. Cox JM, Feller JA: Chiropractic treatment of low back pain: a multicenter descriptive analysis of presentation and outcome in 424 consecutive cases. *J Neuromuscoloskel Sys* 1994, 2:178–190.

36.• Ben Eliyahu DJ: Magnetic resonance imaging and clinical follow-up: study of 27 patients receiving chiropractic care for cervical and lumbar disc herniations. *J Manipulative Physiol Ther* 1996, 19:597–606.

In this small, yet intriguing study, BenEliyahu compared pre- and post-treatment MRI scans of lumbar and cervical disk cases undergoing chiropractic treatment. Of the post-treatment MRI scans, 63% showed herniations either reduced in size or completely resorbed and 80% of patients had a positive clinical response. This is significant as a preliminary exploration of the role of manipulation for disk syndromes.

37. Cassidy JD, Thiel HW, Kirkaldy-Willis WH: Side posture manipulation for lumbar disc herniation. *J Manipulative Physiol Ther* 1993, 16:96–103.

38. Terrett AGJ, Kleynhans AM: Complications from manipulation of the low back. *Chiropr J Aust* 1992, 22:129–140.

39.• Taylor JAM, Clopton P, Bosch E, et al.: Interpretation of abnormal lumbosacral radiographs: a test comparing students, clinicians, radiology residents, and radiologists in medicine and chiropractic. *Spine* 1995, 20:1147–1154.

In this comparison of chiropractic and medical students, clinicians, radiology residents, and radiologists, no significant differences were found between chiropractic and medical radiologists or between chiropractic and medical clinicians or students. This study should allay fears that chiropractors are more likely than medical physicians to miss key diagnoses and thus delay needed care.

40. Jarvis KB, Phillips RB, Morris EK: Cost per case comparison of back injury claims of chiropractic versus medical management for conditions with identical diagnostic codes. *J Occup Med* 1991, 33:847–852.

41. Nyiendo J, Lamm L: Disability low back Oregon workers' compensation of claims. Part I: methodology and clinical categorization of chiropractic and medical cases. *J Manipulative Physiol Ther* 1991, 14:177–184.

42. Nyiendo J: Disability low back Oregon workers' compensation of claims. Part II: time loss. *J Manipulative Physiol Ther* 1991, 14:231–239.

43. Nyiendo J: Disability low back Oregon workers' compensation of claims. Part III: diagnostic and treatment procedures and associated costs. *J Manipulative Physiol Ther* 1991, 14:287–297.

44. Johnson MR: A comparison of chiropractic, medical and osteopathic care for work-related sprains/strains. *J Manipulative Physiol Ther* 1989,12:335–344.

45. Bergmann BW, Cichoke AJ: Cost-effectiveness of chiropractic treatment of low-back injuries. *J Manipulative Physiol Ther* 1980, 3:143–147.

46. Duffey DJ: *A Study of Wisconsin Industrial Back Injury Cases*. Madison, WI: University of Wisconsin Market Research; 1978.

47. Manga P, Angur D, Papadopoulos C, Swan W: *The Effectiveness and Cost-Effectiveness of Chiropractic Management of Low-Back Pain*. Richmond Hill, ON: Kenilworth; 1993.

48. Stano M: The economic role of chiropractic: further analysis of relative insurance costs for low back care. *J Neuromusculoskel Sys* 1995, 3:139–144.

49. Curtis P, Bove G: Family physicians, chiropractors, and back pain. *J Fam Pract* 1992, 35:551–555.

50. Redwood D: Pathways for an evolving profession. In *Contemporary Chiropractic*. Edited by Redwood D. New York: Churchill Livingstone; 1997.

51. Gellert G: Global explanations and the credibility problem of alternative medicine. *Adv J Mind Body Med* 1994,10:60–67.

52. Office of Technology Assessment: *Assessing the Efficacy and Safety of Medical Technologies*. Washington DC: US Government Printing Office; 1978.

53. Smith R: Where is the wisdom . . . ? the poverty of medical evidence. *Br Med J* 1991, 303:798.

Current Controversies in Therapeutic Touch

Eric Leskowitz

OVERVIEW OF ALTERNATIVE MEDICINE

Alternative medicine (or complementary and alternative medicine [CAM], as it is more commonly called), is a multifaceted field, as evidenced by the wide array of subjects addressed in this book. However, some alternative therapies are more *alternative* than others—some are contained within the standard allopathic medical model, whereas others are so different that they require a new paradigm to include them. The topic of this chapter, *Therapeutic Touch* (TT), is just such an alternative, because it appears to be inexplicable within the standard biomedical model of physiology. TT is a widely used nursing technique in which the nurse/healer uses his or her hands to smooth out a "subtle energy field" that surrounds the patient, thereby calming the patient and facilitating healing. This idea of a human energy field has been at the center of controversy in scientific circles for decades, if not centuries, but is fundamentally incompatible with allopathic or Western medicine.

Before addressing directly the full TT controversy, we must put this technique into context by outlining the spectrum of healing techniques that are included in *alternative medicine* and define the role of TT in CAM.

The key feature of standard Western medicine is its belief that human health and illness can be reduced to aspects of biology and cellular physiology. This biomedical reductionism has led to great triumphs, such as antibiotics, surgery, and magnetic resonance imaging, but is often accused of reducing human beings to complex machines. For this reason, the new field of mind/body medicine (comprehensively called *psycho-neuro-immunology* [PNI]) delves into the mechanisms by which more subjective processes like emotions and thought patterns affect the human body. The stress response of Selye and techniques that elicit a counterbalancing *relaxation response* have been at the forefront of mind/body medicine. New approaches that reverse heart disease [1] and improve cancer survival [2] are striking, but PNI can be explained with reference to the workings of the brain and its connections to the central nervous system and the endocrine system.

However, no direct physiologic explanation is available for truly alternative therapies, such as acupuncture, homeopathy, and energy healing (*ie*, the laying-on of hands). All three of these techniques assert the existence of a subtle, circulating human energy field that is not affected by standard medical interventions (or even detectable by current medical instrumentation). This perspective requires specific new techniques to manipulate and balance the human energy field. Although a full discussion of these *energy medicine* techniques is beyond the scope of this chapter, it seems clear from emerging scientific literature [3] that all three techniques can produce reliable, replicable clinical effects on human and animal systems, effects that cannot simply be ascribed to the placebo effect or the powers of suggestion. Rather, it appears that human beings must be considered multilayered or multidimensional organisms, with health and disease arising from dysfunction or imbalances on any and all levels. These levels are commonly referred to as physical, emotional, mental and spiritual. Allopathic medicine deals only with the first level; mind/body medicine incorporates the first three levels, and the outer fringes of CAM deal with the last level. In other words, alternative medical practices such as herbal medicine or nutritional supplementations are essentially biochemical manipulations of the physical or biologic level, and thus blend well with allopathic medicine. Meditation, hypnosis, biofeedback, expressive psychotherapies, and movement-based therapies such as yoga and Feldenkrais integrate physical structure with emotional and mental levels (*ie*, by noticing what memories or types of emotions are triggered by specific body postures), and the spiritual dimension of subtle energy is addressed most directly by techniques such as acupuncture, homeopathy, prayer, psychic healing and hands-on energy healing.

SUBTLE ENERGY

Western allopathic medicine is the world's only healing tradition that does not invoke the theory of subtle energy. This notion, which underlies TT in the form of the human energy field, is found in every culture and world view except that of the Western European intellectual tradition. The Cartesian emphasis on intellectual rigor set up a mind/body split that prevents Western scientists from examining subjective internal phenomena, such as energy flow, that are the basis of traditional Chinese medicine (*qi*) and Ayurvedic or yoga philosophy (*prana*). Modern medicine looks to biochemistry or molecular genetics to explain the concept of *homeostasis*, which is the closest we come to a balanced energy flow. Still, an undercurrent of interest in subtle energy has always existed in the West. For example, Franz Anton Mesmer was the first Westerner to seek analogues to *qi* or *prana*. Although he did not appear to be aware of these Eastern traditions, he built on the rising tide of interest in electromagnetism, labeling his interactional field "animal magnetism." He was followed by such controversial scientists as Henri Bergson (*élan vital*), Sigmund Freud (libido), Wilhelm Reich (orgone), and modern biomagnetic theorists Harold Saxton Burr and Robert Becker.

The recent development of refined technologies to measure and manipulate electromagnetic fields has, in fact, led to a resurgence of interest in biomagnetism. It now appears that physiologic processes such as limb regeneration, cell division, wound healing, and sleep–wake cycles are regulated by electromagnetic fields [4]. Technologies to manipulate these processes have become accepted (*eg*, the transcutaneous electrical nerve stimulation device to control chronic pain and the external pulsed magnetic field generator to speed up the healing of bone fractures). Measurements of skin surface resistance have shown that acupuncture points of traditional Chinese medicine have different electrical properties than neighboring skin, with their measurably lowered electrical resistance possibly being the electromagnetic correlate of the subtle energy flow described by acupuncturists. Becker's work [4] is highly recommended as a readable summary of this fascinating field.

HISTORY OF THERAPEUTIC TOUCH

The history of TT usually begins with the colorful life of clairvoyant Dora Kunz, who observed that life was an interplay of subtle energies. Her story of the development of her own intuitive gifts is a fascinating one, and her later collaboration with American nurse Delores Krieger to develop the technique now known as TT is noteworthy [5•]. The true origins of TT, however, can be traced to 200 years earlier. The discredited theories of animal magnetism propounded by Mesmer foretold three important aspects of the modern TT phenomenon: the European scientific tradition's development of a "subtle energy" theory; an awareness of the important role interpersonal relationships play in healing interactions; and the never-ending conflict between scientific orthodoxy and paradigm-breaking theories.

Mesmer was greatly influenced by the European intellectual renaissance of the 1700s. Science was beginning to make sense of electromagnetism, and lodestones and batteries were being explored for their therapeutic potential. Mesmer's speculations about "animal magnetism" were in keeping with the intellectual ferment of the times. He attempted to stimulate this interconnecting "fluidium" by using externally applied magnets; by passing on his own healing magnetism through a water-filled tub that large groups of people could access at once; with mirrors; and most famously by direct personal touch. This latter technique is most relevant to this chapter because Mesmer developed a system of passing his hands several inches from the patient's body in long flowing sweeps that clearly resemble modern TT (*see* Ellenberger [6] for more details).

Historical accounts of Mesmer's actual clinical practice describe the importance of his personal charisma and striking interpersonal dynamic of power and adoration as a key element in his healing technique. The attitude in TT practice today is exactly opposite, stressing respect and compassion rather than flamboyance and manipulation. It is significant, however, that Mesmer recognized that his attitude toward his patients and their attitudes toward him were vital to healing. He thus moved beyond the prevailing view of humans as machines and considered the importance of interpersonal interaction. Similarly, TT requires the cultivation of a particular form of interpersonal connection as a foundational element of treatment.

Mesmer's success in attracting wealthy Parisians to his healing demonstrations incurred the jealousy of the medical establishment. A committee was appointed by King Louis XVI to investigate his work, and the leading scientists of the day were included (Lavoisier, who discovered oxygen; Franklin, the US ambassador; and the surgeon Guillotine). Their report, released in 1784, acknowledged significant clinical improvements in Mesmer's patients as a result of his unorthodox treatments, but ascribed these changes to the power of suggestion. They found no evidence for the existence of his magnetic powers. Mesmer left Paris in disgrace and was never able to regain his prominence. However, a follow-up commission 40 years later fully vindicated Mesmer's theories, which is not usually mentioned in historical accounts. The first commission's tests did not actually involve Mesmer himself, who never had the opportunity to meet with any of the committee members. Rather, one of his students (with whom he had recently split) was the designated healer for the study. How might this evident bias have affected the findings of the commission? Biased experimental conditions skew outcomes as much today as they did 200 years ago.

A recently published study [7••] reported negative findings about TT and the human energy field, although leading TT practitioners were neither consulted nor observed in action. These negative findings were given the support of the medical establishment, despite available contradictory findings. An accompanying editorial made reference to a profit motive that supposedly drove TT practitioners to build up their "international business"; this echoes the French Renaissance concern that the economic position of the medical society was being challenged by Mesmer.

Thus, in the use of subtle energy concepts, the focus on the healer/patient relationship, and the attendant political controversies surrounding its practice, Mesmerism presaged TT.

THE TECHNIQUE OF THERAPEUTIC TOUCH

Therapeutic touch was developed by Dora Kunz after observing the work of several naturally gifted energy healers. In conjunction with Delores Krieger at the New York University School of Nursing, she adapted energy healing procedures into a standardized process that has been taught to tens of thousands of nurses in America and abroad since its introduction in 1969. Nearly 100 schools of nursing offer TT training in their curriculum.

The basic technique of therapeutic touch is deceptively simple. There are three phases to the standard TT process: centering, assessment, and active treatment [8•]. Several superficially similar holistic therapies include some but not all of these elements and thus cannot rightfully be considered to be TT, including healing touch, touch for health, laying-on of hands techniques like Reiki or psychic healing, and external *qi gong*. Similarly, attempts to scientifically assess the efficacy of TT must include all three elements in the treatment protocol to ensure validity.

Centering is the process by which the TT practitioner refocuses attention to an inner state of calm balance, independent of the vagaries of the external environment. This is done by developing an attitude of compassionate intent to be of service to the patient, independent of personal wishes or ideas of what might be best for the patient. This state may be facilitated by a brief internal meditation or simply by taking some deep, relaxing breaths. Experienced practitioners can attain this state within a matter of seconds, whereas novices may need to spend several minutes cultivating this quiet frame of mind.

In the assessment phase, the nurse practitioner uses his or her own hands as sensing or measuring devices to gauge the nature of the patient's energy field dynamics. The practitioner's hands are placed several inches from the patient's body, palms facing the patient, and moved over the surface of the patient's body, attending to fairly subtle sensory cues. Feelings range from warmth and tingling to numbness and heaviness, and are noted as part of an inventory of the patient's energy field. Areas of imbalance or impeded energy flow are presumed to be reflections of underlying symptoms, and are returned to during the subsequent treatment phase. Assessments may take only a few minutes to complete.

Active treatment involves repatterning areas of imbalanced or distorted energy flow, using the hands as instruments of rebalancing. A series of slow, gentle, downward strokes on both sides of the patient are used to "unruffle" and smooth out the energy field. Focus is then placed on localized areas of abnormal sensation in an attempt to bring them into balance, whether from the right to the left side or with increased circulation into the affected area. Direct physical contact occasionally is used, but the nurse's hands typically stay 3 to 6 inches away from the fully-clothed body of the patient. Treatments generally last about 10 minutes, and the practitioner usually stops when a change is perceived in the field characteristics initially detected during the assessment phase.

RELEVANT RESEARCH

The list of conditions in which TT has been used is staggering, but the research literature on TT is characterized by varying claims about its efficacy and by studies of widely varying methodologic rigor. Several good literature reviews are now available [8•,9•], and more than 100 studies have appeared in the literature, largely in nursing journals and published doctoral theses. Many of these reports are statistically uncontrolled, anecdotal studies that offer provocative hints about potential efficacy in situations such as stimulating growth in premature neonates, enhancing immune function in AIDS patients, minimizing anxiety, and treating symptoms like pain and insomnia. The number of tightly controlled studies of TT is surprisingly limited.

Double-blind clinical studies are considered the standard criterion of clinical research, and treatments that have not proved efficacious when using this methodology can never hope to gain acceptance in the medical community. However, one aspect of TT cannot be controlled in double-blind protocol—the intent of the healer. It is not difficult to devise a sham TT procedure that can mimic true TT; nurses who are untutored in TT can be shown how to move their hands in a pattern that looks to the observer like true TT but does not encompass either healing intent or energetic sensitivity. This "false" TT has been used experimentally with some success; patients can reliably sense the difference between mimic TT and real TT [10]. In the standard double-blind approach, however, the person administering the treatment should not know whether he or she is providing the active or placebo therapy. However, in TT the intent of the practitioner cannot be separated from the energetic aspects of the treatment, making TT inappropriate for the double-blind protocol. This research dilemma is shared by other CAM interventions and has been addressed in some detail by Dossey [11] and Schlitz and Braud [12•].

These warnings notwithstanding, one study by Turner *et al.* [13] demonstrates partial efficacy for TT as an adjuvant to pain relief when used in conjunction with opiates for acute pain due to burns. Results with several postoperative populations have also not been clear cut [14]. Tension headaches seem to be more amenable to TT [15], as is anxiety resulting from several clinical situations [16]. However, solid studies of physiologic change due to TT are hard to come by. Some attempts to demonstrate alterations in cellular immune function have demonstrated inconsistent results, with increases in some immune parameters and decreases in others [17]. Perhaps the most telling study of TT's physiologic efficacy is the study by Wirth [18], who tested the rate of skin-wound healing under fairly rigorous experimental conditions.

Volunteers in the Wirth [18] study had standardized punch biopsies taken of their forearm skin. These arm wounds were measured daily to monitor the rate of tissue healing. Measurements were taken while the arm was placed through a barrier, allowing photographic measurements to be made (and TT to be administered) outside of the subject's awareness. One group of patients received TT while their wounds were being measured, whereas the control group had no treatments during the measurement process. Hence, no placebo or expectancy differential existed between the two groups. The TT groups healed much more rapidly than the control groups; by day 16, none of the 23 control patients' wounds had healed, whereas 13 of the 23 TT recipients' wounds had healed ($P < 0.001$).

Unfortunately, no other research group has reproduced these findings, and Wirth's own subsequent replications are not directly relevant to this discussion because he modified the original TT approach into an altogether divergent technique. Further, he has not publicly presented his work at scientific meetings and several methodologic questions have thus never been adequately resolved. However, his experimental protocol could be readily adapted by a researcher interested in pursuing this matter further.

CLINICAL APPLICATIONS

The following clinical vignettes describe the use of TT in the pain management program at Spaulding Rehabilitation Hospital, where the clinical focus is on maximizing function by teaching self-management techniques for dealing with chronic, nonmalignant pain. Specific syndromes treated with TT include AIDS neuropathy, phantom limb pain, and general anxiety induced by pain.

Neuropathic Pain

Anne, a woman aged 65 years, suffered inadvertent damage to her femoral nerve during unrelated hip surgery performed 1 year prior to presentation and had experienced persistent burning thigh pain. She benefited indirectly by increasing her level of aerobic conditioning and her awareness of body mechanics. Stress management training helped her feel less anxious, but her pain persisted despite a regimen of tricyclic antidepressants and opiates. A trial of noncontact TT was initiated because she had been unwilling to pursue desensitization physical therapy to her thigh. She would not permit any therapist to touch the affected area because direct contact was simply too painful to tolerate.

She was surprised to find that TT somehow "defused" the discomfort in her thigh, allowing for the first tentative contact by a rehabilitation therapist. As she continued with regular TT sessions, she began to experience significant reductions in the level of her neuropathic pain for the first time; however, these respites lasted only a few hours after each session. She worked further with a psychotherapist to discharge her resentment toward the surgeon who had damaged her nerve. Her TT benefits lasted longer once she was able recognize and discharge her anger. She soon ended treatment, with a significant improvement over baseline, but with residual resentment and pain that she was unable to transform.

Phantom Pain

Joe, who was 73 years of age at presentation, had lost the lower half of his right leg as a result of peripheral vascular disease secondary to diabetes. The surgery had saved his life, but left him with residual phantom pain in his missing leg. In this condition, he experienced intense pain that appeared to come from the absent, or "phantom," limb. No pharmacologic intervention helped, including opiates. He was receptive to TT, but neither of us was prepared for the dramatic results that followed. We could both sense when my hand came into contact with his phantom limb in space. As I began to stroke the phantom limb with downward TT passes, he felt immediately that the pain in his knee was flowing down and out through his missing foot. Within moments, he was without pain for the first time in years. He remained comfortable until the night before his next appointment, when he had a pain flare-up. Another TT session relieved the pain, and he described how stressful situations (including worrying about whether he would arrive on time to scheduled meetings) typically worsened his pain. He was taught a simple relaxation technique to practice between TT sessions and thus gradually learned to prevent flare-ups of his phantom pain.

A RECENT CONTROVERSY

The most controversial situation involving TT was generated by the previously mentioned article published in the *Journal of the American Medical Association* (*JAMA*)[7]. Entitled "A Close Look at Therapeutic Touch," the article at first appeared to debunk the therapeutic claims of TT, using statistics, diagrams, and an editorial note from George Lindberg, Senior Editor of *JAMA*. He claimed that "such a (human energy) field does not exist," and that patients should "refuse to pay for this procedure until or unless additional honest experimentation demonstrates an actual effect." Major media outlets were swept up in this story as the medical news event of the week. Closer examination of the study, however, reveals as much about the true nature of TT as it does about medical politics in the United States as it approaches the millennium. The composition of the research team, a critical analysis of the study's statistics and conclusions, and the political aspects of the article's extensive coverage in the general media are issues of note. The reader is urged to keep Mesmer's experiences in mind.

The Research Team

The paper itself is a rewritten version of an elementary school science fair project. No physicians were directly involved in the design or implementation of the study, and the professional affiliations of the authors include membership in organizations such as Quackwatch, Inc. and National Council Against Health Fraud. These are well-known advocacy groups that do not conduct independent research but use media access to regularly debunk holistic medicine and the National Institutes of Health's Office of Alternative Medicine, among others. Two of the paper's coauthors are the parents of the student, Emily Rosa, and the only physician involved rewrote the science fair project in medical jargon after the fact. Because Emily Rosa, the principal investigator, was only 11 years of age when she did this work, she quickly became the subject of media attention, not only as the youngest person ever to have a paper published in *JAMA*, but also as the administrator of an apparently devastating final blow to the theory of the human energy field and the entire field of energy medicine itself.

The Study's Conclusions

What did the study actually demonstrate? The experimental protocol is actually quite elegant in its simplicity. The goal was to assess whether practitioners of TT could actually detect an energy field surrounding human subjects, an indirect test of the assessment phase of TT. The nurse subjects were effectively blindfolded, sitting behind a cardboard barrier that shielded them from Rosa and allowed only their hands to project forth through holes in the barrier. The nurses' upturned hands rested on the table top, outside of their view, and directly in front of Rosa, who would then hold her own hand 1 ft away from either the right or left hand of the nurse (whichever hand had been randomly chosen). The nurse would try to detect which of her hands was being approached by the hand of the experimenter. The logic was that if energy fields existed, the nurses would be able to sense the energy field of Rosa's hand, and correctly guess which of their own hands was being approached. However, the results seemed to show that the nurses fared no better than chance in guessing where the experimenter's hand was being placed.

What does this finding mean? The study claimed to prove that "the human energy field does not exist," but in fact it demonstrated only that this particular protocol did not detect the energy field. One wonders what would have happened if top TT practitioners had been used as subjects (rather than recruits from newspaper advertisements—nurses of widely varying TT experience) and if Rosa had been impartial (assuming, perhaps unfairly, that the child shared her parents' biases against TT). If the experimenter had instead been a master energy healer or a martial arts expert—someone who has or claims to have the ability to manipulate the human energy field—the chances of the project's protocol having detected the presence of such a field would have been greatly magnified. An earlier study that was not referenced in the article, in fact, found that volunteers could reliably detect the hands of unbiased experimenters at an accuracy rate of over 65% [19].

The volunteers in the Rosa study were incorrect more often (56%) than the 50% chance level to which truly random guessing would lead. This data suggests that Rosa's own skeptical attitude may have unconsciously created negative results. Experimenter intentionality [12•] was not controlled for in the study, and skepticism may have unconsciously influenced Rosa's own energy field to minimize, rather than maximize, the experimental findings. In other words, these apparently negative results may actually demonstrate that human energy fields do exist but were simply manipulated in the "wrong" direction in this study. It was logically inconsistent for the authors of the article and the *JAMA* editor to state that TT is clinically useless because TT's clinical effects were not tested in the study. Opposing studies have been presented in greater detail elsewhere [20,21].

Conclusions

TT is a controversial healing technique with deep roots. It is an energy-based view of health and disease that is common in many cultures but seemingly alien to the Western medical model. When viewed through the lens of modern biomagnetism, a plausible case for TT's mechanism of action can be made. Relevant research suggests powerful therapeutic effects, but this research is not yet of iron-clad quality. A recent attempt in *JAMA* to debunk TT has been shown to be logically inconsistent and of no scientific merit. Several case examples from the field of pain management have shown how TT potentially may be used in the clinical setting, and further research will undoubtedly answer some of the remaining questions about this intriguing therapeutic modality.

References and Recommended Reading

Recently published papers of particular interest have been highlighted as:
• Of interest
•• Of outstanding interest

1. Ornish D: Can lifestyle changes reverse coronary heart disease? *Lancet* 1990, 336:129–133.
2. Spiegel D: Effect of psychosocial treatment on survival of patients with metastatic breast cancer. *Lancet* 1989, 2:888–891.
3. Benor D: *Healing Research*. Munich: Helix Press; 1997.
4. Becker R: *Cross Currents: The Promise of Electromedicine, the Perils of Electropollution*. Los Angeles: J Tarcher; 1990.
5.• Wager S: *A Doctor's Guide to Therapeutic Touch*. New York: Perigee Books; 1996.

An easy-to-read overview of TT, including its history and development, clinical applications, and a review of research.

6. Ellenberger H: *The Discovery of the Unconscious*. New York: Basic Books; 1970.
7.•• Rosa E, Sarner L, Barrett S: A close look at therapeutic touch. *JAMA* 1998, 279:1005–1010.

This article triggered the current controversy over TT. The reader can readily judge the objectivity of the study and of the accompanying editorial comments.

8.• Meehan T: Therapeutic touch as a nursing intervention. *J Adv Nurs* 1998, 28:117–125.

An even-handed critical review of TT studies highlighting the methodological problems encountered by TT researchers.

9.• Mulloney S, Wells-Federman C: Therapeutic touch: a healing modality. *Cardiovasc Nurs* 1996, 10:27–49.

Another excellent review of the clinical and research aspects of TT.

10. Kreiger D: Therapeutic touch: the imprimatur of nursing. *Am J Nurs* 1985, 75:784–787.
11. Dossey L: The return of prayer [editorial]. *Alt Ther* 1997, 3:10–17.
12.• Schlitz M, Braud W: Distant intentionality and healing: assessing the evidence. *Altern Ther* 1997, 3:62–73.

An important and subtle topic often overlooked by mainstream medicine in its insistence on the double-blind protocol as the standard criterion of research.

13. Turner J, Clark A, Gauthier D, Williams M: The effect of therapeutic touch on pain and anxiety in burn patients. *J Adv Nurs* 1998, 28:10–20.
14. Heidt P: Effect of therapeutic touch on anxiety level of hospitalized patients. *Nurs Res* 1981, 30:33–37.
15. Keller E, Bzdek V: Effects of therapeutic touch on tension headache pain. *Nurs Res* 1986, 35:101–106.
16. Quinn J: Therapeutic touch as energy exchange: testing the hypothesis. *Adv Nurs Sci* 1984, 6:42–49.
17. Olson M, Sneed N, LaVia M, *et al.*: Stress-induced immunosuppression and therapeutic touch. *Altern Ther* 1997, 3:68–74, 1997.
18. Wirth D: The effect of noncontact therapeutic touch on the rate of healing of full thickness dermal wounds. *Subtle Energies* 1990, 1:1–21.
19. Schwartz G, Russek L, Beltrani J: Interpersonal hand-energy registration: evidence for implicit performance and perception. *Subtle Energies*. 1995, 6:183–200.
20. Achterberg J: Clearing the air in the therapeutic touch controversy. *Altern Ther* 1998, 4:100–101.
21. Leskowitz E: Un-debunking therapeutic touch. *Altern Ther* 1998, 4:101–102.

Chelation Therapy: Cardiovascular Cure or Heavy Metal Hype?

Steven C. Halbert

The primary U.S. Food and Drug Administration (FDA)-approved use for chelation therapy with EDTA is the treatment of lead intoxication. Nevertheless, for over three decades, chelation therapy has been widely used by practitioners of alternative medicine as a treatment for atherosclerotic disease and other degenerative conditions [1]. It is estimated that over 500,000 patients undergo chelation therapy annually for unapproved conditions. Thus, more patients are treated with EDTA chelation for atherosclerosis each year than those who undergo coronary artery bypass grafting.

What factors have combined to create such an interest and demand for an "off-label" use of EDTA chelation therapy that remains rejected by the conventional medical community? The literature supporting off-label use of EDTA consists largely of patient testimonials, case reports, and uncontrolled retrospective clinical trials. Although most publications report favorably on the use of EDTA for atherosclerotic vascular disease, critics are quick to point out the poor scientific quality and lack of peer review of these reports. Advocates and critics of chelation therapy hold strong and biased opinions based on limited scientific data. Viewed as an "alternative" therapy, the perhaps reflexive tendency of mainstream medicine is to equate this treatment with quackery.

This review puts chelation therapy into perspective for the primary care clinician in a manner that enables the physician to inform patients as to the value of chelation and how it might integrate with other, more traditional forms of vascular disease management. Topics addressed in this chapter include a brief history of use of EDTA as a chelating agent and therapy for atherosclerotic disease, theoretical mechanisms of action, clinical applications, contraindications, and toxicity.

HISTORY

EDTA is an amino acid first synthesized in 1930 (Figure 10-1). It is currently approved by the FDA for removal of toxic metal cations, such as lead. The term *chelation* derives from the Greek *chele*, which refers to the claws of a crab or a lobster. Chelation is the chemical reaction in which a molecule surrounds and bonds with a metal cation to form a heterocyclic structure (Figure 10-2). The compound resulting from a chelating agent and a metal is described as a metal chelate. Metal chelates are widely represented in biologic systems (*eg,* hemoglobin, chlorophyll, and vitamin B_{12} are metal chelates of iron, magnesium, and cobalt, respectively). EDTA binds with divalent and trivalent metal cations, such as iron, copper, calcium, magnesium, zinc, mercury, aluminum, and lead. These chelates are then excreted in the urine. Calcium EDTA is used for lead toxicity, whereas disodium EDTA is used for treating atherosclerosis.

In 1955, Clarke *et al.* [2] suggested that atherosclerosis could be treated with EDTA. He observed that patients treated for lead toxicity who had concomitant atherosclerosis experienced improvements in their vascular disease. Clarke later reported on the successful use of EDTA in the management of angina pectoris and occlusive vascular disease [3,4]. Kitchell *et al.* [5,6] and Meltzer *et al.* [7] initially

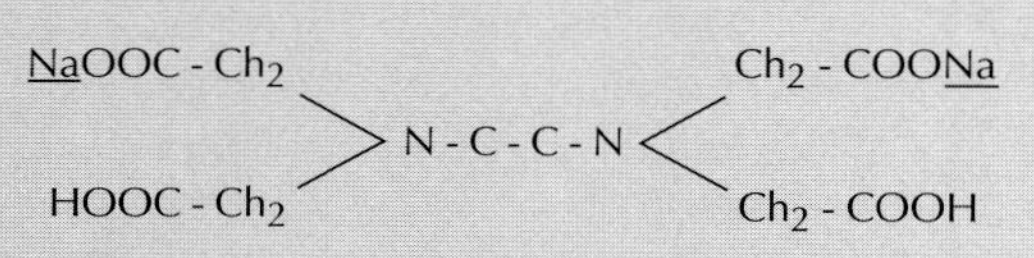

FIGURE 10-1. Disodium EDTA.

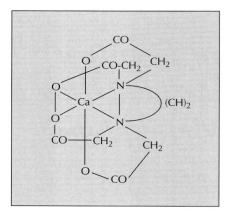

FIGURE 10-2. Calcium ion chelated with EDTA.

confirmed Clarke's work. Later, in 1963, after further investigation, they concluded that chelation therapy was not any more beneficial than traditional therapeutics for coronary artery disease. This small trial of 38 patients, which had no objective endpoints, is currently the only prospective double-blind trial studying chelation therapy for angina pectoris. Academic researchers no longer pursued investigating EDTA chelation therapy for vascular disease after publication of the study.

Subsequent published experiences with EDTA chelation therapy for arteriosclerotic vascular disease, although quite favorable, consist largely of testimonials, case reports, and uncontrolled retrospective clinical series. A large, retrospective analysis of 2870 patients with vascular and other degenerative diseases was reported by Olszewer and Carter [8] that suggested a beneficial effect of chelation therapy. Chappell and Stahl [9] conducted a meta-analysis covering 19 studies and a total of 22,765 patients with vascular disease that were treated with EDTA chelation. This study revealed a measurable improvement in approximately 87% of patients, an analysis that has been criticized for including two large, uncontrolled, retrospective studies, the scale of which dwarfed the other 17 studies in the assessment. It also involved patients with coronary artery disease, peripheral vascular disease, and cerebrovascular disease, which makes the results difficult to interpret for any single condition.

Two prospective trials conducted by vascular surgeons in Denmark and New Zealand have evaluated the use of EDTA in peripheral vascular disease [10–12]. In 1992, the Danish trial randomized 153 patients with stable intermittent claudication to receive either EDTA or placebo [10,11]. The primary endpoints were walking distance (subjective) and ankle/brachial pressures. At 6 months, no intergroup differences were noted. However, the blinding protocol was violated and the Danish Committee on Scientific Dishonesty criticized various aspects of the study [13••]. In 1994, the New Zealand group [12] randomized 32 patients and compared EDTA with placebo in the treatment of stable intermittent claudication. Both EDTA and placebo groups improved. On closer analysis of the placebo group, however, much of the improvement found could be attributed to one patient. Therefore, if this patient were removed from the analysis, EDTA chelation did improve walking distance. This trial also reported on a statistically significant improvement in resting ankle/brachial pressure indices for the EDTA-treated group. Despite the quality of this study, the small population of patients enrolled precludes any definitive assessment as to the value of chelation therapy for peripheral vascular disease.

Currently, large prospective trials using chelation therapy for various manifestations of atherosclerotic vascular disease are sorely needed. Ideally, both short-term and long-term improvement should be evaluated. Unfortunately, the patent on EDTA has expired, which has eliminated financial incentives for pharmaceutical funding. This funding will therefore need to come from government, institutional, and private sources. In the short term, prospective patient outcome studies should help define the direction of future investigations.

MECHANISMS OF ACTION

Several theoretical mechanisms exist by which EDTA chelation can prevent the development and clinical manifestations of atherosclerotic disease. The mechanism most commonly invoked involves the ability of heavy metals to contribute to in vivo oxidation of low density lipoprotein (LDL) cholesterol. Present theories of atherosclerosis cite a key role for oxidized LDLs in the evolution of coronary artery disease from a fatty streak to a fibrous cap overlying a necrotic lipid core with subsequent rupture and thrombosis [14,15]. Metal cations, such as copper and iron, are in vitro catalysts for oxidation of LDL cholesterol and may therefore have a significant impact on the subsequent initiation and progression of atherosclerosis [16]. It has been demonstrated that EDTA inhibits copper-catalyzed LDL oxidation in vitro [17]. Therefore, the inactivation and excretion of copper and iron cations by EDTA may favorably affect the progression of atherosclerosis.

EDTA may also favorably influence endothelial function. Oxidized LDL may significantly limit the half-life of nitric oxide, the mediator of endothelial relaxation [18]. Impairing endothelial relaxation may exacerbate angina pectoris by altering the relationship of coronary blood supply to demand. To the extent that EDTA inhibits in vivo LDL oxidation, it will favorably impact on endothelial relaxation.

Apart from its ability to bind metal cations, EDTA possesses multiple and complex pharmacologic actions, some of which may, in theory, render it effective for treatment of atherosclerosis. EDTA has been shown to reverse plaque formation in animal models of atherosclerosis [19]. It mobilizes calcium from atherosclerotic plaque in cadaveric coronary and iliac arteries [20,21]. Reports have demonstrated the ability of EDTA to lower plasma cholesterol levels in humans [22]. Other reported mechanisms of action that may affect the progression of atherosclerosis include inhibition of platelet aggregation, reduction of blood pressure, and improved glucose control in type II diabetes mellitus [23–26].

CLINICAL APPLICATIONS OF CHELATION THERAPY

It is known that up to 40% of the U.S. population uses some form of alternative therapy. However, most of these individuals are not forthcoming about such treatment in discussions with their primary care physician [27]. Awareness of this dichotomy has prompted many primary care clinicians to inquire directly about their patient's use of alternative healing modalities. Increasingly, it is likely that the clinician will encounter questions from their patients regarding EDTA chelation therapy for atherosclerosis. Therefore, this section is intended to provide the primary care physician with an understanding of the clinical applications of EDTA chelation therapy.

Coronary Artery Disease

Chelation therapy is not indicated as a treatment for unstable angina. EDTA chelation requires between 3 and 6 months of weekly intravenous infusions to produce what may be described as clinical benefit. Those patients who have spontaneous or provokable ischemia, in the face of reasonable medical therapy, are candidates for angiography and possibly coronary revascularization, not chelation therapy.

Recent reports have supported a conservative medical strategy in acute coronary syndromes [28–30]. These reports demonstrate that, in those patients with unstable angina in whom medical therapy controls symptoms, clinical outcomes are comparable with those of clinically similar patients undergoing angiography and revascularization. In this subset of patients, it is reasonable to add chelation therapy once the patient has been stabilized.

Patients with chronic stable angina that is well controlled on medical therapy without evidence of left ventricular dysfunction are candidates for EDTA chelation therapy. In contrast, those individuals who have high-risk coronary disease suggested by significant left main coronary disease, three-vessel disease with left ventricular dysfunction, and two vessel disease with proximal left anterior descending artery involvement are clearly candidates for surgical revascularization. These patients often have had coronary angiography occasioned by failure of medical therapy or high risk predicted by clinical findings or stress testing. Patients who refuse angiography for these indications may inquire about chelation therapy as a therapeutic alternative. This is a difficult situation because the patients may have high-risk disease. In this circumstance, it is best to avoid EDTA chelation therapy and encourage the patient to proceed with angiography.

Patients with stable angina and significant left ventricular dysfunction should avoid chelation therapy. The additional sodium and fluid load imposed by chelation can cause left ventricular decompensation. Additionally, a subset of these patients may benefit from revascularization.

Peripheral Vascular Disease

Patients with *acute* limb ischemia should not be managed with chelation therapy. This subgroup requires prompt angiography and definitive endovascular or surgical intervention. In *chronic* peripheral arterial occlusive disease, patients may inquire about chelation therapy as a nonsurgical option. Symptoms range from stable intermittent claudication to more severe symptoms of disabling claudication and rest pain. At present, other than cessation of smoking and exercise conditioning, little evidence suggests that medical interventions improve outcomes or relieve symptoms in peripheral vascular disease. A large retrospective analysis of over 2800 patients who were receiving chelation therapy reported marked improvement in 91% of those with peripheral vascular disease as opposed to 77% of those with coronary artery disease and only 24% with cerebrovascular disease [31]. My experience with EDTA chelation therapy also suggests that in the spectrum of atherosclerotic disease, the most marked clinical improvement is seen in patients with peripheral vascular disease.

CONTRAINDICATIONS AND TOXICITY

Despite concerns to the contrary, EDTA chelation therapy, when used by physicians properly trained in its use, has a low morbidity rate. Renal toxicity is directly related to the rate and dose of EDTA infused. Adherence to dosing protocols based on lean body mass, creatinine clearance, and infusion rate minimizes toxicity [32]. Liberal fluid intake is encouraged to reduce the risk of renal injury. Nephrotoxicity is reversible and responds promptly to cessation of EDTA treatment. A prudent clinical approach is to advise patients with a serum creatinine level above 2.5 mg/dl to avoid chelation therapy.

Patients with congestive heart failure are at risk for decompensation as a result of fluid and sodium overload or as a result of the negative inotropic effect of transient hypocalcemia induced by EDTA. Patients with mild compensated congestive heart failure can be managed successfully by paying attention to restricting intravenous fluid volume and by providing additional diuretic therapy when necessary. However, with severe left ventricular dysfunction, it is best to avoid EDTA chelation therapy.

Patients who are receiving anticoagulant therapy with warfarin can safely receive chelation therapy. Pregnancy, known allergy to EDTA, and active liver disease represent contraindications. A summary of these and other contraindications to EDTA chelation therapy is shown in Table 10-1.

Toxicity of EDTA chelation therapy, apart from its potential for nephrotoxicity, remains minimal. Relatively common symptoms during a course of treatment include fatigue and muscle cramping. Correcting mineral deficiencies usually alleviates these symptoms. Mild hypocalcemia is also particularly common. Hypoglycemia may occur during treatment, especially in patients who do not eat before receiving their infusion. Transient hypocalcemia induced by chelation has the potential to induce arrhythmias; however, this is rarely observed clinically.

TABLE 10-1. CONTRAINDICATIONS TO EDTA CHELATION THERAPY

Acute coronary syndromes
Acute limb ischemia
Severe left venticular (LV) dysfunction with LV ejection fraction below 30%
Angiographic indications for coronary revascularization
    Left main coronary disease
    Two vessels coronary disease with proximal left anterior descending artery involvement
    Three vessels coronary disease with LV dysfunction
Serum creatinine level above 2.5 mg/dl
Pregnancy
Active hepatic disease
Allergy to EDTA

TREATMENT PROTOCOL

A treatment course of chelation therapy usually consists of a series of between 30 and 40 intravenous infusions of disodium magnesium EDTA, adjusted for appropriate osmolality and buffered with sodium bicarbonate. The most common solution contains 3 g (or 50 mg/kg) of EDTA in 500 mL of sterile water, which is infused over 3 hours and administered weekly. Alternative regimens have included 1.5 g of EDTA in 250 mL of sterile water administered over 1.5 hours [33••]. Typically, 2 g magnesium chloride and 7 g vitamin C are added to the standard chelation therapy infusion. Patients who improve often receive monthly "maintenance" treatments for an indefinite period following the initial course of treatment. The optimal frequency and duration of treatment have not been studied.

Patients who are considering EDTA therapy should be encouraged to consult with a physician who has received training in EDTA chelation protocols through the American College for Advancement in Medicine (ACAM). Further credentials include Diplomate status obtained by passing written and oral examinations administered by the American Board of Chelation Therapy.

CONCLUSIONS

For 40 years, EDTA chelation therapy for vascular disease has remained controversial and of unproven clinical benefit. Hundreds of thousands of Americans expose themselves to treatment with EDTA chelation therapy yearly. If this therapy proves helpful, then additional, as yet untreated patients may be able to benefit from it. Conversely, if EDTA chelation were without clinical merit, then physicians, administrators, and regulatory authorities would be able to reject it on solid scientific evidence. The few double-blind prospective trials that have been performed are methodologically flawed. At a time when the number of position statements regarding EDTA chelation therapy far surpasses the number of quality scientific studies, more rigorous research is essential. Until such trials are completed, physicians can intelligently counsel patients wishing to integrate EDTA chelation therapy into their current therapeutic regimen by adhering to the guidelines presented here.

REFERENCES AND RECOMMENDED READING

Recently published papers of particular interest have been highlighted as:
- Of interest
- •• Of outstanding interest

1. Grier MT, Meyers DG: So much writing, so little science: a review of 37 years of literature on edetate sodium chelation therapy. *Ann Pharmacother* 1993, 27:1504–1509.
2. Clarke NE Sr, Clarke NE Jr, Mosher RE: The "in vivo" dissolution of metastatic calcium: an approach to atherosclerosis. *Am J Med Sci* 1955, 229:142–149.
3. Clarke NE: Treatment of angina pectoris with disodium EDTA. *Am J Med Sci* 1956, 232:654–666.
4. Clarke NE: Atherosclerosis, occlusive vascular disease and EDTA. *Am J Cardiol* 1960, 6:233–235.
5. Kitchell JR, Meltzer LE, Seven MJ: Potential uses of chelation methods in the treatment of cardiovascular diseases. *Prog Cardiol Dis* 1961, 3:338–349.
6. Kitchell JR, Palmon F, Aytan N, Meltzer L: The treatment of coronary artery disease with disodium EDTA: a reappraisal. *Am J Cardiol* 1963, 11:501–506.
7. Meltzer LE, Kitchell JR, Palmon F Jr: The long term use, side effects and toxicity of disodium ethylenediamine tetraacetic acid (EDTA). *Am J Med Sci* 1961, 242:51–57.
8. Olszewer E, Carter JP: EDTA chelation therapy in chronic degenerative disease. *Med Hypotheses* 1988, 27:41–49.
9. Chappell LT, Stahl JP: The correlation between EDTA chelation therapy and improvement in cardiovascular function: a meta-analysis. *J Adv Med* 1993, 6:139–160.
10. Sloth-Nielson J, Guldager B, Mouritzen C, *et al.*: Arteriographic findings in EDTA chelation therapy on peripheral arteriosclerosis. *Am J Surg* 1991, 162:122–125.
11. Guldager B, Jelnes R, Jorgensen SJ, *et al.*: EDTA treatment of intermittent claudication: a double-blind, placebo-controlled study. *J Int Med* 1992, 231–267.
12. Van Rij AM, Solomon C, Packer SGK, Hopkins WG: Chelation therapy for intermittent claudication: a double-blind, randomized, controlled trial. *Circulation* 1994, 1194–1199.
13.•• Chappell LT, Maargolis S: Point/counterpoint. *Alt Therap* 1995, 2:53–56.
This paper offers two perspectives on EDTA chelation therapy, one from an advocate and the other from a critic. Rather than drawing definitive conclusions, this article makes it clear why EDTA chelation therapy for vascular disease is controversial.
14. Steinberg D, Lewis A: Conner memorial lecture: oxidative modification of LDL and atherogenesis. *Circulation* 1997, 95:1062–1071.
15. O'Keefe J, Conn R, Lavie C, Bateman T: The new paradigm for coronary artery disease: altering risk factors, atherosclerotic plaques and clinical prognosis. *Mayo Clin Proc* 1996, 71:957–965.
16. Schwartz CJ, Valente AJ, Sprague EA: A modern view of atherogenesis. *Am J Cardiol* 1993, 71:9B–14B.
17. Lamb DJ, Leake DS: The effect of EDTA on the oxidation of low density lipoprotein. *Atherosclerosis* 1992, 94:35–42.
18. Harrison DG, Ohara Y: Physiologic consequences of increased vascular oxidant stresses in hypercholesterolemia and atherosclerosis: implications for impaired vasomotion. *Am J Cardiol* 1995, 75:75B–81B.

19. Wartman A, Lampe TL, McCann DS, Boyle AJ: Plaque reversal with MgEDTA in experimental atherosclerosis elastin and collagen metabolism. *J Atherosclerosis Res* 1967, 7:331–341.
20. Bolick LE, Blankenhorn DH: A quantitative study of coronary arterial calcification. *Am J Path* 1961, 39:511.
21. Wilder L, DeJode L, Milstein SR: Mobilization of atherosclerotic plaque calcium with EDTA utilizing the isolation-perfusion principle. *Surgery* 1962, 52:793–795.
22. Olwin J, Koppel J: Reduction of elevated plasma lipid levels in atherosclerosis following EDTA therapy. *Proc Soc Exp Biol Med* 1968, 128:1137–1140.
23. Schroeder H: A practical method for the reduction of plasma cholesterol in man. *J Chron Dis* 1956, 4:461–468.
24. Suvarov A, Markosyan R: Some mechanisms of EDTA on platelet aggregation. *Byall Eksp Biol Med* 1981, 5:587.
25. Lamar CP: Chelation endarterectomy for occlusive atherosclerosis. *J Am Geriatr Soc* 1966, 14:272–294.
26. Meltzer LE, Palmon FJ, Kitchell JR: Hypoglycemia induced by disodium ethylenediamine tetra-acetic acid. *Lancet* 1961, 2:637–638.
27. Lamar CP: Chelation therapy of occlusive arteriosclerosis in diabetic patients. *Angiology* 1964, 15:379–395.
28. Astin, JA: Why patients use alternative medicine: results of a national study. *JAMA* 1998, 279:1548–1553.
29. Boden WE, O'Rourke RA, Crawford MH, *et al.*: Outcomes in patients with acute non-Q-wave myocardial infarction randomly assigned to an invasive as compared with a conservative management strategy. *N Engl J Med* 1998, 338:1785–1792.
30. Williams DO, Braunwald E, Thompson B, *et al.*: Results of percutaneous transluminal coronary angioplasty in unstable angina and non-Q-wave myocardial infarction: observations from the TIMI IIIB trial. *Circulation* 1996, 94:2749–2755.
31. Anderson HV, Cannon CP, Stone PH, *et al.*: One-year results of the Thrombolysis in Myocardial Infarction (TIMI) IIIB clinical trial: a randomized comparison of tissue-type plasminogen activator versus placebo and early invasive versus early conservative strategies in unstable angina and non-Q-wave myocardial infarction. *J Am Coll Cardiol* 1995, 26:1643–1650.
32. Olszewer F, Carter JP: EDTA chelation therapy: a retrospective study of 2870 patients. *J Adv Med* 1989, 2:197–211.
33.•• Rosema T: The protocol for safe and effective administration of EDTA and other chelation agents for vascular disease, degenerative disease and metal toxicity. *J Adv Med* 1997, 10:5–100.

This is an updated revision of the EDTA chelation protocol approved by the American College for Advancement in Medicine. It is a useful guide for the safe and effective clinical application of EDTA chelation in vascular disease.

Intensive Lifestyle Intervention for Coronary Artery Disease: Alternative Medicine or Common Sense?

Lee Lipsenthal and Dean Ornish

The medical approach toward treatment of most diseases has become highly reductionistic. For example, in the 1950s, it was noted that excess weight increased the risk of coronary artery disease (CAD). In the 1960s and 1970s, CAD was seen to be more strongly associated with elevated cholesterol levels than with weight. In the 1980s, the low-density lipoprotein (LDL) cholesterol component was most suspect and it was determined that high LDL levels were associated with familial tendencies. Thus it was presumed that a genetic predisposition toward the production of LDL-C or inability to metabolize LDL-C was a prominent cause of CAD. In the 1990s, small, dense LDL was described as the most atherogenic subfraction of LDL and that endothelial inflammation was the root process of atherogenesis. If you follow this train of thought to its "logical" end, it would seem that the treatment of CAD must depend on decreasing serum levels of small, dense LDL combined with genetic manipulation of LDL receptors to enhance the liver's capacity to take up and break down LDL. The ultimate treatment might be a "magic bullet" pharmaceutic that decreases our arterial susceptibility to small, dense LDL and other detrimental agents. These would all have some effectiveness; however, this overly reductionistic approach is often only partially useful and generally very expensive, especially when applied to the treatment of a large population at risk. It also does not necessarily address the root cause of the problem. By analogy, it would be like taking an aspirin to diminish a headache, when it might make more sense to eliminate the hammer that is hitting you on the head.

How did we get to this style of thinking? The "magic bullet" mentality of medicine began with, or was enhanced by, the advent of antibiotics. An antibiotic drug would often eliminate a health problem, in some cases overnight, with minimal, if any, harm to the patient. Although this is not a holistic approach, it is often reasonable and lifesaving. A brief course of pills is also much less expensive than a hospital stay for pneumonia and any subsequent adverse health outcomes of a serious infection. Using pharmaceuticals and, later, high-tech treatments in this very focused fashion, clinicians had success in eliminating or decreasing adverse outcomes in multiple disease states. Physicians and patients enjoyed this success, as did the pharmaceutical firms. Thus was the stage set for the search for a "magic bullet" cure for all diseases.

The problem in approaching CAD this way is that CAD is multifactorial. The contributors to the process (that we understand) are a mix of genetic and environmental factors and include diet, physical activity, emotional make-up, smoking, diabetes, and many others. We have tried the "magic bullets" of coronary artery bypass graft (CABG), percutaneous transluminal coronary angioplasty (PTCA), β-blockers, nitrates, statins, and other therapies only to find partial success in the treatment of CAD while simultaneously creating a very expensive treatment system.

Many of the risks for CAD are related to lifestyle, and therefore, patients can be empowered to treat or "cure" themselves of these risks. This allows for a true treatment partnership between physician and patient. Difficulties arise because we, as clinicians, are not accustomed to being or willing to be partners. Many patients want to relinquish the responsibility of their health care to their physician. Many physicians have trouble sharing this responsibility with their patients because it puts them in a fallible, less than "divine" role. It may be time to create a new model of care, but first let us review where we are today in the treatment of CAD.

HEART DISEASE IN THE UNITED STATES

More than 500,000 Americans die annually as a result of CAD, making it the leading cause of death in the United States. At present, 5 to 6 million Americans are afflicted with CAD and present an occurrence rate of 1.5 million heart attacks per year. Approximately 500,000 CABG operations and approximately 600,000 PTCAs were performed in the United States in 1994 at a combined cost of approximately $15.6 billion, which exceeds the aggregate cost for any other surgical procedure. At that time, the American Heart Association [1] estimated the cost of treatment of CAD in the United States to be $56.3 billion. A potential for significant cost savings exists if safe and comparably effective but less expensive alternative interventions can be implemented.

REVASCULARIZATION PROCEDURES

Developed in the 1960s, CABG was the first successful therapy to improve blood flow to the heart in patients with coronary heart disease. Research showed that CABG is effective in reducing angina and improving cardiac function. However, when compared with medical therapy and followed for 16 years, CABG improved survival only in a select subgroup of patients—those with reduced left ventricular (LV) function and stenotic lesions of the left main coronary artery of over 59%. Median survival was not prolonged in patients with left main CAD below 60% and normal LV function even when a significant right coronary artery stenosis at or above 70% was also present [2–4].

A meta-analysis of seven randomized trials comparing CABG with medical therapy reported lower mortality from CABG than from medical therapy [5], but the benefits were not evident for at least 2 years; after 12 years, no significant difference in survival was found between the two groups. Excluding left main disease and left main equivalent, no benefit in survival rates is proven. Benefit was greater in more severe subgroups, especially in significant left main disease, but patients with three-vessel disease extended survival by only 6 months after 10 years of follow-up. In addition, patients aged more than 65 years were excluded from these clinical trials, and only 3% of the cohort were women. This meta-analysis did not take into account the potentially confounding roles of intensive risk factor modification, aspirin, β-blockers, calcium channel blockers, lipid-lowering drugs, angiotensin-converting enzyme (ACE) inhibitors (of particular value in patients with poor LV function), and other advances in medical therapy.

The strongest evidence is gained from individual randomized controlled trials. In the Coronary Artery Surgery Study (CASS)[6], for example, median survival was 14.3 years in the surgical group and 14.2 years in the medical group (P = not significant) after 15 years, due to a disproportionate increase in the late surgical group mortality. This survival advantage was due to improved mortality in 2.1% of the study population. This suggests that bypass surgery may temporarily benefit a small subset of patients: those with severe, unstable CAD. This is not, however, necessarily representative of current community-based practice of CAD. Medical therapy including intensive risk-factor modification may be necessary to prevent later reocclusion in those who receive bypass, and it may be the treatment of choice in the 97.9% of the population that do not require bypass.

Minimally invasive coronary bypass may not be a step in the right direction toward improved mortality and toward containing the costs related to CABG procedures. It has allowed more frequent single-vessel grafting. Patients with single graft treatment are either not unstable enough to benefit from CABG or, if unstable, may not be appropriately revascularized [7]. This may eventually lead to a greater number of inappropriate bypasses in the United States.

In this way, PTCA was developed with the hope of providing a less invasive, lower-risk approach to the management of CAD and its symptoms. Over the past 15 years, technical advances in PTCA have led to significant improvements in procedural success and safety despite the application of this technique to increasingly challenging lesions. Although widely used, no randomized trials exist comparing PTCA with medical therapy in stable patients with CAD; therefore, the improvement ratios in mortality and morbidity of PTCA remain unknown.

The major obstacle to the success of PTCA has been the high rate of restenosis (ie, reclosure of the vessel after successful PTCA), which is likely due to an inflammatory response of intimal tissue leading to spasm of the vessel, thickening of the arterial wall, and, possibly, accelerated reformation of the plaque [8–12]. Restenosis occurs in 30% to 50% of angioplastied lesions within 6 months of initial treatment [13] and in 63% of patients necessitates a second procedure, either CABG (22%) or PTCA (41%), within 3 years [14]. Restenosis and its subsequent treatment increases the long-term cost of PTCA to nearly that of a CABG [15]. PCTA has failed to surpass bypass surgery in terms of long-term morbidity and mortality rates.

Other related procedures, such as laser atherectomy or rotational atherectomy, have not reduced the long-term restenosis rate in two controlled trials [16,17]. The value of these newer procedures awaits further study.

Coronary stenting (ie, the insertion of a mesh brace into the lumen of the coronary artery during angioplasty) has reduced the short-term restenosis rate compared with conventional balloon angioplasty for patients undergoing elective, single-vessel coronary revascularization [18,19]. No randomized, controlled trial data support long-term efficacy of this approach. Stent procedures are hindered by a longer hospital stay and the accompanying higher likelihood of complication. They also cost more initially, but after 3 years the costs are comparable to those of PTCA due to the lower restenosis rate [20–22]. Further studies are necessary to determine whether ongoing refinements in stent design, irradiation, implantation techniques, and anticoagulation regimens can narrow this cost difference further by reducing stent-related complications or length of stay.

Most adverse events related to CAD—myocardial infarction, sudden death syndrome, and unstable angina—are due to the rupture of an atherosclerotic plaque of less than 40% to 60% stenosis. This often occurs in the setting of vessel spasm and results in thrombosis and occlusion of the vessel [23–27]. Bypass surgery and angioplasty do not affect nonbypassed or nondilated lesions, whereas comprehensive lifestyle changes (or lipid-lowering drugs) may help stabilize all lesions, including mild lesions (*ie*, less than 50% stenosis).

CHOLESTEROL-LOWERING THERAPY

The limitations of revascularization procedures suggest that the more reasonable goal in treating CAD in the stable patient may be stabilizing all existing plaque by modifying its components and addressing the abnormal vascular tone associated with CAD. This has been demonstrated to lower cholesterol levels in animal studies and trials [25,28–36]. These cholesterol-lowering trials, which used medications alone or combined with lifestyle modifications, have demonstrated significant reductions in morbidity and mortality in cardiac-related diseases. In the Scandinavian Simvastatin Survival Study [36], 4444 men and women with CAD were randomly assigned to receive either simvastatin or a placebo. The study demonstrated a 42% lower mortality from CAD and 30% lower mortality from all causes after 5.4 years of treatment in the group receiving simvastatin.

Of these studies, those using cardiac catheterization as endpoint measures have demonstrated cessation of progression or partial regression of disease in up to 80% of study subjects. Although the magnitude of regression is small (*ie*, 3 to 10 absolute percentage points of lumen diameter), it is statistically significant compared with the control subjects' disease progression. This modest regression, associated with dramatic improvement in mortality and morbidity, makes sense in light of the stabilized plaque and normalized vasomotor tone demonstrated with lipid-lowering therapy [37–49].

Use of lipid-lowering therapy would certainly be warranted in those patients with CAD and hyperlipidemia who are already on a low-fat diet and exercise program; however, use of this lipid therapy for primary prevention remains controversial. Studies by Shepard *et al.* [50] and Downs *et al.* [51] suggest the validity of wide-scale, primary, preventive lipid-reduction treatment. The expense of treating a large population would be exorbitant and the potential risk of liver disease and cancer from taking these medications is not negligible, especially when used for prolonged periods [52].

LIFESTYLE MODIFICATION

These mechanisms and study results help to explain the outcomes of our own earlier randomized study, the Lifestyle Heart Trial [53]. Within a few weeks after making comprehensive lifestyle changes (including a low-fat vegetarian diet, exercise, stress management, and psychosocial support) the patients in the intervention group reported a 91% average reduction in the frequency of angina. Most of the patients became essentially pain-free, including those who had been unable to work or engage in daily activities because of severe chest pain. These clinical improvements are not likely to be the result of rapid regression of blockages but more probably reflect improvements in vasomotor tone and thrombotic state.

In this group, the progression of coronary atherosclerosis began to reverse after 1 year (4.4% improvement in absolute percentage of diameter stenosis). This finding was statistically significant in comparison with that of the control group. These patients demonstrated even greater improvement after 4 years (7.8% improvement in absolute percentage of diameter stenosis) than after 1 year. Cardiac positron emission tomography (PET) scans after 4 years revealed that even the relatively small improvements in percentage of diameter stenosis by quantitative coronary arteriography significantly improved myocardial perfusion. These changes were associated with a 37% decrease in LDL cholesterol levels achieved at 1 year without lipid-lowering medication. In contrast, control group patients who made only moderate lifestyle changes worsened after 1 year and became even worse after 4 years in both percentage of diameter stenosis and myocardial perfusion [54]. These findings suggest that the beneficial effects of diet and lifestyle change may be comparable to those provided by cholesterol-lowering medications in achieving clinical benefit without the associated costs and potential short-term and long-term side effects of such pharmacotherapy.

DIET

It is estimated that diet and lifestyle modification could halve the rate of congestive heart disease (CHD) [55] and the impact of this behavioral change would also benefit the elderly [56–58]. However, the current dietary guidelines of the American Heart Association (30% fat, 200 to 300 mg dietary cholesterol) may not be sufficient to stop the progression of CHD. Hunninghake *et al.* [59] demonstrated only a 5% improvement in LDL cholesterol from a step-2 American Heart Association diet compared with 27% improvement from lovastatin in the same patients. Patients randomly assigned to the control group in several regression trials were consuming a step-1 or step-2 diet; however, most of these patients continued to show progression of disease. However, regression of coronary atherosclerosis may result when dietary intake of fat and cholesterol are much lower [39,53,54].

Dietary intake of fat and cholesterol may have short-term as well as long-term effects, for better and for worse. Even a single high-fat, high cholesterol meal may cause acute enhancement of platelet reactivity [60] as well as sludging in arterial beds [61]. These changes may result from a shift in the thromboxane–prostacyclin balance to favor thromboxane production. Cholesterol-enriched platelets release more arachidonic acid from platelet phospholipids than cholesterol-depleted platelets do, and conversion of released arachidonic acid to platelet thromboxane is higher in cholesterol-rich platelets than in those that are cholesterol-depleted [62]. In animals with atherosclerosis induced by high-cholesterol diets, platelets synthesize thromboxane A_2 in increased amounts [63]. Because cholesterol is contained only in foods of animal origin, a vegetarian diet may shift the balance away from thromboxane formation, which would make both coronary spasm and platelet aggregation less likely.

Other benefits of consuming a vegetarian diet exist, beyond changes in thrombotic potential. A diet high in fat and meat products is also high in oxidants and may promote oxidation of LDL, thus making LDL more atherogenic [64]. Oxidized LDL particles are more readily taken up by macrophages, which, in turn, become foam cells, the progenitor of the fatty streak [65]. Additionally, a high intake of heme iron, largely from red meat, has been suggested to be positively associated with increased risk of myocardial infarction [66]. Antioxidant vitamins C, E, A, and beta carotene, the precursor of vitamin A, appear to retard the oxidative process [67]. The diet recommended in this program is low in oxidants and contains abundant sources of antioxidants as well as bioflavonoids, carotenoids, phytochemicals, and other substances that are at higher levels in a plant-based diet than in a meat-based diet.

The health benefits of fiber in the diet are numerous. Although virtually no dietary fiber is present in meat, high amounts of both soluble and insoluble fiber exist in a plant-based diet. High-fiber diets have been shown to lower blood cholesterol levels and to reduce other cardiac risk factors, such as high blood pressure, diabetes, and obesity [68]. Benefits of fiber with respect to lowering cholesterol and stabilizing blood sugar have also been demonstrated [69]. Some studies have shown that high-fiber diets may reduce or eliminate the need for insulin in some patients with diabetes [70]. Therefore, it is generally accepted that soluble, fiber-rich foods not only improve diabetes, but also may significantly reduce other risk factors for heart disease, such as high cholesterol, LDL, elevated triglycerides, and obesity. The American Cancer Society recommends consumption of 20 to 30 g of fiber daily. The lifestyle change diet contains between 30 to 36 g of fiber daily as compared to the average 7 g consumed by most U.S. citizens.

Several studies suggest that transconfigured fatty acids found in certain meat fats and hydrogenated vegetable oils raise total and LDL cholesterol levels [71]. Because a low-fat vegetarian diet is low in both total fat and saturated fat and contains no added fats and oils, it lacks the detrimental effects associated with trans fatty acids.

Some published evidence suggests that homocysteine, a thiol-containing amino acid derived from methionine, is linked to heart disease [72]. Folic acid keeps homocysteine levels from rising too high. A plant-based diet is abundant in fresh fruits and vegetables, which are significant food sources of folic acid and moreover are low in methionine.

A plant-based diet is recognized as consistent with good nutrition status. This diet is linked not only to lower risks of heart disease and stroke but also to significantly lower rates of the most common cancers, including breast, prostate, colon, lung, and ovarian cancers. Low-fat vegetarian diets also may reduce the incidence of osteoporosis, adult-onset diabetes, hypertension, obesity, and many other illnesses [73–85].

The average American diet is estimated to derive 37% of ingested calories from fat, with heavy emphasis on processed foods; it is less nutritionally adequate than a well-balanced, low-fat vegetarian diet. Analyses of 3-day diet diaries of our study participants have shown that experimental-group patients on this diet have significantly more vitamins A, B_6, C, folic acid, pantothenic acid, fiber, magnesium, and potassium than control group patients on a typical American diet; however, their diets had significantly less vitamin B_{12}. Therefore, we recommend a multivitamin supplement to all program patients.

EXERCISE

The role of exercise in the treatment of CAD is strongly supported by reviews of the literature. Two meta-analyses indicate that the risk of death was doubled in those who were physically inactive when compared with more active individuals [86,87]. This suggests that sedentary lifestyle is a risk factor for CHD. In terms of treatment, rehabilitation programs incorporating exercise also show modest benefits of exercise in preventing recurrent CHD events. None of 22 randomized trials in the meta-analysis had the power to show a significant treatment effect, but in a meta-analysis employing the intention-to-treat analysis, there was a significant reduction of 25% in 1- to 3-year rates of CHD and total mortality in the patients receiving cardiac rehabilitation when compared with control patients [88].

Exercise also appears to play a role in helping to slow or stop the progression of CAD when combined with a low-fat diet. In a randomized study of 62 CHD patients using vigorous exercise and a low-fat diet (20% calories from fat), regression of coronary lesions was observed only in patients expending an average of 2200 kcal per week in leisure time physical activity, amounting to approximately 5 to 6 hours per week of regular physical exercise [89]. Other evidence suggests that exercise benefits other atherosclerotic syndromes. In a meta-analysis of 33 studies using exercise training for the treatment of claudication, a 179% increase was seen in the distance before onset of claudication pain, and the distance to maximal claudication pain increased 122%. A greater frequency and duration of exercise corresponded with a greater reduction in claudication pain [90].

PSYCHOSOCIAL RISK FACTORS

The psychosocial status of the patient must be addressed [91]. The patient's psychologic state may affect his or her ability to adhere to any recommended course of therapy. Moreover, the patient's psychologic status and the subsequent health-enhancing and health-damaging behaviors it promotes may contribute to the pathogenesis of some diseases. For example, in a sample of 5115 adults (ages 18 to 40 years), it was shown that hostility, as measured by the Cook-Medley Hostility Scale, was strongly associated with tobacco and marijuana smoking, increased alcohol consumption, and greater caloric intake in both blacks and whites and in both men and women [92]. In addition, results from a prospective epidemiologic study found hostility measured by the same scale to be related to a higher body mass, a poorer lipid profile, and a greater likelihood of hypertension 20 years later [93]. Treatment of disease may not be as successful without also addressing adverse health risk behaviors and the underlying psychologic causes.

Various psychologic states have been associated with CAD and its prognosis. The relationship between major and minor depression and CHD has been studied for many years, and it is generally accepted that depression, anxiety, and related states are associated with increased risk for the development and progression of CAD [94]. It has been estimated that 33% to 50% of myocardial infarctions were preceded by depression [95], and recent studies have found significant associations between depression and CAD-related morbidity and mortality [96–98]. The mechanism whereby depression places people at increased risk for heart disease is still under investigation; however, because depressed CAD patients are less likely to adhere to prescribed lifestyle modifications, such as diet and exercise, and to their medical regimens, interventions designed to reduce depression may affect their long-term prognosis.

Anger has also been demonstrated to be a trigger for acute myocardial infarction. Men and women with CAD were 230% more likely to have an acute myocardial infarction within 2 hours of an angry episode. This is likely to be triggered by increased catecholamine levels, vasospasm, and plaque disruption as well as increased myocardial oxygen demand [99].

Anxiety and its relation to CAD events has also been evaluated. In a 32-year prospective study of 2271 men, those reporting two or more symptoms of anxiety, such as nervousness, had a 320% increased incidence of fatal CAD and a 573% increased risk of sudden death. This, too, is thought to be mediated by catecholamines and vasospasm [100].

A socially supported lifestyle also appears to be important to the patient with CAD. Deficits in social support have been implicated as likely contributors to CAD morbidity and mortality [101–104]. In an epidemiologic comparison using data from the Alameda County study in California and the North Karelia Study in Eastern Finland, Kaplan [105] found that those who were socially isolated were two to three times more likely to die from ischemic heart disease than those who were more socially connected. In a similar study, Jenkinson *et al.* [106] followed 1376 patients with suspected acute myocardial infarction for a median time of 3 years and found that socially isolated patients were 49% more likely to die after an infarct than were patients classified as not being socially isolated. The mechanism underlying the inverse relationship between social connectedness and heart disease is complex, and no single causal relationship is likely to be found. It is likely, however, that enhancing social support improves an individual's cardiac risk profile by improving his or her ability to cope with stress and to adhere to prescribed lifestyle modifications, as well as by providing a sense of contact, consistency, and safety with others.

The aforementioned psychologic states are not of an extreme or unusual nature. In all the studies cited, subjects were functional and not receiving psychiatric medications. Fortunately, it is clear that these behaviors can be modified through interventions that decrease the risk of adverse events related to CAD. Many of these interventions are typically group based and use various strategies including cognitive-relaxation coping skills [107–109] as well as social and communication skills training [110]. The value of psychosocial interventions is further supported by a recent meta-analysis of 23 randomized controlled trials that evaluated the impact of group-based cardiac rehabilitation programs [111]. Patients who received psychosocial interventions had greater reductions in cholesterol levels, systolic blood pressure, heart rate, and psychologic distress; patients who did not receive psychosocial interventions had greater cardiac recurrence rates and greater mortality during the first 2 years of follow-up.

The group support techniques in our research have evolved over the last 19 years of conducting lifestyle change studies. These techniques have the following objectives: 1) to help patients overcome their sense of isolation; 2) to learn communication techniques; 3) to allow participants to become aware of their feelings; and 4) to facilitate a bonding that would help the patients adhere to the other aspects of the program [112,113].

STRESS AND THE HEART

Emotional stress has long been suspected as a contributor to the pathogenesis of coronary heart disease. Recent studies have shown that myocardial ischemia with or without accompanying chest pain may be caused by emotional stress [114]. Emotional stress may lead to myocardial ischemia both through coronary artery spasm and by increased platelet aggregation within coronary arteries [115]. Stress may lead to coronary spasm mediated either by direct α-adrenergic stimulation or secondary to the release of thromboxane A_2 from platelets, perhaps by increasing circulating catecholamines or other mediators [116]. Both thromboxane A_2 and catecholamines are potent constrictors of arterial smooth muscle and powerful endogenous stimulators of platelet aggregation. Stress management is likely to lower catecholamine levels and diminish this response.

STRESS MANAGEMENT

Stress management techniques that we have employed in all previous lifestyle change studies have been based in part on hatha yoga [53,54,117–119]. These techniques include stretching, progressive relaxation, breathing techniques, meditation, and visualization. Some clinical trials show various physical and psychologic benefits of these techniques, which are sometimes implemented as an intervention separately (*eg*, stretching and meditation) and sometimes used in combination (*eg*, stretching and relaxation). Controlled trials have shown that participants doing hatha yoga (stretching) have lower resting oxygen consumption [120], increased hemoglobin and vital capacity [Dhanaraj, unpublished doctoral dissertation, 1974], decreased plasma renin activity and plasma aldosterone concentration [121], reduced respiration rate, decreased muscular activity, and increased peripheral blood flow [122]. In terms of psychological benefits, Vahia *et al.* [123] used stretching, breathing, and meditation as the intervention and found decreased anxiety, depression, hysteria, and increased ability to concentrate when compared with a group given anxiolytic or antidepressant drugs. These combined benefits should impact significantly on the prognosis of the patient with CAD.

Conclusions

The Secondary Prevention Panel of the American Heart Association and American College of Cardiology [124] reported that "compelling scientific evidence, including data from recent studies in patients with CAD, demonstrate that comprehensive risk factor interventions extend overall survival, improve quality of life, decrease the need for interventional procedures such as angioplasty and bypass grafting, and reduce the incidence of subsequent myocardial infarction." They go on to report that "studies demonstrate that only approximately one third of eligible patients continue risk factor interventions over the long term. However, data also show that this proportion can be significantly increased by a team approach in which health care professionals—including physicians, nurses and dietitians—manage risk reduction therapy." This is an integrated and wise view toward the management of CAD. Medications and revascularization are more effective when combined with a healthy lifestyle.

We have taken this approach in our Lifestyle Heart Trial [53] and our ongoing Multi-Center Lifestyle Heart Trial, currently in its fifth year, in which we have 477 enrollees at eight geographically diverse sites. To date, outcomes have been consistent with our results from the Lifestyle Heart Trial and will be published in 1999.

A recent editorial in *The New England Journal of Medicine* by Angell and Kassirer [125] questioned the value of "alternative medicine": "There is only medicine that has been adequately tested and medicine that has not, medicine that works and medicine that may or may not work. Once a treatment has been tested rigorously, it no longer matters whether it was considered alternative at the outset." In this context, our program of comprehensive lifestyle changes is no longer "alternative medicine" but is "medicine that works."

References and Recommended Reading

Recently published papers of particular interest have been highlighted as:
- Of interest
- Of outstanding interest

1. American Heart Association: *Heart and Stroke Facts: 1995 Statistical Supplement*. Dallas: American Heart Association; 1994.
2. Alderman EL, Bourassa MG, Cohen LS, *et al.*: Ten-year follow up of survival and myocardial infarction in the randomized coronary artery surgical study. *Circulation* 1990, 82:1629–1646.
3. Caracciolo EA, Davis KB, Sopko G, *et al.*: Comparison of surgical and medical group survival in patients with left main coronary artery disease: long-term CASS experience. *Circulation* 1995, 91:2325–2334.
4. Varnauskas E: Twelve-year follow-up of survival in the randomized European Coronary Surgery Study. *N Engl J Med* 1988, 319:332–337.
5. Yusof S, Zucker D, Peduzzi P, *et al.*: Effect of coronary artery bypass graft surgery on survival: overview of 10-year results from randomised trials by the Coronary Artery Bypass Graft Surgery Trials Collaboration. *Lancet* 1994, 344:563–570.
6. Caracciolo EA, Davis KB, Sopko G, *et al.*: Comparison of surgical and medical group survival in patients with left main equivalent coronary artery disease: long-term CASS experience. *Circulation* 1995, 91:2335–2344.
7. Bonchek LI, Ullyot DJ: Minimally invasive coronary bypass: a dissenting opinion. *Circulation* 1998, 98:495–497.
8. Anderson HV, Vignale SJ, Benedict CR, Willerson JR: Restenosis after coronary angioplasty. *J Intervent Cardiol* 1993, 6:189–202.
9. Bauters C, McFadden EP, Lablanche JM, *et al.*: Restenosis rate after multiple percutaneous transluminal coronary angioplasty procedures at the same site. *Circulation* 1993, 88:969–974.
10. Cohen MV, Byrne MJ, Levine B, *et al.*: Low rate of treatment of hypercholesterolemia by cardiologists in patients with suspected and proven coronary artery disease. *Circulation* 1991, 83:1294–1304.
11. Gould KL: Quantitative analysis of coronary artery restenosis after coronary angioplasty: has the rose lost its bloom? *J Am Coll Cardiol* 1992, 19:946–947.
12. Rensing BJ, Hermans WRM, Vos J, *et al.*: Luminal narrowing after percutaneous transluminal coronary angioplasty. *Circulation* 1993, 88:975–985.
13. Hirschfeld JW, Schwartz JS, Jugo R, *et al.*: Restenosis after coronary angioplasty: a multivariate model to relate lesions and procedure variables to restenosis. *J Am Coll Cardiol* 1991, 18:647–656.
14. King SB, Lembo NJ, Weintraub WS, *et al.*: A randomized trial comparing coronary angioplasty with coronary bypass surgery: Emory Angioplasty versus Surgery Trial. *N Engl J Med* 1994, 331:1044–1050.
15. Weintraub WS, Mauldin PD, Becker E, *et al.*: A comparison of the costs of and quality of life after coronary angioplasty or coronary surgery for multivessel coronary artery disease. *Circulation* 1995, 92:2831–2840.
16. Appelman YE, Piek JJ, Strikwerda S, *et al.*: Randomized trial of excimer laser angioplasty versus balloon angioplasty for treatment of obstructive coronary artery disease. *Lancet* 1996, 347:79–84.
17. Strikwerda S, Montauban van Swijndregt E, Foley DP, *et al.*: Immediate and late outcome of excimer laser and balloon coronary angioplasty: a quantitative angiographic comparison based on matched lesions. *J Am Coll Cardiol* 1995, 26:939–946.
18. Serruys PW, de Jaegere P, Kiemeneij F, *et al.*: A comparison of balloon-expandable-stent implantation with balloon angioplasty in patients with coronary artery disease. *N Engl J Med* 1994, 331:489–495.
19. Fischman DL, Leon MB, Baim DS, *et al.*: A randomized comparison of coronary-stent placement and balloon angioplasty in the treatment of coronary artery disease. *N Engl J Med* 1994, 331:496–501.
20. Cohen DJ, Krumholz HM, Sukin CA, *et al.*: In-hospital and one-year economic outcomes after coronary stenting or balloon angioplasty: results from a randomized clinical trial. Stent Restenosis Study Investigators. *Circulation* 1995, 92:2480–2487.
21. Hlatky MA: Analysis of costs associated with CABG and PTCA. *Ann Thorac Surg* 1996, 61:S30–S34.
22. Sherman DL, Ryan TJ: Coronary angioplasty versus bypass grafting: cost–benefit considerations. *Med Clin North Am* 1995, 79:1085–1095.
23. Ambrose JA, Tannenbaum MA, Alexopoulos D, *et al.*: Angiographic progression of coronary artery disease and the development of myocardial infarction. *J Am Coll Cardiol* 1988, 12:56–62.
24. Brown BG, Zhao XQ, Sacco DE, Albers JJ: Lipid lowering and plaque regression: new insights into prevention of plaque disruption and clinical events in coronary artery disease. *Circulation* 1993, 87:1781–1791.

25. Fuster V, Badimon L, Badimon JJ, Chesebro JH: The pathogenesis of coronary artery disease and the acute coronary syndromes. *N Engl J Med* 1992, 326:242–318.
26. Richardson PD, Davies MJ, Born GVR: Influence of plaque configuration and stress distribution on fissuring of coronary atherosclerotic plaques. *Lancet* 1989, 2:941–944.
27. van der Wal AC, Becker AE, van der Loos CM, Das PK: Site of intimal rupture or erosion of thrombosed coronary atherosclerotic plaques is characterized by an inflammatory process irrespective of the dominant plaque morphology. *Circulation* 1994, 89:6–44.
28. Casino PR, Kilcoyne CM, Quyyumi AA, et al.: Investigation of decreased availability of nitric oxide precursor as the mechanism responsible for impaired endothelium-dependent vasodilation in hypercholesterolemic patients. *J Am Coll Cardiol* 1994, 23:844–850.
29. Chilian WM, Dellsperger KC, Layne SM, et al.: Effects of atherosclerosis on the coronary microcirculation. *Am J Physiol* 1990, 258:H529–H539.
30. Harrison DG: Endothelial dysfunction in the coronary microcirculation: a new clinical entity or an experimental finding? *J Clin Invest* 1993, 91:1–2.
31. Harrison DG, Armstrong ML, Freiman PC, Heistad DD: Restoration of endothelium-dependent relaxation by dietary treatment of atherosclerosis. *J Clin Invest* 1987, 80:1801–1811.
32. Kuo L, Davis MJ, Cannon S, Chilian WM: Pathophysiological consequences of atherosclerosis extend into the coronary microcirculation: Restoration of endothelium-dependent responses by l-arginine. *Circ Res* 1992, 70:465–476.
33. Reddy KG, Nair RV, Sheehan HM, Hodgson JM: Evidence that selective endothelial dysfunction may occur in the absence of angiographic or ultrasound atherosclerosis in patients with risk factors for atherosclerosis. *J Am Coll Cardiol* 1994, 23:833–843.
34. Treasure CB, Klein JL, Weintraub WS, et al.: Beneficial effects of cholesterol-lowering therapy on the coronary endothelium in patients with coronary artery disease. *N Engl J Med* 1995, 332:481–487.
35. Uren NG, Marraccini P, Gistri R, et al.: Altered coronary vasodilator reserve and metabolism in myocardium subtended by normal arteries in patients with coronary artery disease. *J Am Coll Cardiol* 1993, 22:650–658.
36. Scandinavian Simvastatin Survival Study Group: Randomized trial of cholesterol-lowering in 4444 patients with coronary heart disease: The Scandinavian Simvastatin Survival Study. *Lancet* 1994, 344:1383–1389.
37. Blankenhorn DH: Angiographic trials testing the efficacy of cholesterol lowering in reducing progression or inducing regression of coronary atherosclerosis. *Coron Artery Dis* 1991, 2:875–879.
38. Blankenhorn DH, Nessim SA, Johnson RL, et al.: Beneficial effects of combined colestipol-niacin therapy on coronary atherosclerosis and coronary venous bypass grafts. *JAMA* 1987, 257:3233–3240.
39. Brown GB, Albers JJ, Fisher LD, et al.: Niacin or lovastatin combined with colestipol regresses coronary atherosclerosis and prevents clinical events in men with elevated apolipoprotein B. *N Engl J Med* 1990, 323:1289–1298.
40. Buchwald H, Varco RI, Matts JP, et al.: Effect of partial ileal bypass surgery on mortality and morbidity from coronary heart disease in patients with hyperlipidemia. *N Engl J Med* 1990, 323:946–955.
41. Cashin-Hemphill L, Mack WJ, Pogoda JM, :Beneficial effects of colestipol-niacin on coronary atherosclerosis. *JAMA* 1990, 264:3013–3017.
42. Gould KL, Ornish D, Kirkeeide R, et al.: Improved stenosis geometry by quantitative coronary arteriography after vigorous risk factor modification. *Am J Cardiol* 1992, 69:845–853.
43. Haskell WL, Alderman EL, Fair JM, et al.: Effects of intensive multiple risk factor reduction on coronary atherosclerosis and clinical cardiac events in men and women with coronary artery disease: The Stanford Coronary Risk Intervention Project (SCRIP). *Circulation* 1994, 89:975–990.
44. Kane JP, Malloy MJ, Ports TA, et al.: Regression of coronary atherosclerosis during treatment of familial hypercholesterolemia with combined drug regimens. *JAMA* 1990, 264:3007–3012.
45. National Cholesterol Education Program: Second report of the expert panel on detection, evaluation, and treatment of high blood cholesterol in adults (adult treatment panel II). *Circulation* 1994, 89:1329–1445.
46. Schuler G, Hambrecht R, Schlierf G, et al.: Regular physical exercise and low-fat diet: effects on progression of coronary artery disease. *Circulation* 1992, 86:1–11.
47. Schuler G, Hambrecht R, Schlierf G, et al.: Myocardial perfusion and regression of coronary artery disease in patients on a regimen of intensive physical exercise and low-fat diet. *J Am Coll Cardiol* 1992, 19:34–42.
48. Singh RB, Rastogi SS, Verna R, et al.: Randomised controlled trial of cardioprotective diet in patients with recent acute myocardial infarction: results of one-year follow-up. *Br Med J* 1992, 304:1015–1019.
49. Watts GF, Lewis B, Brunt JN, et al.: Effects on coronary artery disease of lipid-lowering diet, or diet plus cholestyramine, in the St. Thomas Atherosclerosis Regression Study (STARS). *Lancet* 1992, 339:563–569.
50. Shepard J, Cobbe SM, Ford I, et al.: Prevention of coronary heart disease with pravastatin in men with hypercholesterolemia: West of Scotland Coronary Prevention Study. *N Engl J Med* 1995, 333:1301–1307.
51. Downs JR, Clearfield M, Weis S, et al.: Primary prevention of acute coronary events with lovastatin in men and women with average cholesterol levels. *JAMA* 1998, 279:1615–1622.
52. Newman TB, Hulley SB: Carcinogenicity of lipid-lowering drugs. *JAMA* 1996, 275:55–60.
53. Ornish D, Brown SE, Scherwitz LW, et al.: Can lifestyle changes reverse coronary heart disease?: The Lifestyle Heart Trial. *Lancet* 1990, 336:129–133.
54. Gould KL, Ornish D, Scherwitz L, et al.: Changes in myocardial perfusion abnormalities by positron emission tomography after long-term intense risk factor modification. *JAMA* 1995, 274:894–901.
55. Denke MA: Diet and lifestyle modification and its relationship to atherosclerosis. *Med Clin North Am* 1994, 78:197–223.
56. Aronow WS: Cardiac risk factors: still important in the elderly. *Geriatrics* 1990, 45:71–80.
57. Carroll JF, Pollack ML: Rehabilitation and life-style modification in the elderly. *Cardiovasc Clin* 1992, 22:209–227.
58. Kannel WB: Epidemiology of cardiovascular disease in the elderly: an assessment of risk factors. *Cardiovasc Clin* 1992, 22:9–22.
59. Hunninghake DB, Stein EA, Dujovne CA, et al.: The efficacy of intensive dietary therapy alone or combined with lovastatin in outpatients with hypercholesterolemia. *N Engl J Med* 1993, 328:1213–1219.
60. Haft JI: Role of blood platelets in coronary artery disease. *Am J Cardiol* 1979, 43:1197–1206.
61. Friedman M, Rosenman RH, Byers SO: Serum lipids and conjunctival circulation after fat ingestion in men exhibiting Type A behavior pattern. *Circulation* 1964, 29:874–886.
62. Stuart MJ, Gerrard JM, White JG: Effects of cholesterol on production of thromboxane B_2 by platelets in vitro. *N Engl J Med* 1980, 302:6–10.
63. Zmuda A, Dembinska-Kiec A, Chytkowski A, Gryglewski RJ: Experimental atherosclerosis in rabbits. *Prostaglandins* 1977, 14:1035–1043.

64. Duthie GG, Wahle KWJ, James WP: Oxidants, antioxidants, and cardiovascular disease. *Nutr Res Rev* 1989, 32:51–62.
65. Steinberg D, Berliner JA, Burton GW, *et al.*: Antioxidants in the prevention of human atherosclerosis: summary of the proceedings of a National Heart, Lung, and Blood Institute Workshop; Bethesda, Maryland. *Circulation* 1991, 85:2338–2345.
66. Ascherio A, Willett WC, Rimm EB, *et al.*: Dietary iron intake and risk of coronary disease among men. *Circulation* 1994, 89:969–1994.
67. Gaziano JM, Manson JE, Buring JE, Hennekens CH: Dietary antioxidants and cardiovascular disease. *Ann NY Acad Sci* 1992, 669:249–259.
68. Ripsin CM, Keenan JM, Jacobs DR, *et al.*: Oat products and lipid lowering: a meta-analysis. *JAMA* 1992, 267:3317–3325.
69. Haskell WL, Spiller GA, Jensen CD, *et al.*: Role of water-soluble dietary fiber in the management of elevated plasma cholesterol in healthy subjects. *Am J Cardiol* 1992, 69:433–439.
70. Anderson JW, Garrity TF, Wood CL, *et al.*: Prospective, randomized, controlled comparison of the effects of low-fat and low-fat plus high fiber diets on serum lipid concentrations. *Am J Clin Nutr* 1992, 56:887–894.
71. Zock P, Katan MB: Hydrogenation alternatives: effects of trans fatty acids and stearic acid versus linoleic acid on serum lipids and lipoproteins in humans. *J Lipid Res* 1992, 33:399–410.
72. Malinow MR: Hyperhomocystinemia: a common and easily reversible risk factor for atherosclerosis. *Circulation* 1991, 81:2004–2006.
73. Anderson JW: Plant fiber and blood pressure. *Ann Intern Med* 1983, 98:842.
74. Armstrong BK, Brown JB, Clarke HT, *et al.*: Diet and reproductive hormones: a study of vegetarian and non-vegetarian postmenopausal women. *J Nat Cancer Inst* 1981, 67:761–767.
75. Brenner BM, Meyer TW, Hostetter TH: Dietary protein intake and the progressive nature of kidney disease. *N Engl J Med* 1982, 307:652–659.
76. Castelli WP: Epidemiology of coronary heart disease: the Framingham study. *Am J Med* 1984, 76:4–12.
77. Ellis FR, Montigriffo VME: Veganism, clinical findings and investigations. *Am J Clin Nutr* 1970, 23:249–255.
78. Ernst E, Pietsch L, Matrai A, Eisenberg J: Blood rheology in vegetarians. *Br Med J* 1987, 294:180.
79. Goldin BR, Adlercreutz H, Gorbach SL, *et al.*: Estrogen excretion patterns and plasma levels in vegetarian and omnivorous women. *N Engl J Med* 1982, 307:1542–1547.
80. Graham S, Haughey B, Marshall J, *et al*: Diet in the epidemiology of carcinoma of the prostate gland. *J Nat Cancer Inst* 1992, 70:687–692.
81. Hardinge MG, Stare FJ: Nutritional studies of vegetarians. *Am J Clin Nutr* 1954, 2:73–82.
82. Marsh AG, Sanchez TV, Mickelsen O, *et al.*: Cortical bone density of adult lacto-ovo-vegetarian and omnivorous women. *J Am Diet Assoc* 1980, 76:148–151.
83. Melby CL, Hyner GC, Zoog B: Blood pressure in vegetarians and nonvegetarians. *Nutr Res* 1985, 5:1077–1082.
84. Schultz Y, Flatt JP, Jequier E: Failure of dietary fat intake to promote fat oxidation: a factor favoring the development of obesity. *Am J Clin Nutr* 1989, 50:307–314.
85. Skoldstam L: Fasting and vegan diet in rheumatoid arthritis. *Scand J Rheumatol* 1986, 15:219–223.
86. Berlin JA, Colditz GA: A meta-analysis of physical activity in the prevention of coronary heart disease. *Am J Epidemiol* 1990, 132:612–628.
87. Powell KE, Thompson PD, Caspersen CJ, Kendrick JS: Physical activity and the incidence of coronary heart disease. *Ann Rev Public Health* 1987, 8:253–287.
88. O'Connor TP, Roebuck BD, Peterson FJ, *et al.*: Effect of dietary omega-3 and omega-6 fatty acids on development of azaserine-induced preneoplastic lesions in rat pancreas. *J Nat Cancer Inst* 1989, 81:858–863.
89. Hambrecht R, Niebauer J, Marburger C, *et al.*: Various intensities of leisure time physical activity in patients with coronary artery disease: effects on cardiorespiratory fitness and progression of coronary atherosclerotic lesions. *J Am Coll Cardiol* 1993, 22:468–477.
90. Gardner AW, Poehlman ET: Exercise rehabilitation programs for the treatment of claudication pain. *JAMA* 1995, 274:975–980.
91. Booth-Kewley S, Friedman HS: Psychological predictors of heart disease: a quantitative review. *Psychol Bull* 1987, 101:343–362.
92. Scherwitz L, Perkins L, Chesney M, *et al.*: Hostility and health behaviors in young adults: the Cardia study. *Am J Epidemiol* 1992, 136:136–145.
93. Siegler IC, Peterson BL, Barefoot JC, Williams RB: Hostility during late adolescence predicts coronary risk factors at mid-life. *Am J Epidemiol* 1992, 136:146–154.
94. Shuster JL, Stern TA, Tesar GD: Psychological problems and their management. In *Rehabilitation of the Coronary Patient* edn 3. Edited by Wenger NK, Hellerstein HK. New York: Churchill Livingstone; 1992:483–510.
95. Wenger NK, Froelicher ES, Smith LK, *et al.*: *Cardiac Rehabilitation*. Clinical Practice Guideline No. 17, AHCPR Publication No. 96-0672. Rockville, MD: US Department of Health and Human Services, Public Health Service, Agency for Health Care Policy and Research and the National Heart, Lung, and Blood Institute; 1995.
96. Carney RM, Freedland KE, Eisen SA, *et al.*: Major depression and medication adherence in elderly patients with coronary artery disease. *Health Psychol* 1995, 14:88–90.
97. Frasure-Smith N, Lesperance F, Talajic M: Depression and 18-month prognosis after myocardial infarction. *Circulation* 1995, 91:999–1005.
98. Frasure-Smith N, Lesperance F, Talajic M: Depression following myocardial infarction: impact on 6-month survival. *JAMA* 1993, 270:1819–1825.
99. Determinants of Myocardial Infarction Onset Study Investigators: Triggering of acute myocardial infarction onset by episodes of anger. *Circulation* 1995, 92:1720–1725.
100. Kawachi I, Sparrow D, Vokonas PS, Weiss ST: Symptoms of anxiety and risk of coronary heart disease. *Circulation* 1994, 90:2225–2229.
101. Orth-Gomer K, Rosengren A, Wilhelmsen L: Lack of social support and incidence of coronary heart disease in middle-aged Swedish men. *Psychosom Med* 1993, 55:37–43.
102. Orth-Gomer K, Unden AL, Edwards ME: Social isolation and mortality in ischemic heart disease. *Acta Medica Scand* 1998, 224:205–215.
103. Ruberman W, Weinblatt E, Goldberg JD, Chaudhary BS: Psychosocial influences on mortality after myocardial infarction. *N Engl J Med* 1984, 311:552–559.
104. Williams RB, Barefoot JC, Califf RM, *et al.*: Prognostic importance of social and economic resources among medically treated patients with angiographically documented coronary artery disease. *JAMA* 1992, 267:520–524.
105. Kaplan GA: Social contacts and ischaemic heart disease. *Ann Clin Res* 1988, 20:131–136.
106. Jenkinson CM, Madeley RJ, Mitchell JR, Turner ID: The influence of psychosocial factors on survival after myocardial. *Public Health* 1993, 107:305–317.
107. Deffenbacher JL: Cognitive-relaxation and social skills treatments of anger: a year later. *J Counsel Psychol* 1988, 35:234–236.
108. Deffenbacher JL: Anger reduction: issues, assessment, and intervention strategies. In *Anger, Hostility, and the Heart*. Edited by Siegman AW, Smith TW. Hillsdale, New Jersey: Lawrence Erlbaum; 1994.

109. Deffenbacher JL: Relaxation and cognitive-relaxation treatments of general anger. *J Counsel Psychol* 1992, 39:158–167.
110. Moon JR, Eisler RM: Anger control: an experimental comparison of three behavioral treatments. *Behav Ther* 1983, 14:493–505.
111. Linden W, Stossel C, Maurice J: Psychosocial interventions for patients with coronary artery disease. *Arch Intern Med* 1996, 156:745–752.
112. Billings J, Scherwitz L, Ornish D, Sullivan R: Lifestyle heart trial: comprehensive treatment and group support therapy. In *Heart and Mind: The Practice of Cardiac Psychology*. Edited by Allan R, Scheidt S. Washington DC: American Psychological Association; 1996: 342–364.
113. Ornish D: *Love & Survival*. New York: HarperCollins; 1998.
114. Deanfield JE, Shea M, Kensett M, *et al.*: Silent myocardial ischaemia due to mental stress. *Lancet* 1984, 2:1001–1005.
115. Oliva PB: Pathophysiology of acute myocardial infarction. *Ann Intern Med* 1981, 94:236–250.
116. Schiffer F, Hartley LH, Schulman CL, Abelman WH: Evidence for emotionally induced coronary arterial spasm in patients with angina pectoris. *Br Heart J* 1980, 44:62–66.
117. Ornish D, Brown S, Billings S, *et al.*: Can lifestyle changes reverse coronary atherosclerosis?: four-year results of the Lifestyle Heart Trial. *Circulation* 1993, 88(suppl):I-7–I-87.
118. Ornish D, Gotto AM, Miller RR, *et al.*: Effects of a vegetarian diet and selected yoga techniques in the treatment of coronary heart disease. *Clin Res* 1979, 27:720A.
119. Ornish DM, Scherwitz LW, Doody RS, *et al.*: Effects of stress management training and dietary changes in treating ischemic heart disease. *J Am Med Assoc* 1983, 249:54–59.
120. Dhanaraj VH, Singh M: *Effects of yoga relaxation and transcendental meditation on metabolic rate*. Paper presented to the First Canadian Congress for Multi-Disciplinary Study of Sport and Physical Activity. Montreal, Quebec, Canada; 1973.
121. Patel C, Marmot MG, Terry DJ, *et al.*: Trial of relaxation in reducing coronary risk: four-year follow-up. *Br Med J* 1985, 290:1103–1106.
122. Gopal KS, Anantharaman V, Nishit SD, Bhatnagar OP: The effect of Yogasan on muscular tone and cardio-respiratory adjustment. *Yoga Life* 1975, 6:3–11.
123. Vahia N, Vinekar S, Doongaji D: Some ancient Indian concepts in the treatment of psychiatric disorders. *Br J Psych* 1966, 112:1089–1096.
124. Secondary Prevention Panel: Preventing heart attack and death in patients with coronary disease. *Circulation* 1995, 92:2–4.
125. Angell M, Kassirer JP: Alternative medicine: the risks of untested and unregulated remedies. *N Engl J Med* 1998; 339:839–841.

Complementary Therapy in HIV Disease: Living Long and Living Well

Mary Lou Galantino

Staggering achievements have been made in the science of AIDS etiology, pathogenesis, and in the development of a series of antiretroviral drugs capable of lowering viral replication to undetectable levels in peripheral blood samples. March, 1996 was a turning point, when triple combination therapy, including protease inhibitors, became the mode of conventional treatment. Long-term survival with HIV disease became an even more definitive reality. But what about those who also incorporated complementary/alternative medicine (CAM) into this "long-term survival" equation? What perspectives on quality of life were gleaned from individuals who engaged in conventional medicine or CAM or both? What evidence supports the efficacy of these complementary interventions? Over the last decade, both the philosophy and some of the technology of CAM have been mainstreamed and incorporated into the health-care system.

Manual therapy, such as massage, acupuncture, and various other hands-on techniques have been reported to decrease pain, improve body awareness, enhance flexibility, and foster greater connection to one's emotional state. Exercise is a good example of a proven behavioral medical intervention that demands establishing new partnerships across various disciplines. Movement therapies can be potential sources of alternative exercise interventions, such as tai chi, yoga, and qigong. This chapter presents a few of the CAM interventions that are currently used by several people living long and living well with HIV disease.

ADDRESSING PAIN SYNDROMES THROUGH COMPLEMENTARY INTERVENTIONS

Advances in the medical management of HIV disease have increased life expectancy of those afflicted. Addressing quality of life becomes increasingly important in all dimensions of work and activities of daily living. Therefore, pain management should be integrated into the total care of patients with HIV disease [1]. The prevalence of pain in HIV-infected individuals varies with the stage of disease but generally ranges from 25% to 80%, with the prevalence of pain increasing as the disease progresses [2]. Studies suggest that approximately 25% to 30% of ambulatory HIV-infected patients with early HIV disease experience clinically significant pain [3]. People living with pain related to AIDS, like their counterparts with cancer pain, typically describe an average of two to three concurrent pains at a time [4].

Opportunistic infections and drug side effects for the treatment of HIV disease can have a direct effect on daily functional activities. Examples include peripheral neuropathy syndrome, rheumatologic complications, Kaposi's sarcoma, and various musculoskeletal alterations. Weakness, pain, and loss of range of motion caused by these conditions can lead to changes in ambulation, loss of function, and decreased quality of life [5]. The role of pain management in the care of these HIV complications may take various forms of pharmacologic and nonpharmacologic approaches.

Federal guidelines developed by the Agency for Health Care Policy and Research (AHCPR) [6] for the management of cancer pain also address pain management in

HIV/AIDS. A multidimensional model acknowledges the interaction of emotional, cognitive, cultural, and environmental aspects of pain. Optimal management of the person experiencing HIV-related pain may require a combination of pharmacologic, cognitive-behavioral, psychologic, psychotherapeutic, anesthetic, neurosurgical, and rehabilitative approaches. This section is concerned with complementary manual therapy approaches of this multimodal intervention. Some various clinical problems often presented to the health care professional are listed in Table 12-1.

The typical description of pain syndromes associated with HIV portrays a disorder that produces a multitude of pathologic changes and deficiencies of the immune system. The possible causes of most associated pain syndromes or sites are complex. The symptom of pain may be overshadowed by a constellation of other overwhelming problems, such as opportunistic infections, diarrhea, dyspnea, anorexia, weight loss, and neuropsychologic symptoms.

A careful history, physical examination, and differential diagnosis are important first steps. The etiology may be multifactorial and the mechanism of pain must be determined before treatment is rendered. Medications, diagnostic procedures, and other interventions may cause pain. Patients may have a preexisting pain syndrome unrelated to the course of HIV disease [7]. Treatment needs to be individualized and must address both pain and functional issues in the HIV-infected population [8].

The musculoskeletal concerns for people living with HIV disease can be orthopedic in nature. Often, patients with associated peripheral neuropathy may incur low back pain. Pain may not be related directly to HIV disease but rather to the aftermath of an opportunistic infection, which may result in muscle spasms and postural changes. A constellation of problems may manifest in altered gait and difficulty with transitional positions. This leads to neuromusculoskeletal dysfunction. Traction produced by postural dysfunction on the sensory nerve elements within the connective tissue system may produce pain.

Soft tissue mobilization can include massage and myofascial release techniques (MFR). Fascial dysfunction due to a number of external and internal insults to the body can contribute to changes in health [9]. Relaxation in the tissue tension results from treatment and heat may thereby be released from the tissues. Another technique for pain management may include trigger point releases and can be included in the repertoire of manual therapy techniques. Strain and counterstrain technique, developed by Lawrence Jones [10], is a positional technique that results in decrease or arrest of inappropriate proprioceptor activity of the muscle spindle. The result of this technique is relaxation and elongation of the muscle fiber, which permits improved articular balance for increased joint mobility and range of motion.

A muscle energy technique developed by Fred Mitchell is a positional modality that facilitates correction of biomechanical dysfunction by normalizing neuromusculoskeletal balance [11]. This technique fosters normalization of the musculoskeletal system and can be taught to the person living with HIV disease for self-correction in a home program.

Visceral manipulation is a manual therapy consisting of light, gentle, specifically placed manual forces that encourage normal mobility, tone, and inherent tissue motion of the viscera and their connective tissue [12,13]. People living with HIV disease experience a host of gastrointestinal problems caused by various opportunistic infections; visceral manipulation may potentiate normal physiologic function of individual organs. These techniques ought not to be done in patients with acute infection, however. Visceral motion can be divided into four categories, according to the bodily system that influences or controls them: 1) somatic nervous system, 2) autonomic nervous system, 3) craniosacral rhythm, and 4) visceral motility.

Craniosacral therapy is a gentle, noninvasive, yet powerful and effective treatment approach that relies primarily on hands-on evaluation and treatment. The hands-on contact is extremely tender and supportive. It is accompanied by a sincere intention to assist the patient in any way possible. In short, the therapist serves primarily as a facilitator to the patient's own healing processes. The rapport that develops during the patient–therapist interaction is excellent and lends itself powerfully to the positive therapeutic effect that most patients experience. This gentle, caring approach is obviously welcomed by most people living with HIV disease [14–16].

ENERGY-BASED SYSTEMS

The field of energy medicine is diverse and ancient, predating our conventional modern Western medicine by thousands of years. Research has demonstrated that the clinician need not physically touch a recipient in order to achieve the desired effects during and following a session [17]. Reiki, a Tibetan–Japanese technique, is an example of such energetic intervention. *Noncontact Therapeutic Touch* (TT) is another modality taught in nursing schools; it was first introduced to health professionals by Dolores Krieger and Dora Kunz. A critical factor in understanding the mechanisms that underlie the effects of TT stems from studies in quantum physics. Efforts to isolate possible mechanisms responsible for relax-

TABLE 12-1. VARIOUS CLINICAL PROBLEMS PRESENTED BY PATIENTS WITH HIV DISEASE

Postural dynamics secondary to weight loss from protein calorie malnutrition
Peripheral neuropathy secondary to drug toxicity and progression of HIV disease
Myopathies secondary to medication and direct HIV involvement
Arthrosis secondary to side effects of medication
Neurologic deficits secondary to central nervous system involvement with resultant neurocognitive and functional changes
Past medical history of previous injuries that may be exacerbated during HIV disease

ation outcomes experienced by recipients of TT can be located in four main categories: 1) electromagnetic field studies, 2) pain studies, 3) stress and anxiety studies, and 4) wound healing [18]. Each of these areas have been studied and their outcomes measured. In a classic study, Krieger [19] reported a significant increase in hemoglobin values in response to therapeutic touch (treatment group) versus routine hospital care (control group). These results have implications for the HIV patient receiving zidovudine therapy who may experience side effects of anemia.

The procedure for conducting TT requires two conditions: 1) intentionality, a form of meditation and a way of calming the mind so that the practitioner is nonjudgmental and intends to help or heal and 2) assessment, performed by scanning over the person's body between 3 and 6 inches away from the skin to detect differences in temperature, electrical potential, or other perceivable sensations. The treatment is the transfer of energy occurring from the practitioner to the patient.

Patients who experience hypersensitivity due to distal sensory peripheral neuropathy can benefit by the hand-mediated energetic healing techniques when direct manual therapy techniques cannot be tolerated by the client. People living with HIV disease have explored these techniques. Because a recipient is not touched during a treatment, these aforementioned techniques cannot be explained directly by physiologic and psychologic effects of physical touch such as those described by psychoneuroimmunology. These techniques and responses suggest a twofold explanation based on electromagnetic and quantum physics and on transpersonal psychology [20].

This section focused on manual and energy-based therapies for the management of pain in patients with HIV disease. However, there are a host of manual therapy techniques beyond the scope of this chapter that can provide beneficial effects for pain management and generalized relaxation. The consumer of manual therapy interventions must understand the specific techniques used during a therapeutic session. Questioning the practitioner and experiencing the physical, psychological, and spiritual effects throughout a session foster greater understanding and future continued intervention with manual therapy.

MOVEMENT THERAPIES IN HIV DISEASE

The HIV epidemic has witnessed increasing use of alternative therapies, some more traditional than others [21]. The exploration outside the medical model has fostered investigations by the Office of Alternative Medicine at the National Institutes of Health [22]. Traditional forms of exercise, such as aerobics and weight training, are incorporated in the medical model through exercise physiology and rehabilitation. However, various movement therapies (eg, martial arts) are often viewed as less traditional and more outside the established medical model.

Substantial evidence suggests that traditional exercise, particularly aerobic exercise, can provide great physiologic and psychologic benefits for most individuals, and especially those with chronic diseases. However, the mode, duration, and intensity of many traditional standardized exercise programs may not always be entirely appropriate during chronic illness. The stage of disease and the type of illness itself may preclude these more strenuous exercise activities at various times. During such times, less traditional movement therapies may prove to be more appropriate and efficacious. In fact, movement therapy includes a number of similar constructs used in physical therapy and can be quite complementary to an individual's program of more traditional exercise.

Depending on the originating discipline of study, there are various types of movement therapy. Eastern thought perspectives dominate this area and some examples include Feldenkrais [23], qigong [24], and tai chi [25,26].

Literature Review on Exercise Studies and HIV Disease

Increases in physical fitness are often associated with improvements in certain chronic diseases, such as coronary heart disease and hypertension [27]. Evidence has shown that exercise also influences the neuroendocrine and immune systems, which results in a potential benefit to those with chronic immunodeficiency diseases [28]. Aerobic exercise training programs may enhance certain critical components of cellular immunity and also act as a buffer for the detrimental mood changes that typically accompany stress, thus providing a behavioral approach for helping HIV-infected individuals [29].

Strength and Cardiopulmonary Enhancement

It is well documented that aerobic activity can enhance the immune status and cardiopulmonary function of HIV positive individuals [29–32]. A progressive resistance exercise program for AIDS patients demonstrated improvements in strength, power, and endurance [33]. A study completed by Olsen et al. [34] found that among HIV-infected patients motivated about and capable of regular strenuous exercise, weight training may offer a salutary benefit that is superior to intense running. Outcomes measures included mean change in CD4+ level percentages over a 24-month period.

Exercise Challenges in the Traditional Mode of Exercise

The end-stage of HIV disease also begins with several years of quality living. However, this period may be replete with various opportunistic infections. Furthermore, patients may not be physically able to maintain an aerobic fitness level to sustain a significant change in the immune system. Only one study investigated the effects of aerobic activity on the moderately to severely immunocompromised AIDS-infected population [31]. Physical function in the advanced disease state varies; only 6 of 25 study subjects were able to complete the 24-week exercise program.

Most exercise studies involve people who had an early diagnosis of HIV, because minimal to no opportunistic infections are encountered by this population [29]. Because greater disability is noted in the progression of HIV disease to AIDS, an adverse impact on quality of life and functional outcomes results from advanced disease. A need exists for further research evaluating the benefits of alternative exercise programs for AIDS-infected individuals who are unable to participate in a rigorous aerobic or progressive resistance exercise program. Exercising in a group fosters various social interactions. Benefits may also be observed through physical and movement therapy interventions. Finally, as the health-care market continues to change, cost-effective measures though group-oriented intervention may better serve this population and our health-care system.

A review of available literature reveals no decline in CD+ cell counts regardless of the initial stage of disease, the level of $CD4^+$ cells, or symptomatology. There is also a trend toward increases in the number of $CD4^+$ cells in all but one study, with more significant increases seen in those patients who are at earlier stages of the disease. Homogeneous study samples are essential when investigating the effects of exercise in a dynamic disease such as HIV/AIDS [35]. From a psychoneuroimmunologic (PNI) perspective, psychological stress has been implicated among the cofactors contributing to immunologic decline in HIV disease. Evidence supports the stress management role of exercise training as a means to explain the buffering of suppressive stressor effects, thereby facilitating a return of the $CD4^+$ cells. Early intervention with exercise, in compliance with guidelines, is most prudent in order to stave off opportunistic infections throughout the spectrum of HIV disease.

MOVEMENT THERAPY

Literature on long-term survivors with AIDS is replete with anecdotal evidence linking survival to one or more of the following: holding a positive attitude toward the illness, participating in health-promoting behaviors, engaging in spiritual activities, and taking part in AIDS-related activities [36–38]. Positive relationships have been demonstrated between hardiness, perception of physical, emotional, and spiritual health, participation in exercise, and the use of special diets [39–41].

A working definition of *movement therapy* includes an array of modalities. It can take the form of a dance therapy program, a particular technique (*eg*, Feldenkrais, Alexander), or a martial art (*eg*, tai chi, qigong). Use of movement therapy has been advocated since the early 1900s. Empiric evidence for its beneficial effects on mood has accumulated slowly. Most relevant data come from studies on the effect of exercise on depression [42].

Use of Tai Chi as a Movement Modality

Eastern cultures have practiced the art of tai chi for centuries. The five schools of tai chi share three essential features: 1) the body is naturally extended and relaxed, giving priority to lissomeness; 2) the mind is tranquil but alert; and 3) body movements are slow, smooth, and well-coordinated throughout the exercise period [26].

A recent study conducted with a group of AIDS patients compared the use of traditional aerobic exercise ($n = 13$) with tai chi ($n = 13$). A control group ($n = 12$) was also included. Outcome measures included the Medical Outcomes Survey (MOS-HIV), whereas the functional measures included the functional reach, sit-up, and sit and reach tests. The physical performance test was used for general function. The MOS-HIV showed a significant greater perception of overall health after the intervention. Significant differences were demonstrated in all functional measures as compared with the controls. Both aerobic and tai chi exercise interventions benefited this group of AIDS patients [43].

Use of Yoga and Qigong as Movement Modalities

The physiologic similarities between the various movement therapies presented and the previous psychoneuroimmunologic perspectives in the traditional use of aerobic exercise must be recognized. Qigong is one of the four aspects of Chinese medicine and is a spontaneous balancing and enhancing of the natural healing resources in the human system. Three areas delineated and enhanced through the use of yoga and qigong include oxygen metabolism, the lymphatic system, and the nervous system. These systems include the use of several activities, such as breath practice, visualization, various postures, concentrated movement, self-massage, relaxation, and meditation.

Progressive relaxation and meditation have been found to alter heart rate, brain wave activity, neurotransmitter profile, skin temperature, and muscle control [44–46]. These features are an integral part of these two movement interventions and both may be influenced by voluntary control of the body's self regulating mechanisms. Moderate body movement occurring within a context of deep relaxation is common to qigong and yoga. Research on exercise, relaxed states, and other triggers of specific physiologic responses are clearly implicated as useful resources that may help build scientific information on the self-applied health maintenance methods of the Asian systems of traditional medicine [47]. Furthermore, research from Asian cultures are still being translated. The First World Conference on Academic Exchange of Medical Qigong was held in 1988 in Beijing, and 128 scientific papers must still be translated into English [48]. Qigong and yoga practice appear to activate mechanisms associated with the lymphatic system. They include lymph generation, lymph propulsion, immune function, cerebrospinal fluid circulation, and nutritive function [47].

Studies conducted on yoga are just beginning to emerge. Rehse [49] presented an experiential workshop at the International Conference on AIDS in 1992 and reported improvements in self-confidence and a return to sport activities following intervention. Applications of yoga in the rehabilitation setting are being explored for several populations, including people living with HIV-related disease [50]. Yoga and qigong have exciting applications in the management of HIV-related disease and further research is warranted to evaluate the physiologic underpinnings in various immunologic markers, physical improvements, and quality-of-life outcomes.

Precautions and Concerns During Exercise

Before beginning any exercise regimen, a differential diagnosis for pain and fatigue must be made, including anemia, low testosterone levels, or specific vitamin deficiencies. Proper caloric intake must set the standard for each type of exercise in order to meet the energy expenditure required for the activity. Seeking the advice of a nutritionist is recommended for proper guidance.

A supervised training program should be consistent with recommendations by the American College of Sports Medicine. Guidelines have been established for the spectrum of the three stages of HIV disease [35]. Exercise is safe and beneficial for most individuals with HIV disease; however, caution is warranted in Stages 2 and 3. Stage 1 (asymptomatic disease) has no limitations on maximum graded exercise testing. In this stage, all metabolic parameters are within normal limits for most individuals. In Stage 2 (symptomatic disease), exercise capacity may be reduced as may VO_2 max and O_2 pulse max levels. Heart rate reserve and breathing reserve may be elevated. Stage 3 (AIDS) presents with dramatically reduced exercise capacity, vital capacity, and VO_2 max and O_2 pulse max levels. Elevated heart rate and breathing reserve persists during this stage. Therefore, careful monitoring of the stage and various other opportunistic infections is an important factor in the comprehensive exercise management.

The quality-of-life issues of people with HIV/AIDS are becoming more complicated as more people with the disease achieve higher $CD4^+$ counts and lower viral load levels. Improvement in health status is directly related to improved effectiveness of newer treatment regimens; many individuals are improving enough to consider reentering the work force. Manual therapy, exercise, and movement therapy may augment the stress and fatigue associated with the adjustment to the workplace.

Complementary therapies as mentioned in this chapter are but a few of the many modalities available for people living with HIV disease. Other interventions include acupuncture, homeopathy, naturopathy, and psychospiritual approaches. The complementary therapy consumer must participate in outcome measurements for the enhancement of research. Careful monitoring is needed when conventional and complementary care is rendered. Further research remains necessary but the present findings are promising for living long and living well with HIV disease.

References and Recommended Reading

Recently published papers of particular interest have been highlighted as
- Of interest
- •• Of outstanding interest

1. Breitbart W, McDonald MV: Pharmacologic pain management in HIV/AIDS. *J Int Assoc Physicians AIDS Care* 1996:17–26.
2. Singer E, Zorilla C, Fahy-Crandon B, *et al.*: Painful syndromes reported for ambulatory HIV-infected men in a longitudinal study. *Pain* 1993, 5:15–19.
3. Breitbart W, Passik S, Bronaugh T: Pain in the ambulatory AIDS patient: prevalence and psychosocial correlates. In Proceedings of the 38th Annual Meeting of the Academy of Psychosomatic Medicine: Atlanta, Georgia, 1991.
4. Breitbart W, Rosenfeld B, Passik S, *et al.*: The undertreatment of pain in ambulatory AIDS patients. *Pain* 1996, 65:239–245.
5. Galantino ML, McCormack G: Pain management. In *Clinical Assessment and Treatment in HIV Disease: Rehabilitation of a Chronic Illness*. Thorofare, NJ: Slack; 1992:101–114.
6. Jacox A, Carr D, Payne R: Clinical practice guideline number 9: management of cancer pain. Washington, DC: Agency for Health Care Policy and Research; 1994:139–141. US Department of Health and Human Services Public Health Service AHCPR Publication no. 94-0592.
7. Muma RD, Boruki MJ, Ayachi S, *et al.*: Diagnosis and treatment of HIV-related conditions. In *HIV Manual for Health Care Professionals*. Edited by Muma RD, Lyons BA, Borucki MJ, *et al.* Stamford, CT: Appleton & Lange; 1997:41–70.
8. O'Dell MW, Dillon ME: Rehabilitation in adults with human immunodeficiency virus-related diseases. *Am J Phys Med Rehabil* 1993, 71:183–190.
9. Barnes J: Myofacial release: the missing link in traditional treatment. In *Complementary Therapies in Rehabilitation*. Edited by Davis C. Thorofare, NJ: Slack; 1997:21–47.
10. Jones L: *Strain and Counterstrain*. Old Westbury, NY: The American Academy of Osteopathy; 1981.
11. Weiselfish S, Kain J: Introduction to developmental manual therapy: an integrated systems approach for structural and functional rehabilitation. *Phys Ther Forum* 1990, 6:4–6.
12. Barral JP: *Visceral Manipulation*. Seattle: Eastland Press; 1987.
13. Barral JP: *Visceral Manipulation II*. Seattle: Eastland Press; 1989.
14. Upledger JE: Thermographic view of autism. *Osteopath Ann* 1983; 118:356–359.
15. Upledger JE: *CranioSacral Therapy II*. Seattle: Eastland Press; 1987.
16. Upledger JE: *SomatoEmotional Release and Beyond*. Palm Beach Gardens: UI Publishing; 1990.
17. Quinn JF: Therapeutic touch as energy exchange: testing the theory. *Adv Nurs Sci* 1984, 6:42–49.
18. Quinn JF: Building a body of knowledge: research on therapeutic touch 1974-1986. *J Holistic Nurs* 1988, 6:37–45.
19. Krieger D: Healing by the "laying on" of hands as a facilitator of bioenergetic change: the response on in-vivo human hemoglobin. *Psychoenergetic Syst* 1979, 1:121–129.
20. Slater VE: Healing touch. In *Fundamentals of Complementary and Alternative Medicine*. Edited by Micozzi M. Philadelphia: Churchill-Livingston; 1996:121–136.
21. Sande MA, Volberding PA: Alternative therapies in HIV. In *Medical Management of AIDS* edn 4. Edited by Sande MA, Volberding PA. Philadelphia: WB Saunders; 1995:25–30.
22. Office of Alternative Medicine: *Functional Description of the Office*. Bethesda, MD: National Institutes of Health; 1993.
23. Jackson O, Gula D, Kire A, Steeves M: *Effects of Feldenkrais Practitioner Training on Motor Abilities: A Video Analysis*. Platform Presentation. Denver, CO: APTA Annual Conference; 1992.
24. Kastner M, Burroughs H: *Alternative Healing: The Complete A-Z Guide to over 160 Different Alternative Therapies*. La Mesa, CA: Halcyon Publishing; 1993.
25. Belyea C: T'ai chi ch'uan. In *A Visual Encyclopedia of Unconventional Medicine*. Edited by Hill A. New York: Crown Publishers; 1978: 10–15.
26. Cheng MC: *Tai Chi: The Supreme Ultimate Exercise for Health, Sport, and Self-Defense*. New York: Prentice Hall; 1986.
27. American College of Sports Medicine: *Guidelines for Exercise Testing and Prescription* edn 5. Philadelphia: Lea & Febiger; 1995:121–158.
28. Mackinnon LT: Clinical implications of exercise. In *Exercise and Immunology*. (Current Issues in Exercise Science Series—Monograph Number 2). Champaign, IL: Human Kinetics; 1992:77–84.
29. LaPerriere A, Fletcher MA, Antoni MH, *et al.*: Aerobic exercise training in an AIDS risk group. *Int J Sports Med* 1991, 12(suppl):S53–S57.

30. LaPerriere A, Ironson G, Antoni MH, *et al.*: Exercise and immunology. *Med Sci Sports Exercise* 1994, 26:182–190.
31. MacArthur RD, Levine SD, Birk TJ: Supervised exercise training improves cardiopulmonary fitness in HIV-infected persons. *Med Sci Sports Exercise* 1992, 25:684–688.
32. Birk T, MacArthur R: Chronic exercise training maintains previously obtained cardiopulmonary fitness in patients seropositive for human immunodeficiency virus type 1. *Sports Med Training Rehabil* 1994, 5:1–6.
33. Spence DW, Galantino ML, Mossberg KA, Zimmerman SO: Progressive resistance exercise: effect on muscle function and anthropometry of a select AIDS population. *Arch Phys Med Rehabil* 1990, 71:644–648.
34. Olsen PE, Wallace MR, Carl M: $CD4^+$ correlates of weight training in HIV-seropositive outpatients. *Natl Con Hum Retroviruses Relat Infect (2nd)* 1995:155.
35. LaPerriere A, Klimas N, Major P, Perry A: Acquired immune deficiency syndrome. In *ASCM's Exercise Management for Persons with Chronic Disease and Disabilities*. Edited by Durstine LJ. Champaign, IL: Human Kinetics; 1997:132–136.
36. Kendall J: Promoting wellness in HIV-support groups. *J Assoc Nurses AIDS Care* 1992, 3:28–38.
37. Lutgendorf S, Antoni MH, Schneiderman N, Fletcher MA: Psychosocial counseling to improve quality of life in HIV infection. *Patient Educ Counseling* 1994, 24:217–235.
38. Nunes JA., Raymond SJ, Nicholas PK, Leuner J: Social support, quality of life, immune function, and health in persons living with HIV. *J Holistic Nurs* 1995, 12:174–198.
39. Belcher AE, Dettmore D, Holzemer SP: Spirituality and sense of well-being in persons with AIDS. *Holistic Nurs Prac* 1989, 3:16–25.
40. Kendall J: Wellness spirituality in homosexual men with HIV infection. *J Assoc Nurses AIDS Care* 1994, 5:28–34.
41. Carson VB: Prayer, meditation, exercise and special diets: behaviors of the hardy person with HIV/AIDS. *J Assoc Nurses AIDS Care* 1993, 4:18–28.
42. Lyons S, Pope M: Constructs in motion. In *Normalities and Abnormalities in Human Movement: Medicine and Science in Sports* vol 26. Edited by Kirkcaldy B. New York: Karger; 1989:147–165.
43. Galantino ML, Findley T, Krafft L, *et al.*: Blending traditional and alternative strategies for rehabilitation: measuring functional outcomes and quality of life issues in an AIDS population: the 8th World Congress of International Rehabilitation Medicine Association. Kyoto, Japan: Monduzzi Editore; 1997:713–716.
44. Benson H: *The Relaxation Response*. New York: Morrow; 1975.
45. Krippner S, Villoldo A: *The Realms of Healing*. Berkeley, CA: Celestial Arts Press; 1976.
46. Green E, Green A: *Beyond Biofeedback*. New York: Delacorte Press; 1977.
47. Jahnke R: Physiological mechanisms operating in the human system during the practice of qigong and pranayama. In *The Most Profound Medicine*. Edited by Jahnke R. Santa Barbara, CA: Health Action Publishers; 1996:135–157.
48. Collected Proceedings: The First World Conference for the Academic Exchange of Medical Qigong. Beijing, China, 1998.
49. Rehse A: Body movement workshop for people with HIV/AIDS [abstract no Pub 7464]. International Conference on AIDS, Amsterdam, 1992.
50. Telles S, Naveen KV: Yoga for rehabilitation: an overview. *Ind J Med Sci* 1997, 51:123–127.

Insurance Coverage for Alternative Therapies

John Weeks

OVERVIEW

This chapter looks at the movement in the insurance industry toward coverage of complementary and alternative medicine (CAM). The first section looks at consumer interests and other forces shaping CAM coverage, followed by a necessarily impressionistic examination of the current extent of coverage offered by insurers and health-care plans. In the third section, models for inclusion or coverage are examined. The chapter concludes with a comment on the two overall coverage strategies that define the intentions of the current effort at integration. One paradigm may best be called CAM-grafting, a process by which a few discrete CAM therapies are added to conventional practice. In another model, CAM is viewed as a distinct method of care that prompts a significant question for American medicine: How do we create health?

FORCES BEHIND THE COVERAGE MOVEMENT

Consumer Interest

Many health-care plans and delivery systems that have been pioneering development of CAM products and services over the past few years began by polling consumers or members. The many purposes for these surveys include gaining an understanding of a specific market; proving to reluctant executives that demand exists; relating local data to national trends; and focusing development of CAM programs to meet identified interests. Interest, clearly strong, is growing dramatically. The most recent survey, from Stanford/American Specialty Health Plans [1], found that 69% of respondents had used some CAM in the previous year. Table 13-1 [2–6] provides some results from consumer surveys on CAM from diverse service areas.

A health maintenance organization (HMO), insurer, or health-care system weighing an investment in CAM might wish to ascertain that use of the adopted therapy will not quickly fade. Evidence suggests that such a concern is not warranted. A notable finding common across these surveys is that interest in potential use is uniformly higher than actual use. The Landmark Healthcare survey [4], for instance, found that over 70% of respondents were "likely to use" chiropractic (73%), massage (80%), herbal medicine (75%), and vitamin therapy (80%). A 1996 survey by Providence GoodHealth Plan [7] found that 40% of members were interested in having access to acupuncture, 50% in naturopathic medicine, and 56% in chiropractic. Significant openness to CAM suggests that interest exists beyond current levels of use. A task force on alternative medicine impaneled by the large health-care supplier Columbia HCA used a series of focus groups to measure the depth of the CAM movement. The committee chair reported the task force's early finding: "This has staying power. People are saying it works. It's not a fad" [8].

Consumer Choice and Covered Complementary and Alternative Medicine Benefits

Some queries in these surveys asked members or potential customers several focused, insurance-related questions. Blue Cross Blue Shield of Colorado, in its exploration for a policy designed for senior citizens, discovered that the top two CAM therapies of interest to this group were chiropractic and acupuncture [6]. Kaiser members in Northern California ranked chiropractic and acupuncture in the one and three spots, respectively, with massage ranking second as a desired covered service [3].

These studies suggest that, for significant numbers of CAM users, their choice of health-care policies may be influenced by whether the insurer covers CAM therapies. Nearly three fourths (71%) of respondents to a survey by Baptist St. Vincent Health System (BSVHS) of Jacksonville, Florida, stated that inclusion of CAM would positively influence their decision making (Personal communication, Joseph DeNucci, Jacksonville, FL, 1998). This finding is nearly identical to that found by Landmark Healthcare (67%) [4] when it posed a similar question in a national survey. Among BSVHS respondents, 41% said they would pay more for a policy that included CAM. The corresponding finding in Landmark's national survey was 35% [4]. HMOs and health-care insurers might thus conclude that, for a significant group of CAM users, adding an additional premium ("rider") to cover CAM would not be an obstacle to selling policies.

Health Plan Perspectives on Consumer Interest

This information on the growing consumer interest in CAM is reaching health-care plans at a time when diverse forces in health care are recognizing the role of the consumer when deciding on a plan. One of the forces behind this is competition. The health-care industry's corporate culture is attempting to understand and adopt a consumer-oriented, retail-like focus. CAM may be viewed by a pioneering insurer as a way to distinguish itself in the marketplace.

However, after one major plan in a given geographic area takes the lead in offering CAM, other plans will begin to see CAM coverage as a necessary step to protect against enrollment losses. This phenomenon commanded closer attention in California in the spring of 1997 when, in the period of a few short months, one after another of the regional and statewide HMOs began to announce acupuncture coverage benefits. United Healthcare, Lifeguard Healthcare, and Health Net were among the plans to announce optional acupuncture benefits. Enrolling a member interested in CAM may be viewed as especially enticing to the HMO or insurers, because this type of member may be viewed as the very best type of enrollee. CAM users tend to have above-average income and education and are more likely to engage in healthful practices.

The renewed interest in understanding the consumer and responding to the consumer's desires may also be viewed as an outgrowth of the American Association of Health Plans' (AAHP, the managed-care industry organization) philosophy of "partnership with patients." The HMO philosophy (if not always the HMO practice) also charges plans with "putting the patient first" [9]. A consumer who takes a more active role in health care, and the health-care plan that helps the consumer do so, are viewed as the foundation for creating optimally effective and cost-effective care. This philosophy suggests that significant patient interest in CAM should be acknowledged in some way in the plan's activity, if not in its benefit structure.

Accreditation standards for health-care plans create avenues for consumer input in policy, and therefore on medical alternatives. The "patient" becomes a "member" of the HMO. Standards require health-care plans to guarantee their members certain rights and responsibilities. Members must be surveyed for their input and involved in certain processes. This

TABLE 13-1. DATA FROM NINE SURVEYS ON CONSUMER USE OF COMPLEMENTARY AND ALTERNATIVE MEDICINE IN THE UNITED STATES

Surveyor	Year	Scope	Survey Type	CAM use, % (duration)
Eisenberg et al. [2]	1990	National	Telephone	34 (1 year)
The Alternare Group*	1994	Portland, OR	Telephone	35 (2 years)
Oxford Health Plans†	1995–1996	CT, NY, NJ	Telephone (plan members)	33 (2 years)
Presbyterian Healthcare System‡	1996	NM	Telephone	33 (1 year)
Kaiser Northern California [3]	1996	Northern CA	Mail	31 (1 year)
Landmark Healthcare [4]	1997	National	Telephone	42 (1 year)
Eisenberg et al. [5]	1997	National	Telephone	42 (1 year)
Stanford University/ASHP [1]	1998	National	Telephone	69 (1 year)
Blue Cross Blue Shield of Colorado [6]	1998	CO	Telephone (senior citizens)	48 (1 year)

*Commercial survey; The Alternare Group, Portland, OR
†Commercial survey; Oxford Health Plans, Norwalk, CT
‡Commercial survey; Presbyterian Healthcare System, Rio Rancho, NM
ASHP—American Specialty Health Plans; CAM—complementary and alternative medicine.

enhanced philosophic respect for the consumer is underwriting plan surveys on CAM and may reasonably be expected to affect the role of CAM in future coverage decisions by health-care suppliers.

Mandates: Consumers Provide Grassroots Backing for Complementary and Alternative Medicine Profession Initiatives

Another key motivator for CAM inclusion is the legislated mandate. Over 40 states have mandates regarding provision of some chiropractic services, eight states mandate for acupuncture coverage, and three mandate for coverage of naturopathic medical services. Although the legislative lobby behind these mandates is often composed of organized chiropractors, acupuncturists, or other CAM health-care professionals, their campaigns are usually linked to grass-roots lobbying efforts among the consumers of their services. These mandates may then be appropriately viewed as expressions of consumer demand as mediated by both the CAM professional organizations and the elected officials.

The most influential mandate in the CAM integration experience is a sweeping measure in the state of Washington that took effect in 1996, which requires health-care plans to include all provider categories. This includes massage practitioners, chiropractors, naturopathic physicians, acupuncturists, and direct-entry licensed midwives. The state has been called the "epicenter" of CAM integration experience, partly as a result of subsequent experience [10]. Following the mandate, the state's plans discovered the relative simplicity of primary credentialing of licensed CAM providers. Some concerns over significant cost increases following CAM coverage have been allayed. For instance, actuaries working with PREMERA Blue Cross anticipated that costs might rise as high as 11% under fee-for-service plans. Actual experience in the first year was less than 1% [11]. Reported experience to date under the Washington mandate, which allowed plans to manage CAM services through such tools as provider selection and use review, has generally been reassuring to CAM integration explorers in other markets.

The Purchasers: Functionality, Productivity, and Satisfaction Outcomes

Although consumer use of CAM is of interest to insurers, only a few policy decisions are made by individual consumers. The key players in health-care purchasing are private employers and government entities. Some recent evidence suggests that both of these purchasers are either increasing their investigation of CAM or are directly expanding their covered CAM offerings.

The best data on CAM in benefits policies of private employers come from an annual survey conducted by *Business and Health* [12], a leading monthly magazine that targets human resources personnel. Chiropractic was found to be a benefit covered by over 70% of employers with more than 500 employees. For all respondents, the figure was between 55% and 60% for coverage between 1996 and 1997. However, a separate question regarding coverage of "alternative medicine" showed a significant upward trend. This category was described by the magazine's editors as including such therapies as massage, acupuncture, and relaxation techniques. For all employers, the percentage offering some coverage of CAM jumped from 8% to 16% between 1996 and 1997. Among large employers, the increase was more dramatic, from 8% to 24%. To a health-care insurer or HMO, these findings indicate that interest in CAM exists. An important segment of their potential or present client base is increasingly asking for some expansion of CAM benefits.

An upward trend in CAM interest is also emerging among the other major purchaser of health care—the federal government. Numerous purchasing-related explorations have commenced. Following Congressional action, the U.S. Department of Defense began looking at chiropractic therapy for back pain and later at mind–body programs for risk of cardiac disease [13]. In 1997, the U.S. Bureau of Primary Health Care began an examination of the potential value of CAM in services provided by the nation's community and migrant health clinics. That same year, officials of the Health Care Financing Administration initiated a pilot research project on mind–body interventions as related to cardiac disease risk. Within 6 months, the Veterans Administration (VA) authorized a $250,000 contract to examine and propose the present and future use of CAM within the entire VA system. A quiet exploration of the role of CAM in disability cases began within the Social Security Administration 6 months after the VA contract was authorized.

Although these federal government actions may not directly or immediately produce any impact on insurer activity, the potential for increased coverage of CAM may grow out of any of these initiatives. At this time, however, the only CAM routinely covered in a major federal program is a provision for up to 12 chiropractic visits for low-back pain under Medicare.

Many CAM advocates view the purchaser as the most significant factor in the emerging discussion about CAM coverage. The reasoning goes beyond mere check writing. CAM advocates suggest that cost–benefit analysis of CAM interventions may best be measured by looking at the overall costs to purchasers of a health-care strategy and not merely the medical costs [14]. Advocates believe that when factors such as productivity, absenteeism, patient satisfaction, and quality-of-life considerations are added to direct health-care costs, CAM presents its best face in a head-to-head cost comparison with conventional treatment.

Physician Perceptions

The shadow side of consumer leadership in prompting coverage decisions is that medical directors for HMOs and insurers do not tend to be these leaders. Few coverage or inclusion decisions are made because of the efforts of an HMO medical director who convinced an internal team that CAM coverage would lead to more effective or cost-effective care. CAM is generally not viewed by conventional medical directors as being valuable, for instance, in disease-management strategy or in finding cost-savings for care of prioritized medical conditions. Despite the findings of consumer polls, CAM remains a second-class adjunct to clinical care. The consumer may be viewed as the *driver* of CAM coverage decisions but in reality the consumer's role may best be described as *back-seat driving*.

Recent surveys of physicians show that interest in CAM is penetrating the conventional medical profession. A significant percentage of physicians shows interest; others are currently referring patients for some CAM services. A national survey of primary care doctors found that roughly half would use acupuncture (48.7%), relaxation techniques (47.6%), meditation (43%), hypnotherapy (48%), and massage (31%) in their practices [15]. Among Kaiser physicians in Northern California, 84% wanted the HMO to have acupuncture available to members, 63% wanted acupressure, 52% wanted chiropractic, 44% wanted massage, 80% wanted biofeedback, 57% wanted hypnosis, and 49% wanted yoga coverage [3].

Perhaps more significant are the subsets of physicians who view increased use of CAM as potentially valuable in the core business of creating more effective and cost-effective care. Over two thirds of responding physicians in the BSVHS survey from Jacksonville, Florida, ranked the following as "effective" or "very effective": chiropractic (79%), acupuncture (75%), massage (84%), meditation (69%), biofeedback (86%), and hypnosis (71%). A 1996 survey in the area around Puget Sound, Washington, by Medalia Healthcare asked primary care providers a series of specific hypothetical questions regarding the possible outcomes of greater integration of CAM into their services [16]. In that study, 39% reported that they believed better CAM integration would lead to "more effective care." Nearly one third of respondents (30%) believed appropriate CAM integration would lead to "more cost-effective care." In Jacksonville, 73% of the physicians interviewed in the BSVHS survey stated that better CAM integration could be "valuable" or "very valuable" in creating "more effective care," and 59% in creating "more cost-effective care."

Data from these surveys suggest that although physician beliefs about the core clinical value of CAM may not currently be the dominant influences in CAM benefit design, an undercurrent of belief holds that certain CAM interventions deserve a more prominent spot in the benefits hierarchy. These opinions might be expected to emerge as key factors in CAM coverage decisions as experience deepens, comfort builds, and the CAM integration process matures.

Summary of Motivators and Obstacles to Coverage

Health-care plan motivations for developing CAM benefits may be summarized as the "four Ms": mission, marketplace, mandates, and medicine. A list of factors important to plans was developed by Pelletier *et al.* [17] at Stanford University following a survey of plans and hospitals offering CAM. This list included attracting new enrollees, retaining existing enrollees, attracting distinct populations (such as Hispanic or Asian individuals who may value traditional CAM approaches like acupuncture and herbal medicine), distinguishing the plan in the marketplace; evaluating perceived or possible cost-effectiveness; providing potentially less-invasive care (with fewer adverse effects), satisfying demands from purchasers, and personal CAM therapy experience among plan executives.

Plans weighed these potential benefits against various counterbalancing influences. One major factor is the upward trend in health-care costs, which may be viewed as a disincentive to adding new benefits. Lovelace Health System pulled back on its CAM pilot due to escalation in core benefit costs when a lead purchaser stalled on adding a surcharge for new CAM services [18]. In addition, any downward trend in the general economy away from the growth that has dominated the 1990s may have a negative impact on purchaser decisions. For example, if unemployment levels begin to increase, thus providing a supply of people seeking work, employers may be less likely to add new benefits because the competition for employees would be reduced.

Research by Pelletier *et al.* [17] found the following problematic factors in CAM coverage for HMOs: the need for further research on efficacy; the cost of new benefits; internal ignorance about CAM; provider competition (mainstream versus CAM); the need for CAM standards; fear of change; and cultural biases. However, most of these obstacles may be viewed as part of the start-up process and can be resolved through increased familiarity and experience. Examination of longer-term trends—including shifts in physician education, research trends, capital investment, and CAM infrastructure development—suggests that the movement toward increased CAM coverage and integration is robust [19].

CURRENT EXTENT OF COMPLEMENTARY AND ALTERNATIVE MEDICINE INTEGRATION

By early 1999, the status of CAM integration into benefit designs in the United States may be summarized, in absolute terms, as extremely limited. In relative terms, however, compared with the polarized perspectives on CAM that prevailed through the early 1990s, a dynamic process of investigation and exploration is underway. Yet no definitive study of health-care plans and HMOs has been published that provides quantitative, detailed data on the CAM products or programs that HMOs and insurers already have in place. This absence is due to the very recent growth in CAM interest, the rapidity with which the environment is changing, and the complexity of the question. Although not yet available, HMO analyst group InterStudy reportedly asked a whole series of CAM-related questions in its late-1998 industry survey [20]. A plan that covers CAM is a difficult entity to define. Table 13-2 lists the different ways that CAM can be said, or believed, to be covered.

Given the ambiguity of what we mean by the terms *CAM* and *coverage,* the present status of CAM coverage must be presented in a somewhat impressionistic manner.

Two useful data points are from a 1996 survey by Landmark Healthcare (Sacramento, CA) of HMOs in states in which there is substantial HMO presence: 1) in the previous year, over 70% of the HMOs had seen an increase in requests for alternative medicine coverage and 2) 58% of HMOs planned to increase their CAM offerings in the subsequent 2 years. Table 13-3 includes impressionistic data based on numerous feature stories in the mainstream and industrry media, plus my own continuous tracking of these developments as publisher and editor (since June 1996) of *The Integrator for the Business of Alternative Medicine*, a monthly newsletter devoted to these topics.

Additional indicators of increased CAM interest are the number of features, focused publications, and focused conferences that target CAM coverage and integration issues. In November 1998, *JAMA, Healthcare Forum Journal,* and *The Physician Executive* all devoted a significant portion of their editorial space to CAM-related articles. By mid-1999, there will be at least three new newsletters serving managed-care readers working with CAM coverage issues. Many health-care conference organizations have added CAM coverage to their stable of conferences. The National Managed Health Care Congress, which pioneered the theme of integrating CAM into managed care through 2-day seminars and preconference workshops between 1996 and 1998, elevated CAM to an entire track at its annual spring meeting in 1999, the managed care industry's largest gathering [21].

SELECTING AND DEFINING A COMPLEMENTARY AND ALTERNATIVE MEDICINE BENEFIT

A frequently told story about what makes insurance companies and managed-care organizations run uses the metaphor of driving an automobile. The marketing director is said to have his foot on the gas, while the chief financial officer's foot is slammed on the brake. The car's direction is guided by the actuary who, basing decisions on historical data, is looking out the back window. This story relates to CAM coverage discussions because organized American medicine does not yet have enough experience with developing,

TABLE 13-2. COMPLEMENTARY AND ALTERNATIVE MEDICINE COVERAGE OFFERED BY SOME INSURANCE POLICIES

A plan may:
- Offer CAM, but only subsequent to a state mandate, and therefore without any internal, pro-active process
- Include direct access to numerous CAM services, but only for worker's compensation claims
- Have CAM services, but in only one or two of perhaps two dozen distinct insurance or HMO "products" it offers purchasers
- Promote a CAM program, but only to its group purchasers and not to individuals
- Administer an insurance policy for a self-insured company that has some CAM coverage, but the plan does not offer the coverage
- Allow conventional providers to offer certain CAM therapies but not cover those services when provided by members of distinct CAM professions
- Have an offering for which the purchaser has to pay more ("rider") and that is outsourced to a CAM network but has little to no internal expertise in CAM
- Create a program that allows members to access CAM services on a discounted basis but not as a covered benefit
- Cover a certain provider category, such as chiropractor, for only very limited conditions, such as low back pain

CAM—complementary and alternative medicine; HMO—health maintenance organization.

TABLE 13-3. IMPROVEMENTS IN COMPLEMENTARY AND ALTERNATIVE MEDICINE COVERAGE

- Most national plans, including United Healthcare, Aetna-US Healthcare, CIGNA, Kaiser, and Blue Cross Blue Shield either have a CAM product or have an ad hoc team working on a CAM strategy.
- Regional plans in many areas of the country, such as Oxford, Matthew Thornton, Lifeguard, and Providence GoodHealth Plan have jumped into CAM offerings.
- Representatives of the Preventive Medicine Research Institute, which promotes a mind–body approach to reversing coronary artery disease, claim that 30 to 40 insurers have covered their multiweek mind–body program.
- Acupuncture is joining chiropractic as an offering among California's health plans.
- The late 1990s witnessed burgeoning growth in the number of businesses established to credential and lease networks of CAM providers to healthplans and other payers.

CAM—complementary and alternative medicine.

pricing, offering, and managing CAM benefits. The actuary tends to side with the chief financial officer (put on the brakes!); to move ahead with CAM, the actuary has to take an uncharacteristic "leap of faith" [22].

Credentialing Providers of Complementary and Alternative Medicine

The remainder of this chapter reviews the types of benefits that plans are offering in this context. Attention is focused on the key interests of plans that approach CAM: Who will provide CAM services? What training and licensing programs exist to educate the provider? Health-care plan credentialing is a core standard on which health plans are judged. Credentialing is a fundamentally protective function. The health plan, through credentialing, ensures its members that all providers meet minimal requirements. Leading criteria include licensing, education, and proof of malpractice insurance. Accrediting bodies require these claims to be independently verified.

In practical terms, credentialing criteria suggest that distinct, regulated CAM professional associations—chiropractors, acupuncturists, massage practitioners, naturopathic physicians—are the optimal providers with which to work in the states in which they are licensed. Licensing is based on educational criteria and, generally, success in passing an examination. Professional licensing requirements exist for chiropractors in 50 states. Licensing for acupuncturists is available in 33 states, for naturopathic physicians in 11 states, and for massage practitioners in 28 states. These three professions are all actively promoting expansion of licensing. The chiropractors, acupuncturists, and naturopathic physicians have each established an accrediting agency that has successfully gained approval from the U.S. Department of Education. In recent years, malpractice insurers have extended policies to licensed acupuncturists, naturopaths, massage practitioners, and even licensed but direct-entry (non-nurse) midwives. In short, intensive work over the past 15 to 25 years has put these providers on the doorstep of health-care plans with their credentials largely in order.

Yoga practitioners, herbalists, specialized body workers, and indigenous healers who are not regulated by states are much more difficult to credential. Some plans deal with this issue by requiring that practitioners of these services also have an accepted medical degree, such as physician, nurse, mental health counselor, or physical therapist. Others have created internal credentialing criteria, based largely on recommendations of advisory boards that include leaders of the various professions involved.

Another potentially difficult, and as yet unresolved, area for credentialing is the conventional provider who has gained some experience or expertise in offering one or more CAM treatment modality. Although this provider may be easily credentialed under his or her conventional license, the lack of formal standards to define an integrative or wholistic medicine practitioner makes it difficult for the plan to ensure the consumer that the provider meets a certain standard of education or licensing in the CAM field. For example, one such practitioner may have developed a passion for European phytomedicine (herbal medicine), but possesses little knowledge of mind–body literature or approaches. Another conventional physician may be a student of homeopathy and other energy medicine but have little interest in therapeutic nutrition. Each may have some CAM expertise, even in numerous modalities, whereas training programs are generally ad hoc, individualized, do not have third party review, and are difficult to verify independently. The exception is acupuncture, in which a 200-hour training program (significantly below the 3000 hours in an accredited acupuncture school) is a de facto standard for physicians practicing acupuncture [23]. Significant efforts to set standards in this area may be expected over the next decade.

Affinity Products: Discounting Complementary and Alternative Medicine Services Not Covered by Health-Care Plans

One direction some plans and purchasers are taking is to offer members benefits that do not put the plans themselves at any risk [24]. This model, called an "affinity product," is favorably recommended as a starting point by a medical director with the National Blue Cross Blue Shield Association. With affinity programs, the plan gives members access to uncovered services at a discount. These discount programs have been developed in recent years for conventional treatments, such as eye care or cosmetic surgery, and are now an easy niche for CAM services. In the affinity-product design, the HMO or insurer contracts with a network of credentialed providers who agree to give the plan's members a discount on available services. Most plans contract these network services to a specialty firm. The discount usually varies from 10% to 30%.

Oxford Health Plans was among the first providers to offer an affinity CAM benefit to its members, beginning in early 1997. In 1999, California Blue Cross chose to add an affinity dimension to the chiropractic and acupuncture services that the plan already included as a CAM offering. Table 13-4 describes the "Healthy Extensions" affinity product developed by California Blue Cross. Interestingly, this product was developed subsequent to the plan's offering covered chiropractic and acupuncture benefits.

Whereas some HMOs, such as Oxford, choose to contract with providers directly, most companies contract through a specialty organization. For instance, Blue Shield of California, a pioneer of this CAM strategy on the West Coast, partnered with Consensus Health, whose network providers agreed to offer their services at a 25% discount. In 1998, the Shield organization took the unusual step, also in partnership with Consensus, of offering the CAM discount program to all Californians who chose to sign up on the firm's website. The Consensus network includes stress management programs and fitness centers as well as acupuncturists and body workers. With the 1999 year, Georgia Blue Cross Blue Shield and Anthem Blue Cross Blue Shield each began similar products, contracting with external CAM networks Holisticos and The Alternare Group, respectively. Another significant HMO, Minnesota's Health Partners, began a similar program with CAM services organization InfiniteHealth. Health-care plans

TABLE 13-4. BLUE CROSS OF CALIFORNIA COVERED COMPLEMENTARY AND ALTERNATIVE MEDICINE SERVICES

Healthy extensions: affinity product
Self-referred access
Discounted direct pay
Massage, yoga, hypnotherapy, and fitness practitioner services
Pritikin and nutrition programs
Everlife Store*, Home Fitness Club, NordicTrack[†], other books, tapes, and memberships
Essential and EverLife supplements
Direct contract network plus ASHP
Implemented in individual and small group plans (large group by first quarter 1999)
Currently 4.4 million members

CAM services already offered in core benefit
Chiropractic (covered for 8 years)
Acupuncture (covered for 5 years)
Chiropractor and licensed acupuncturist networks (ASHP)

*EverLife Stores are a division of Holisticos, Atlanta, GA
[†]Minneapolis, MN
ASHP—American Specialty Health Plans; CAM—complementary and alternative medicine.

typically contract for access to these services on a per-member per-month (PMPM) or per-member per-year (PMPY) basis. Although little published data exist, purchasers are said to be paying between a few cents and $2.50 PMPM.

This HMO and third-party-payer interest in affinity products has led to a vast expansion of the number and reach of the businesses offering these services to plans, employers, and directly to individuals. By late 1998, one New York-based entrepreneur had woven a national network of 13 regional CAM networks to be positioned to service national insurance contracts [25]. All these regional businesses were developed specifically to meet the needs of the affinity market. A survey of executives at the top 15 CAM networks that were organized principally to manage covered CAM benefits, however, revealed that most of these firms also rent their networks to service affinity products [26].

Table 13-5 examines the characteristics of seven CAM services organizations that offer affinity products. As the chart reveals, most of the firms offering these discounted services also sell their networks directly to individuals through discount cards. Others see direct sales to employers as their principal market. This affinity strategy is viewed as a winning one for all parties involved, because the plan gains a new, consumer-oriented feature without assuming substantial additional financial risk; the member gets a discount on CAM, as well as reassurance that the CAM provider meets a credentialing standard; and the CAM provider gains some additional recognition by being included in a the plan's list of providers, which may in turn increase his or her business.

One additional potential value of the affinity product is the potential for insurance providers to obtain experience with CAM providers and vice versa, thus opening up opportunities to create even newer products and approaches from an informed perspective. In short, the experience of setting up affinity programs becomes a baseline from which the plan can better estimate the cost of offering an actual CAM benefit. A significant question remains as to whether such data will be gathered, or can be gathered, when the provider, CAM network, health-care plan, and group purchaser are not bound by the exchange of benefit-derived dollars.

The Complementary and Alternative Medicine "Rider"

In the present situation, in which relatively few data are available, health-care plans tend to look at what they believe to be services or policies similar to those with which they have some experience. For health-care plans, the two services that are most closely aligned are behavioral health and chiropractic care. These services are not generally well understood nor highly respected by most medical directors, nor have they historically been viewed as core benefits. Instead, these services are widely offered through what the industry terms a *rider*. The rider is the dominant method by which CAM services are offered as a covered benefit. Typical CAM rider characteristics are listed in Table 13-6. Acupuncture is the CAM service of most significant interest to plans under the rider strategy, after chiropractic. These services are followed by those offered by naturopathic physicians (in states where naturopaths are licensed). Other plans may cover massage or body work.

A survey of CAM network executives in the December 1998 issue of *The Integrator for the Business of Alternative Medicine* [27] found that many HMOs and insurers are contracting for new CAM services through the same businesses with which they contract to manage their chiropractic benefits. The first strong sign of this development was in California in the spring of 1997 when American Chiropractic Health Plan, a chiropractic HMO with contracts with seven of California's 10 largest HMOs, changed its name to American Specialty Health Plan. This new name reflected the group's decision to develop networks of acupuncturists, massage practitioners, naturopathic physicians, and others. Other firms have followed a similar pattern. ChiroNet, which dominates the Oregon market for managed chiropractic, and Wisconsin-based Chiropractic Health Partners re-emerged as Complementary Healthcare Plans and American WholeHealth Networks, respectively, following creation of new CAM provider panels. American Specialty Health Plans inked its first contracts for acupuncture with United Healthcare, Health Net, and Blue Cross of California within the next months. Chiropractic Health Partners initiated broader CAM deals with Kaiser and Providence, whereas American WholeHealth Networks began moving into the broader CAM arena with contracts in Washington state with Group Health Cooperative of Puget Sound and in Arizona with Intergroup.

This concept of "carving-out" a niche in the market is attractive to plans that perceive a lack in internal competency in a given area or in a plan to develop it. If the organization that wins the carve-out contract builds an agreeable track

TABLE 13-5. CHARACTERISTICS OF COMPLEMENTARY AND ALTERNATIVE MEDICINE NETWORKS OFFERING DISCOUNTED "AFFINITY" SERVICES

Policy Features	Health and Healing Card	Alternative Medicine Referral Services	Vitality Access	Health and Healing Trust	Consensus Health	Alternare	Infinite Health
Location	Greater San Francisco	Greater Washington, DC	Denver and Boulder, CO	NY, NJ, CT, Mid-Atlantic states	California	Oregon	Minneapolis and St. Paul, MN
Individual membership option	Yes	Yes	Yes	Yes	No	No (but individuals can purchase)	Yes
Annual individual member fees	$60	$49	$72	$79	—	$35	$30
Total members	800	1000 (awaiting processing)	Just starting	2000 (includes groups)	1.3 million HMO members	30,000 HMO members	200–300
Provider discount	15%–25%	20%	10%–20%	20%	25%	15%	15%
DC, LAc, ND, massage, bodywork	Yes	Yes	Yes	Yes	Yes (except ND)	Yes	Yes
CAM-MD	Yes	Yes	Yes	Yes	Yes (acupuncture only)	No	Yes
Fitness/health club	Yes	Yes	Personal trainers; club planned	Yes	Yes (includes personal trainer)	Yes	No
Natural products (herbs, vitamins)	Developing	Considering	Yes	Considering	?	Yes (mail order)	No
Health food store	Yes	No	Yes	Yes	No	Yes	Not for natural products
Directory	Written, online Wide provider range includes homeopathy, hypnotherapy, herbalists	Toll-free phone number Triage to providers; education; developing website	Written, online Website w/ forum; CDC's Personal Health Profile"; mail order catalog, book on herbs and vitamins; seminars planned	Planned Discounted seminars, 24 h audio library (1200 topics)	? Wellness services; guided imagery; stress management	Yes Nurse-based information services; web resources; special wellness (yoga, bodywork)	Yes Website in development; consumer health education, stress reduction
Other							
Credentialing fee	No	$95	No	No	No	No	$150
Annual provider fees for participation	Directory advertising $35 for 50 words, $50 for website profile	$360–$2700/y	No	No	No	No	$100–$300
Network size	900	120 completed	> 100	1600	700	300 (in Oregon)	110

Continued

TABLE 13-5. CHARACTERISTICS OF COMPLEMENTARY AND ALTERNATIVE MEDICINE NETWORKS OFFERING DISCOUNTED "AFFINITY" SERVICES (CONTINUED)

Policy Features	Health and Healing Card	Alternative Medicine Referral Services	Vitality Access	Health and Healing Trust	Consensus Health	Altermare	Infinite Health
Representative plan contracts	Not planned	Not initially	Not initially	Core Strategy (under discussion with others)	California Blue Shield (1998 exclusive)	QualMed of Oregon, Pacificare Secure Horizons	Relationship with Health Partners
Group fee (plan or employer)	$2.90–$5 PMPM ($15/y less for spouse, $1.70/mo for kids)	Down to $2 PMPM	$6 PMPM (plus $0.50 PMPM for each dependent)	$3–$4 PMPM/PEPM	Volume driven	Discount off $35 rate	$30 cafeteria; $18 up front, 100% participation; 60%–99% $21/y
Representative employer contracts	Core strategy, TriNet	Assessing	Core Strategy	24 small firms	Assessing	Yes (United Way agencies)	Randy Sanitation, Select Comfort
Network includes insured benefits	Partner with AcuPlan	Assessing	Unsure	In strategy	In strategy	Yes	Assessing

CAM-MD—complementary and alternative medicine medical doctor; CDC—Centers for Disease Control and Prevention; DC—doctor of chiropractic (chiropractor); HMO—health maintenance organization; LAc—licensed acupunturist; ND—naturopathic doctor; PEPM—per employee per month; PMPM—per member per month;

---

record in managing chiropractic, for instance, the health-care plan may deem it reasonable to go to the same firm to create and provide additional CAM benefits. For the provider of acupuncture, massage, or naturopathic services, the model may be acceptable merely because these professions, as a rule, have neither the infrastructure nor the capital to create their own networks or independent practitioner associations.

Is a Rider an Integrated Benefit?

Proponents of CAM riders argue that these benefits are a good way to begin covering CAM services. The argument runs that, after the plan has gained experience in this context of diminished financial risk, the HMO can begin to consider offering CAM as a part of a core benefit. The rider may also be created in a way that allows the consumer to access the CAM provider without referral from a conventional doctor. The consumer can thus avoid conflicts with conventional providers who may oppose the decision to use CAM. In these ways, the acupuncture, chiropractic, or other CAM benefit that is purchased through a rider may seem more "integrated" to the customer.

From the perspectives of payment and care delivery, however, the rider may be viewed as an essentially nonintegrated product. It is usually not clinically integrated, because often no referral or reporting is required. The rider is not economically integrated, because payment for services comes from a separate fund—the additional PMPM payment of the rider—rather than from base premiums. The rider is frequently not organizationally integrated because the benefit has often been carved-out to a specialty organization or alternate provider.

Unless organizations develop policies to mitigate these nonintegration tendencies, the following can be viewed as expected side effects of using the rider as a mechanism for offering CAM services: 1) neither conventional nor CAM providers, because they may be in separate organizations, have substantial organizational incentives to learn to work closely and understand when CAM is most appropriate; 2) if the outside contractor does a good job, CAM will not receive much internal attention and thus little internal knowledge of CAM will accrue to the HMO or insurer; 3) leadership of the health-care plan will have little reason to assess whether CAM actually replaces or limits conventional services—and thus might be best considered as a core benefit—or is merely an add-on benefit, and thus reasonably paid for by additional fees.

Interestingly, CAM providers and many CAM consumers believe that better integration of CAM will lead to more cost-effective treatment. They believe that CAM methods can guide the health-care system toward a more fundamental, health-oriented focus that they believe is true reform. However, these characteristics of the typical organization of a CAM benefit suggest that the rider may limit the extent to which the health-care payment and delivery system discovers and optimizes CAM in delivery of effective and cost-effective care. Table 13-7 describes two CAM benefits with distinct design features. In one case, the employer, Lotus, is at risk on services provided by an internal network credentialed by Lotus' third-party administrator, Tufts Health Plan. In the

Table 13-6. Typical Characteristics of Complementary and Alternative Medicine Riders

Provision of services by a credentialed network of providers that is either contracted directly by the plan or rented through an external network on a per member/per month basis

Contracted CAM providers offer services at a discounted rate

External contracting network may handle a range of services, from billing and provider education to assuming full risk on the CAM services

Generally only offered to groups in order to cut down on "adverse selection" (only being purchased by individuals who are high users of the specific service)

Often allow the consumer or member direct access to the provider without referral from a primary care physician

Limitation on the benefit (either a total annual dollar figure, typically $500 to $2000, or total annual number of visits, typically 12 to 20)

Additional fee, generally paid by the group on a per member/per month or per employee/per month basis (a rider for chiropractic may run $0.50-$4 per month/per member depending on the benefit)

In some cases, a higher than usual co-pay is required, perhaps up to 50%

CAM—complementary and alternative medicine.

Table 13-7. Two Complementary and Alternative Medicine Benefits Designs

Features	Colorado Blue Cross Blue Shield Senior, with Landmark Healthcare	Lotus Development, with Tufts Health Plans
Members	12,000 seniors	2200 in greater Boston
Acupuncture and chiropractic visits	Up to 12/yr (combined)	Up to 20/y (combined)
Massage	Noncovered, discount cash basis	Up to 6/y
Natural products	10% discount on Amrion's HealthSmart catalog	None
Mind–body program	—	Specific conditions, referral required
Other CAM therapies	24 types, discounted cash basis through WellCall	—
Access	Self-referred	Self-referred
Payment	$15/visit (member pays remainder)	$10 point of sale co-pay, $5 HMO
Visits beyond policy limits	—	Paid cash, at negotiated PPO rates
At risk?	Landmark Healthcare	Lotus Development
CAM network	Landmark Healthcare	Tufts Health Plans

CAM—complementary and alternative medicine; HMO—health maintenance organization; PPO—preferred provider organization.

other case, Landmark Healthcare, the CAM services organization, is at risk rather than Colorado Blue Cross Blue Shield, the employer. Interestingly, Colorado Blue Cross Blue Shield chose to offer these services as part of their core benefit.

Other Covered Complementary and Alternative Medicine Benefits

As previously noted, coverage of CAM can also be restricted to specific programs. An example is Mutual of Omaha's coverage of a specific CAM-oriented, multiweek program for controlling and reversing coronary artery disease. Mutual's coverage decision was pursuant to extensive published research that produced an anticipation of substantial savings in the area of foregone treatments, surgeries, and hospital stays for this costly medical condition. Condition-specific, multiweek CAM programs developed through Harvard's MindBody Medical Institute and its affiliates are also finding some success in gaining increased coverage, particularly from HMOs. However, as recently as early 1998, most third-party payments for these services were available only through structuring the group encounter around a billable physician visit [28].

The difficulty in covering integrative medicine services as provided by conventional physicians has been described by a former health-care plan chief executive officer who also served as an executive with a leading Phoenix-based, integrative medicine clinic [29]. A primary care model for CAM service delivery counteracts with managed care's time constraints on primary care physician visits, which do not allow for the additional time costs associated with the complex intervention of many whole-person–oriented CAM services. Securing a steady stream of referrals for specialty services from physicians who may be ignorant of the potential value of the CAM services or opposed to them is a time-consuming educational process at best. Early data from a benchmarking survey on integrative clinics run by medical doctors and osteopaths, which are being created inside health-care systems and hospitals, suggest that many are simply choosing to pursue the cash-paying client more aggressively [30]. Both physician referrals and HMO contracting tend to rank low on the priority list for generating patient flow and income.

One coverage strategy that is emerging from the integrative clinic environment is a condition-specific, program-based, multipractitioner approach. In this situation, the group of practitioners seeks a fee for managing patients with a certain condition and may go at risk for all patients managed with the given conditions. CAM advocates of this coverage approach tend to favor working directly with employers, targeting conditions that are significant factors in absenteeism and declines in productivity. The fee may then also be measured against overall savings to the purchaser rather than the strictly medical costs of the HMO or insurer.

Complementary and Alternative Medicine as Core Benefit: "Add-on" or "Replacement?"

Ultimately, CAM is rolled into a core benefit only if the plan is willing to consider CAM a marketing loss-leader to lure in new members (*ie,* the Colorado Blue Cross Blue Shield program for senior citizens in Table 13-7); if a mandate requires it (Washington state's experience); if an extraordinarily high level of data argues for inclusion (*eg,* potential addition of certain botanicals to a formulary, as is being explored by Kaiser Northern California); if a decision is made to include CAM following a practice guideline process or inclusion of acupuncture for certain nausea, based on the NIH Consensus conference on acupuncture [30]; or executives believe that doing so is a calculated risk that will return significant cost benefits. The core question in deciding whether to charge extra (on a rider basis) for CAM services is: are these services an "add-on" to conventional treatment, which reasonably require additional fees, or do they replace other services? In the latter case, the plan then has cost offsets that may make the services either cost-neutral or cost-beneficial (Table 13-8).

A growing body of data suggests that, from the perspective of CAM users, between 30% and 65% of CAM interventions diminish the use of conventional services. The potential credibility of these perceptions is underlined by data from the Stanford/American Specialty Health Plan survey [1], which found a dose–response relationship between the intensity of CAM intervention and the perception that the CAM therapy replaced conventional treatment (Table 13-9). For instance, vitamin therapy, which is generally self-administered, replaced other care only 21% of the time, whereas patients who visited chiropractors or acupuncturists perceived that their treatment replaced conventional services about 60% of the time.

These consumer data would be expected to be biased upward, necessarily tentative, and in need of comparison against actual claims data. Ultimately, such a study should be

TABLE 13-8. IS COMPLEMENTARY AND ALTERNATIVE MEDICINE AN "ADD-ON" OR REPLACEMENT FOR CONVENTIONAL MEDICINE? DATA FROM THREE SURVEYS

Study	Year	Question	Yes, %
Landmark Healthcare [7]	1997	Decreased visits to conventional physician	30
Alternare Health Services [3]	1997	Decreased use of conventional services	55
		Decreased use of prescription drugs	61
Stanford/American Health Specialty Plans [1]	1998	Decreased use of conventional services	55

TABLE 13-9. A DOSE–RESPONSE RELATIONSHIP?

CAM Therapy	In Addition to Conventional Medicine, %	In Place of Conventional Medicine, %
Vitamins	79	21
Medication	76	24
Relaxation	75	25
Herbal medicine	59	41
Massage	50	50
Acupuncture	44	57
Chiropractic	36	64
Chinese medicine	36	64

CAM—complementary and alternative medicine.
Data from Stanford University/American Specialty Health Plans [1].

conducted over a long period of time to determine whether the use of CAM either created additional long-term costs or significantly limited use of conventional services. The dose–response pattern, which has been found in other studies, suggests that some CAM services may well have some significant cost offsets and even cost savings.

Some evidence suggests that these perceptions are shared by at least some employers. An east coast HMO study using a focus group of manufacturers found that "manufacturing organizations, which have a great deal of experience dealing with workers' compensation injuries, believe chiropractic will get people back to work faster than traditional medicine" [31]. Some perceive that drug expenditures will decrease if access to complementary medicine increases. If these consumer and purchaser perspectives hold, various CAM services should arguably move into core benefit packages.

COMPLEMENTARY AND ALTERNATIVE MEDICINE: GRAFTING OR HEALTH CREATION?

The present exploration of CAM by industry leaders is taking place at a moment when managed care's initial economic success in controlling health care costs is eroding with rising costs and the limitations of the new system. Has health-care reform been more than reform of the payment system? An article by Richard Service in *Business and Health* [32] captures the moment this way: "A decade into the process of restructuring, we are still tinkering with—and deriving cost savings from—the mechanics of a system that is peerless in its ability to cure disease. We have yet to address the more important question, 'How shall we deliver health?'."

For many consumers and providers of CAM services, CAM approaches are viewed as an answer to this question. CAM is presented as a health-oriented, patient-centered paradigm. It is compared favorably by these advocates to the reactive, disease-oriented, and more vertical physician–patient orientation of conventional treatment. Thus, if the experiences of these consumers and providers is to be honored, leaders of the dominant system who are also asking how to "deliver health" may wisely look at CAM as a partner in this system-wide exploratory venture. When coupled with the health-care plan's principle of actively partnering with patients—a principle actively promoted by the American Association of Health Plans—an avenue of shared interest appears to suggest a direction toward a healthier future.

It is fair to say, however, that most health-care plans that have begun offering CAM benefits view CAM as an answer to more restrictive questions. They ask an economic question: How shall we deliver consumers (into our plan)? Or if the question is clinical, its boundaries are significantly more limited: Which of these agents and therapies should we add to those we are already offering? What CAM service can we readily graft on to our current way of doing business? Most plans are not taking this consumer-driven interest into the heart of their thinking about health care. Neither do they look excitedly on the potential for cost-savings as suggested by the CAM user perception that CAM services significantly impact their use of conventional services or pharmacies. Rather, the dominant mode for management, payment, and offering of CAM services—the benefit rider managed by an outside contractor—tends to effectively externalize CAM.

Keeping CAM in a separate but unequal position is an easy solution for the medical mainstream. As long as CAM is externalized, however, the challenging opportunity to actually deliver health-care to the populations served may thereby be missed. The consumer, who has made CAM therapies a challenge for the mainstream payment system, may have to continue with advocacy to be certain that, when appropriate, CAM becomes part of the mainstream conventional health-care benefit design.

REFERENCES AND RECOMMENDED READING

Recently published papers of particular interest have been highlighted as:
- Of interest
- Of outstanding interest

1. Stanford University/American Specialty Health Plans: Understanding consumer trends in complementary and alternative medicine: a national survey. Presented at a conference at Stanford University, September 18, 1998.
2. Eisenberg DM, Kessler RC, Foster C, *et al.*: Unconventional medicine in the United States: prevalence, costs, and patterns of use. *N Engl J Med* 1993, 328:246–252.
3. Gordon NP, Sobel DS, Tarazona EZ: Use of and interest in alternative therapies among adult primary care clinicians and adult members in a large health maintenance organization. *West J Med* 1998, 169:153–161.
4. Landmark Healthcare: *The Landmark Report on Public Perceptions of Alternative Care.* Sacramento, CA: Landmark Healthcare; 1998.
5. Eisenberg DM, Davis RB, Ettner SL, *et al.*: Trends in alternative medicine use in the United States, 1990–1997: results of a follow-up national survey. *JAMA* 1998, 280:1569–1575.
6. Weeks J: Open enrollment: two sample new products. *The Integrator for the Business of Alternative Medicine* 1998, 3:8–12.
7. Weeks J: Oregon survey on CAM interest. *St. Anthony's Business Report on Alternative and Complementary Medicine* 1997, 1:7.
8. Blecher MB: Gold in Goldenseal. *Hospitals and Health Networks* 1997: 50–52.
9. American Association of Health Plans: Statement of Principles. Washington, DC: American Association of Health Plans; 1996.
10. Eisenberg DM: Presentation at Virginia Mason Medical Center, Seattle, WA, May 1, 1998.
11. West D: MCOs integrating alternative care. *National Underwriter* 1997:58.
12. Lippman H: Can employers see beyond price? *Business and Health* 1997:44–47.
13. Gillert DJ: Is a chiropractor in your future? *Defense Press Service* 1998.
14. Weeks J: Integrative clinics: condition-based clinical programs with global, in-house fees and codes. *The Integrator for the Business of Alternative Medicine* 1998, 3:6.
15. Berman BM, Singh BB, Hartnall SM, *et al.*: Primary care physicians and complementary–alternative medicine: training, attitudes, and practice patterns. *J Am Board Fam Pract* 1998, 11:272–281.
16. Weeks J, Layton R: Integration as community organizing: toward a model for optimizing relationships between networks of conventional and alternative providers. *Int Med* 1998, 1:15–25.
17. Pelletier KR, Marie A, Krasner M, *et al.*: Current trends in the integration and reimbursement of complementary and alternative medicine by managed care, insurance carriers, and hospital providers. *Am J Health Promot* 1997, 12:112–122.

18. Weeks J: CAM programs: last hired, first fired? *The Integrator for the Business of Alternative Medicine* 1998, 3:1–2.
19. Weeks J: On the outside moving in: will the alternative medicine movement shape U.S. Healthcare? *Healthcare Forum Journal* 1998:14–18.
20. Weber DO: Considering the alternatives. *The Physician Executive* 1998, 24:6–14.
21. National Managed Health Care Congress, Georgia World Congress Center, Atlanta, GA. March 29–April 1, 1999.
22. Weeks J: Operational issues in incorporating complementary and alternative therapies and providers in benefit plans and managed care organizations. Washington, DC: National Institutes of Health Office of Alternative Medicine and the U.S. Agency for Health Care Policy and Research; 1996.
23. Weeks J: Challenges in credentialing MDs for the practice of alternative medicine. *The Integrator for the Business of Alternative Medicine* 1998, 2:1–6.
24. Brown E: The daunting challenge. *The Physician Executive* 1998, 24:16–21.
25. *Newsletter from N-CAM: An Independent Cooperative CAM Network* Cochecton, NY: N-CAM;1998.
26. Weeks J: *The Integrator* 1998 CAM network executive survey, part 1. *The Integrator for the Business of Alternative Medicine* 1998, 3:1–7.
27. Weeks J: Group delivered mind-body medical interventions: the state of coverage and physician acceptance. *The Integrator for the Business of Alternative Medicine* 1998, 2:1–6.
28. Biedess P: Integrating alternative medicine into managed care. National Managed Health Care Congress Preconference Workshop, Los Angeles, CA, November 3, 1997.
29. Weeks J: *The Integrator* special project: benchmarking clinic development, report #1. *The Integrator for the Business of Alternative Medicine* 1998, 3:1–5.
30. National Institutes of Health: Consensus development conference on acupuncture. Washington, DC, November 3–5, 1997.
31. Zablocki E: Health plans, providers struggle with quality in alternative medicine. *The Quality Letter for Healthcare Leaders* 1998, 10:1–13.
32. Service R: What we think. *Business and Health* 1997:6.

Business Aspects of Building an Integrative Medical Practice

David Edelberg

As an internist in a large multi-specialty group practice, I cared for patients with acute and chronic conditions according to accepted allopathic standards of practice. While handling several chronically ill patients, I noticed that they were getting better in a manner unrelated to what I was prescribing. When I discovered that these patients had been to alternative healers, I began calling these practitioners to thank them for their success with *our* patient. I met with several alternative practitioners and studied their methods. Many initially regarded me with both skepticism and trepidation because they were so used to receiving criticism and hostility from the allopathic medicine community. At many offices I was the first allopathic physician to request information, and some practitioners suspected that I was part of an "investigation."

When I thought I had established a comfortable understanding of alternative medicine, I began referring patients to alternative healers. Many patients were pleased, and I was surprised by the number of my patients who were well-versed in alternative modalities. They seemed to appreciate my "open-mindedness." Most patients responded by getting better, although I cannot be sure whether this was due to the alternative therapy or simply to the change of venue. In addition, the HMO was not displeased with my referrals because alternative therapies are not covered; the patients were paying for the treatments themselves.

A 1991 article on alternative medicine described the healthcare center of the future as an integrated facility "where conventional doctors and alternative healers practice under one roof" [1]. Reading this inspired me to think seriously about my observations and reassess how I really wanted to use my medical training and skills. After a typical morning of rounds filled with the usual conflicts over patient discharges, I wondered what had happened to put the patients in hospital beds in the first place. Of the 10 charts I studied, eight patients were admitted as a consequence of preventable illnesses, such as emphysema, cirrhosis of the liver, HIV infection, cancer, and heart disease. The other two patients were recovering from complications of conventional care, such as drug reactions, slowly healing surgical wounds, and drug-resistant bacteria. I grew more concerned about the current system, in which the hospital administrator wants the beds full and the HMO wants the same beds empty. In addition, this illness-based system provides little more than cursory advice to patients and fails to prevent these tragedies from happening; when the disaster occurs, we mobilize complex, invasive, and expensive resources.

ALTERNATIVE MEDICINE

Alternative practitioners emphasize patient empowerment, prevention, and self-care. Their collective philosophy is to "heal by strengthening the body's own self-healing capabilities," an idea that conventional practitioners often do not appreciate. For instance, antibiotics are not always used to kill bacteria; occasionally, echinacea is prescribed to strengthen the immune system. Acupuncture, naturopathy, and homeopathy use the healing powers within the patient. This approach expects patient participation by means of a healthy diet, stress reduction, and regular exercise.

The Integrated Practice

While continuing to work full-time as an internist, I began to form ideas about the best way to deliver integrated health care. I did not know whether comparable centers existed; I later learned that some had been in operation successfully for years whereas others had fallen apart after only a few months of business. I made the assumption that most patients who would want alternative therapies would still prefer to have an allopathic physician nearby supervising their overall care. In addition, after speaking with several good alternative practitioners, I discovered that their knowledge of pathophysiology, pharmacology, and other basic concepts of allopathic medicine was incomplete. Thus, an integrated center required a physician trained in conventional medicine. Although this may seem obvious, there are many "integrated" centers still today in which the most highly trained health-care professional is a chiropractor or naturopath.

With these factors in mind, I interviewed dozens of practitioners throughout 1992. They were subjected to approximately the same process of credential verification that I had used for new allopathic physicians joining my medical group. I looked for qualified practitioners who thought their own therapies were incomplete and wanted to work with a conventional physician in an integrated setting. In January 1993, I opened the Chicago Holistic Center. The weekend before the center opened, a major Chicago newspaper ran a prominent article on alternative medicine in Chicago and featured our office. We soon realized that we had not anticipated the citywide enthusiasm for our endeavor and that our space was far too small to meet the needs of the dozens of patients who were making appointments daily. The success of this first center led to a second in Denver and to the development of American WholeHealth, a company dedicated to the creation of integrated centers nationwide. We now have four centers in Chicago, two each in the Denver and Washington, DC areas, one in Boston, and a corporate headquarters in Reston, Virginia.

For the integrated practice to have a chance of long-term success, it must be based on a for-profit model in which fiscal responsibility to investors drives a streamlined, efficient practice. However, the real philosophy behind the business is a holistic approach to the patient. This means that each person is treated as a unique individual, and that issues of health and disease are a function of physical, emotional, and spiritual factors. By incorporating the best of science, mind–body healing, and nutrition, we can truly focus on the patient and not just the disease. The best health care draws on the broadest range of tools when addressing the factors that influence health. Humans have an inherent ability to assist in their own healing. Western healing is based on doing something to the body to reverse disease processes. Non-Western healing traditions are based on the idea of unleashing the body's own self-healing abilities. A health-care center that honors the patient's own value system and right to self-determination will be more effective in engaging the patient in his or her own healing process.

The model of practice we have established is more than a loose affiliation of allopathic and alternative practitioners. We are a tightly integrated multispecialty group of physicians and practitioners that practice in one location under the supervision of conventionally trained physicians experienced in integrative medicine. The physicians are board certified in primary care medicine and are also trained in integrative medicine so that they feel equally comfortable using fluoxetine, St. John's wort, or acupuncture for depression. They thus have access to a full range of therapeutic and health promotion possibilities and can to work with a multidisciplinary team to identify the best treatment choices, including chiropractic, acupuncture, massage therapy, nutritional counseling, herbal pharmacology, and clinical counseling.

Staff Selection and Evaluation

Our physicians use the "biography before biology" approach when developing a customized "healing path" for each patient. They spend approximately three times longer with a patient than conventional practitioners when taking a medical history because they believe that many chronic conditions are rooted in a patient's personal biography and are more effectively treated by addressing root causes rather than symptoms alone. When selecting physicians and practitioners, we look for a blend of training, skills, philosophy, and personal caring attitudes that we believe our clients need and deserve. We do not expect physicians to arrive skilled in integrative medicine; we have developed extensive training that includes reading material, audio- and videotapes, clinical protocols, and one-on-one mentoring. The medical director of a center has experience in primary care as well as a background in the science and philosophy of complementary therapies. The team thus has a leader with whom other practitioners can quickly establish a comfort level. Complementary-therapy practitioners must not only be certified in their respective fields but must also be observed clinically by senior practitioners in the field. These senior practitioners thoroughly evaluate a candidate's level of expertise before accepting the candidate for the center's staff.

Practice Environment

In addition to the evaluation process, a center's entire staff is oriented and trained in delivering "hospitality-based" service to all clients. In the welcome area, a variety of healthful drinks are provided; in the reading room, clients can peruse relevant literature; and in the natural pharmacy area, selected high-quality dietary supplements and herbal products are offered for sale. Our educational outreach to the community includes seminars and workshops for professionals and the general public. A series of lectures is planned 3 to 6 months in advance and announced through the media. Most presentations are given by center staff; the "health practitioner as educator" concept is a central part of our care delivery framework.

Practice Management

Each center has a practice manager that coordinates all activities and is responsible to the medical director for day-to-day management. Charges for services are made to the individual and help is available for processing reimbursement claims. As health insurance plans continue to add coverage for complementary therapies, we will investigate the best system for our clients and for our practice. Quality documentation and reviews are led by the medical director, who reports to a national medical director. Thorough documentation, informed client choices, evidence-based care, and knowledge of the best practice protocols are integral parts of our quality control process.

THE FUTURE OF INTEGRATED MEDICINE

What should a physician tell patients about alternative medicine? Many physicians do not have the time to ask questions themselves. However, knowing what alternatives patients have tried or are trying and what supplements and herbal medicines they may be taking is becoming a more common part of practice. It should become a part of the documentation and the primary care physician should be a trusted source of knowledge for patients' questions. At the very least, the physician should have sources of reliable information readily available for recommendation.

I am encouraged that changes in our health care model have a real chance to affect medical protocol in this country. The integration of alternative therapies and routine health care must now proceed on a scientific basis. The research centers established by the National Institutes of Health (NIH) Office of Alternative Medicine help to move this along, but more needs to be done. The use of alternative therapies and products appears to be increasing more rapidly than appropriate supporting scientific studies can be conducted. I would support major NIH training grants, similar to those given to the basic sciences in the 1960s and 1970s, for training and supporting physicians in tracking and collecting data that are clinically available. Definitive studies are not required; as patients continue to use alternative therapies on their own, we can track what happens at the care delivery level and perhaps discover positive or negative outcomes to guide further studies. Time and resources are the problem—who will fund these efforts to obtain clinical documentation?

We must exercise greater care and caution when deciding to use alternative therapies in vulnerable populations. These include children, pregnant and lactating women, HIV-infected patients, and the elderly. Science-based studies should be the guide, but what is the physician's responsibility if studies are not yet available and consumers are using unsubstantiated procedures or products? The practices being used and the advice and recommendations being given, including referral to sources of reliable information, should be documented.

PROBLEMS AND FINANCIAL ASPECTS OF THE INTEGRATED PRACTICE

Problems

As medical director of a large, multispecialty group, I had helped open a dozen primary care offices around Chicago, so I was not a novice in how to open an office. However, I was utterly unprepared for the seemingly endless number of problems that needed prompt resolution, including training the practitioners in the office to record coherent data in a progress note; many did not know what a progress note even was. Insurance companies were also a problem. They would often deny claims, explaining that their policies did not cover holistic medicine. We even had medical staff in a shared, hospital-owned office space tell us that they would "walk out forever" if a chiropractor joined our staff.

Financial Aspects

I opened the original Chicago Holistic Center using my own funds. The success of this center spurred me to open more centers across the nation. With the help of a nonmedical acupuncturist who had some business experience, I opened a second center in Denver, again using my personal funds. I soon realized that I could not continue refinancing my house indefinitely. My partner and I drew up a business plan and circulated it to venture capital groups. I later learned that these groups had been exploring the concept of integrated centers based on Eisenberg's [2] article. One group offered to fund the expansion of the company, on the condition that we hire professional business management. We agreed, and in 1996 the company's name changed to American WholeHealth, Inc. (although I act as vice-chairman of the board of directors and senior clinician in our Lincoln Park, Chicago office, I am not and prefer not to be an administrator. Almost my entire day is spent in patient care).

Can integrative medicine boost income? When moving towards the integrative medical model, the time and resources it takes to educate patients in prevention, wellness, and appropriate use of complementary therapies must be considered. The level of reimbursement by health plans does not cover the resources expended. One population of patients willing to pay out-of-pocket for this brand of medicine, the now-aging "baby boomers," may be expanding; however, many in this group have employer health plan coverage, which means many HMO participants. Thus, although an integrative practice can be both successful and profitable, increase in income should not be the primary motive. However, integrative medicine provides the opportunity to affect the health-care model by moving away from illness-based, interventional care and toward preventive care, wellness, and whole-health promotion using a full range of appropriate therapeutic tools in a hospitable atmosphere [3,4,5•].

REFERENCES AND RECOMMENDED READING

Recently published papers of particular interest have been highlighted as:
• Of interest
•• Of outstanding interest

1. Wallis C: Why New Age medicine is catching on. *Time* 1991, 138:68–75.
2. Eisenberg DM, Kessler RC, Foster C, *et al.*: Unconventional medicine in the United States: prevalence, costs, and patterns of use. *N Engl J Med* 1993, 328:246–252.
3. Northrup C: *Women's Bodies, Women's Wisdom*. New York: Bantam Doubleday; 1998.
4. Shealy CN, Myss C: *The Creation of Health*. Boston, VA: Three Rivers Press; 1998.
5.• Davis-Floyd R, St. John G: *From Doctor to Healer: The Transformative Journey*. New Brunswick, NJ: Rutgers University Press; 1998.
This is a comprehensive study (interestingly classified as "cultural anthropology") of physicians who leave the conventional system and enter into integrative medicine.

Designing a Healing Clinical Office Environment: Creating Healing Spaces

15

Annette Ridenour

BACKGROUND

Alternative medicine provides clinicians with an opportunity to develop a wholistic philosophy for designing healing health-care facilities that should be applied to all institutions. Yet, for the most part, leaders of traditional health-care institutions are not ready to adopt these principles as universal design guidelines. Either they do not see a reason to change or they perceive wholistic design to be too expensive or too difficult.

As traditional medical providers embrace alternative medicine and open new facilities, not only will major changes take place in how health-care is practiced, but the profession is bound to look different as well. These changes will be interesting to chronicle in the future. In the meantime, alternative and integrated medicine provides us with a unique office design and business opportunity—one that is much different than creating a traditional medical office.

CREATING A BUSINESS PLAN

Alternative medical centers are being designed in many different ways. Those built in the next 5 years will all be models. At present, there are no tried and true formulas for success. Providers are racing to create them as fast as they can, and few models are being replicated.

In some ways, this situation is similar to the development of women's centers in the mid-1980s. Those facilities were new and different and satisfied a public demand. However, unlike alternative medicine, treatment of women's health as a specialty was more accepted by physicians and insurance companies.

Today, too many administrators are scrambling to open alternative medicine facilities without doing their homework and creating a sound business plan for how they might work in their community. It is not enough to speculate on how many people would potentially flock to a center for a set of services based on demographics. It is far better to research a plan of how a center would serve the specific needs of the community by participating and integrating itself into the community. Once the actual needs have been determined, programs can be established to fit those needs and real income and cost budgets can be extrapolated.

Alternative medicine centers of the future need to generate income as adjunct healing modalities to traditional Western medicine. Patients are experiencing relief from symptoms of chronic diseases through a variety of alternative therapies. Local hospitals, physician groups, and employers need to create partnerships and establish programs that truly meet the needs of the patient population.

DESIGN

Philosophy

To paraphrase Joseph Campbell [1], St. Thomas Aquinas attributes art with three characteristics: integrity, harmony, and clarity. Our design philosophy for creating healing spaces encompasses those same principles. Integrity represents unity—that the entire office be felt as one space. A resonance of all the elements within the space creates a sense of wholeness. Harmony represents the rhythmic arrangement of each part to the other and to the whole. When this is done well, clarity and radiance of experience create an aesthetic sense of arrest. This is what we aspire to do in our design.

Process

The process of designing alternative medicine centers involves empowering patients and staff to participate in the healing process. This is done by creating an experience for the patients that is a unification of all elements. How they experience the environment of care is directly relevant to their perception of the quality of care they are receiving. What is more, true healing centers need to function as healthy communities first. And healthy communities share vision and values.

The Circle of Design process (Table 15-1) provides an opportunity for the health-care team to establish a shared vision and values that will become the guidelines for how the alternative medicine center looks and operates. Symbols representing the vision and values for the community begin to emerge, and become a central point from which to start planning colors, themes, and artwork for the facility. Some universal design considerations are listed in Table 15-2 and illustrated in Figures 15-1 and 15-2.

Details

Have you ever walked into a hospital and realized that it could be located anywhere in the country? That it had no unique bond to the community? Each community has a regional sense of design that is specific to its geography and patient population. What is unique about the neighborhood? Is it a farming community or a mountainous area with lakes and forests? Are there many crafts people in the community? Does it have an interesting history? These questions should be considered when developing an office design.

Artwork is one way of creating a space that is harmonious with its community. In addition, finishes, materials, and colors should also reflect the community. Whenever possible,

TABLE 15-1. THE CIRCLE OF DESIGN PROCESS

All practitioners and support staff including administrators, designers, architects, construction managers, and even long-term patients should participate.

Send an invitation to each person introducing the process, setting the intention for the experience, and asking him or her to bring a personal symbol of healing to the group.

At the first meeting, assemble the group in a circle. Introduce group members and ask them to explain why they are stakeholders in the project, what their individual visions for the center are, and what they feel are their individual symbols of healing.

Show images of different buildings and other sites around the world and discuss what is healing about each of them.

Take participants on a guided imagery experience in which they can focus on their own personal places of healing.

Have them share their experiences with the group and write them down. Review and discuss these to reach a common vision and values.

TABLE 15-2. UNIVERSAL DESIGN CONSIDERATIONS

Each facility is unique to its owners, but there are several universal design considerations that characterize a healing environment.

Upon arrival, patients should feel like they just entered a facility that will support and nurture them, a place where they would want to go for renewal.

Materials should be natural in color, texture, and makeup. There should be adequate areas for privacy and contemplation.

Areas for interfacing with staff members should be intimate and inviting.

The plan of the space should feel open yet engaging.

Views of nature and the inclusion of the four elements—water, fire, earth, and air—should be part of all public spaces.

A full-spectrum color palette and lighting should be designed into all spaces.

The plan of the space should flow naturally without creating nooks and corners that feel disconnected from the rest of the space.

The senses of sound, smell, and touch need to be engaged through the introduction of appropriate music, aromatherapy, and tactile materials.

The design of the environment should be environmentally conscious, using nontoxic and recyclable materials. It should be energy efficient.

The environment needs to reflect the culture of the community through its colors and design style.

The art should be engaging, meaningful, and tell stories of healing.

Gardens and fountains need to be integrated into the waiting and treatment areas.

A resource center offering books, tapes, videos, and products should be accessible to patients.

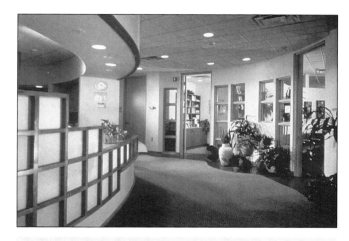

FIGURE 15-1. A small garden and fountain that provide the soothing sounds of water welcome everyone at the entry of the Arizona Center for Health and Medicine, a center offering Western and alternative medicine.

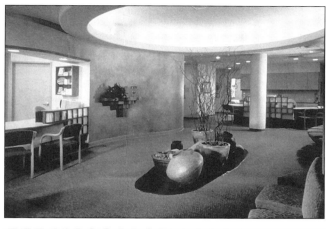

FIGURE 15-2. A central area, the heart of the office and home to a meditation garden, radiates with the intensity of green walls. Color and intensity change as one moves toward treatment areas.

artwork should be created by local artists. Patients and local artists can be asked to tell their stories of healing and express them through paintings, illustrations, poems, sculptures, or quilts. Each of these expressions engages patients in thought about their own personal healing.

It is also important to establish a philosophy of healing, which can be accomplished through artwork and other design elements. For example, when Saint Mary's Hospital and Health Center in Grand Rapids, Michigan, was developing its new Wege Center for Health and Learning several years ago, an overall theme of "wholism" and healing was established. Several subthemes were developed for different floors, such as nature as a healer, spirituality and healing, journeys, and communities. Local artists were asked to create individual pieces based on these subthemes. They wrote explanations of their pieces, which were hung beside the works. Photographs of the region, a mandala quilt, a large heart made of palm leaves and bark, a spiritual fountain with the Mercy Values engraved in the spiral, a sound sculpture, a wind sculpture of the Golden Mean, and special three-dimensional music composed to reflect the Golden Mean are some of the ways these themes were expressed.

How people feel in a given space is a reflection of its harmony. The space plan is a very critical element of why environments "feel" the way that they do. People are used to being in health-care facilities with endless corridors of rooms and corridors branching out from other corridors. Unfortunately, this is the most economical use of space; yet, when calculating usable square footage, it is important to maximize the billable space. When designing a healing environment, the goal is to achieve the maximum billable space while creating an environment that remains inspirational. There will be less usable space, but it will be more productive. Staff will tire less easily and patients will want to come back.

The first introduction to the space should provide people with a balanced experience by using all four elements. Water should be present in some kind of recirculating fountain. Natural light can be brought in, either through windows or views to light in the distance. Wood can be integrated with materials and fire can be introduced using warm tones.

Another way to make a space look less clinical is to add homelike amenities to clinical areas. Freestanding furniture, custom-designed armoires, hampers, and trash receptacles made of wood or laminate make a clinical space more homelike. Special touches, such as soft, comfortable custom gowns and robes, cloth hand towels, and tabletop water fountains, are appreciated by patients.

More studies have been devoted to the healing effects of music than any other of the arts. Many composers create music intended to soothe and relax the listener. Artists are making music therapeutic by composing specific music to assist with different conditions and to complement different therapies. This method is being explored and tested around the country. Patients in waiting rooms benefit from nature sounds and specially composed music. Individual treatment spaces may be outfitted with systems to allow individual choices for patients.

Many practitioners are also using aromatherapy to complement different treatments. Installation of individual diffusers in each space allows for maximum flow and responsiveness to each patient.

Designing Healthy Buildings

Healthy buildings, sometimes called green buildings, are defined in a variety of different ways and address not only health, but ecologic and social issues as well. Buildings should not make people sick, especially those that they visit for medical treatment. Many patients coming to alternative medicine centers already have compromised immune systems because they may be undergoing complementary therapies in conjunction with chemotherapy, dialysis, or radiation therapy. Patients with severe allergies also come in for alternative treatments. For all patients, it is a comfort to know they are being treated in a space that is nontoxic and maintains a high standard of infection control.

The building should be as energy efficient as possible. Use of natural light, appropriate window coverings, ceiling tiles, and insulation will maximize energy efficiently. Having energy-efficient light fixtures and movement sensors also help to save energy. Using recycled material is also important. Carpets are currently available that are made from 95% recycled material.

Often, health-care designers and facility managers select materials for interior finishes based on cost and ease of cleaning. Alternative medicine centers do not get the same level of abuse and foot traffic, which can allow the introduction of more natural interior finishes, thus making patients feel more comfortable.

The American Society of Heating and Refrigeration and Air Conditioning Applications 1995 Handbook [2] explains that "sick building syndrome" occurs when interior air pollutants are released into the interior atmosphere of a building. The air becomes contaminated with disease-causing mold, bacteria, and fungus that can tire people out, cause headaches, lead to lack of ability to concentrate, and cause muscle tension. Therefore, proper air filtration and location and quantity of air-handling vents are critical, especially when aromatherapy and moxibustion are being used in treatment.

A clean, nontoxic, energy-efficient environment can be created by specifying the right materials and planning electrical, heat, ventilation, and air conditioning systems. The construction process should be monitored and the results measured. The most common sources of indoor pollution in health-care facilities, according to Carron [3], are shown in Table 15-3.

Conclusions

All of the design elements discussed in this chapter are individually and collectively important. However, many providers will use these as a menu of desirable items that gradually are cut as budgets are finalized.

Table 15-3. Common Sources of Indoor Pollution in Health-Care Facilities

Construction materials, such as particle board, chipboard, plywood, polyurethane, ocms or fiberglass insulation, floor materials, synthetic wallpaper, sealers, adhesives, lacquers, paints, varnishes, and wood impregnates. It is sometimes unsafe for people to occupy spaces built with these materials and finishes until after a month after construction completion. Outgassing can continue at minor levels affecting sensitive patients and staff for years.
Office and support products, such as electrical and photographic equipment, office materials, glues, lubricants.
Housecleaning products, such as detergents, cleansers, deodorizers, mothballs, floor waxes, polishes, and sprays. Once a facility is open, it is important to sit down with the cleaning contractors to review and eliminate any potentially toxic chemical use.
Hospital and human systems, including HVAC systems, ductwork, combustion appliances, furnishings, tobacco, outside pollutants and soil gases, bioeffluents from humans and animals, and microbial contamination.

HVAC—heating, ventilation, and air conditioning.

Designing alternative medicine centers with a higher level of finishes and details does cost more. How much more, however, varies with the design, designer, and contractor. Facilities with nice features can be built for under $100 per square foot, but it is a challenge! Placing a value on many of the items discussed in this chapter depends on how they support the individual practice. Generally, practitioners who have experienced the difference of working in a nurturing, supportive environment understand the value this type of environment has for their patients.

This is clearly evident at the Arizona Center for Health and Medicine in Phoenix. Shortly after the facility was built and began operation, a patient survey was conducted to ask the following questions: "What was your reaction to the physical environment? How did this compare to other physician offices that you have been to? What were standouts in terms of either real positives or real negatives? What effect did it have on you as an individual?" Most patients responded that the center was "calming and pleasant," and thought it was different from other physician offices. The artwork and colors were distinguishing features, as was the feeling of spaciousness. No matter how many people were waiting in the clinic, or how busy the staff seemed, the facility did not give them the feeling of pressure or the need to move faster.

In a study sponsored by The Center for Health Design [4], researchers at The Picker Institute have identified seven dimensions of the built environment that matter to patients. Focus-group discussions with patients in ambulatory, acute, and long-term care settings revealed that they want 1) an environment that facilitates a connection to staff and caregivers; 2) is conducive to a sense of well-being; 3) is convenient and accessible; 4) promotes confidentiality and privacy; 5) cares for the family; 6) is considerate of impairments; and 7) is close to nature and the outside world.

It is not hard to build a case for using sensitive, thoughtful design when constructing an alternative medicine center. It makes sense for patients, for staff, and for business.

References and Recommended Reading

Recently published papers of particular interest have been highlighted as:
- Of interest
- •• Of outstanding interest

1. Campbell J: *The Way of Art* [lecture series]. New York: Sound Horizons Audio Video; 1990.
2. The American Society of Heating, Refrigerating, and Air Conditioning : *ASHRE Handbook: Heating, Ventilating, and Air Conditioning Applications.* Atlanta, GA: ASHRE; 1995.
3. Shepley M, Fournier M, McDougal K: *Healthcare Environments for Children and Their Families.* Dubuque, IA: Kendall/Hunt Publishing; 1998.
4. MacRae SK, Michel MJ: *Journal of Healthcare Design: Proceedings from the Tenth Symposium on Healthcare Design. Plenary Session: Consumer Perceptions of the Healthcare Environment—An Investigation to Determine What Matters.* Martinez, CA: The Center for Health Design; 1998.

Selected Bibliography

Barrie T: *Spiritual Path...Sacred Place: Myth, Ritual, and Meaning in Architecture*. Boston: SHAMBHALA Publications; 1996.

Bush CA: *Healing Imagery and Music: Pathways to the Inner Self*. Portland, OR: Pudra Press; 1995.

Colby B: *Color and Light: Influences and Impact*. Glendale, CA: Barbara Colby; 1990.

Day C: *Places of the Soul: Architecture and Environmental Design as a Healing Art*. Frome, Somerset, UK: Butler and Tanner Limited; 1990.

Korp M: *Sacred Art of the Earth: Ancient and Contemporary Earthworks*. New York: Continuum Publishing; 1997.

Rossbach S: *Interior Design with Feng Shui*. New York: EP Dutton; 1987.

Rossbach S, Yun L: *Living Color: Master Lin Yun's Guide to Feng Shui and the Art of Color*. New York: Kodansha America, Inc.; 1994.

Swan JA: *Sacred Places: How the Living Earth Seeks Our Friendship*. Santa Fe, NM: Bear & Company Publishing; 1990.

Swan JA: *The Power of Place: Sacred Ground in Natural and Human Environments*. Wheaton IL: Quest Books; 1991.

Tisserand RB: *The Art of Aromatherapy: The Healing and Beautifying Properties of the Essential Oils of Flowers and Herbs*. Rochester, VT: Destiny Books; 1977.

Venolia CA: *Healing Environments: Your Guide to Indoor Well-Being*. Berkeley, CA: Celestial Arts; 1988.

Continuing Educational Opportunities in Complementary Medicine

George R. Haynes

Several years ago I presented a proposed continuing medical education (CME) program to a group of physicians who voted to approve or deny my request. Unexpectedly, the conversation ventured into the realm of complementary medicine. One member shared an anecdote about a patient who had asked him for his thoughts and recommendations. With a tone of disdain in his voice (coupled with an effort to humor the group), he said that he referred the patient to a local health food store and offered to send his medical records to the same address. Later, at the same meeting, in a more serious tone, members of the group asked if I could recommend a reputable person to present a course in complementary medicine to the physicians on staff at the hospital.

This seemingly paradoxical example of physicians' attitudes toward complementary medicine is indicative of the current struggles as well as the ongoing learning that is essential to physicians, their patients, and the health-care organizations. Fortunately, medicine, with its many conventional and complementary components, is slowly beginning to consider and integrate new dynamic healing possibilities. However, many obstacles restrict this process. Laurens Van der Post describes part of our dilemma:

> [O]ne of the tragedies of modern man is that he is cut off from experiencing [the] immense dynamic pattern of renewal deep in himself. It is one of the laws of life that the new meaning must be lived before it can be known, and in some mysterious way modern man knows so much that he is the prisoner of his knowledge. The old dynamic conception of the human spirit as something living always on the frontiers of human knowledge has gone. We hide behind what we know. And there is an extraordinarily angry and aggressive quality in the knowledge of modern man; he is angry with what he does not know; he hates and rejects it. He has lost the sense of wonder about the unknown and he treats it as an enemy. The experience, which is before knowing, which would enflame his life with new meaning, is cut off from him. Curiously enough, it has never been studied more closely. People have measured the mechanics of it, and the rhythm, but somehow they do not experience it. [1]

PERSPECTIVE

For 8 years, I served as the director of education for two distinct, comprehensive medical rehabilitation centers. Both were substantial facilities with over 100 inpatient beds. One was a free-standing facility and the other was part of a much larger integrated health-care system. My role in designing and presenting CME programs as well as working closely with many physicians on numerous organizational initiatives and goals (both professional and personal) was both challenging and personally satisfying. Complementary and integrative medicine were of particular interest to me, and I strove through educational initiatives, small group discussions, and actual practices to help influence organizational decisions. In the process, I relearned the importance of individual stories, which have the potential to celebrate our uniqueness, to transcend our isolation, and the power to initiate or quicken the healing process as we come to better understand ourselves and those whose stories we hear.

Most stories, however, require time to listen and reflect and wonder. Rachel Naomi Remen insightfully writes that:

> Life rushes us along and few people are strong enough to stop on their own....Because we have stopped listening to each other we may even have forgotten how to listen, stopped learning how to recognize meaning and fill ourselves from the ordinary events of our lives. We have become solitary; readers and watchers rather than sharers and participants [2••].

We have also lost much of our capacity as healers—for those we serve as well as ourselves. The following three examples reflect physicians' struggles and the potential for renewal.

A neurologist with whom I worked closely had, for many years, treated diabetics and thought himself to be knowledgeable in his practice. This perception changed dramatically when he himself was diagnosed with diabetes. He discovered how much he did not know about this condition. Since that time, his personal experiences and additional research have greatly expanded his insight and knowledge. He has become more compassionate with his patients and has established a specialty center where he shares his own challenges and lifestyle changes.

Another physician friend is an academic who has been interested in complementary medicine for many years and is a recognized authority. Although his research and knowledge are extensive, his personal integration of this knowledge into his life was limited until he was diagnosed with fibromyalgia. Seeking guidance and relief, he was advised to change his eating patterns, exercise daily, reduce and better manage stress, and receive acupuncture treatments and regular body massages. Today, he has greatly improved and adheres almost religiously to these prescriptions, which were recommended by a holistic and alternative medicine physician.

At a recent national conference on integrative medicine, I had the opportunity to spend several hours with one of the presenters, a recognized and influential authority in the area of integrative medicine. One of the questions that I asked focused on the extent to which she was able to incorporate balance (see Johnson [3••]) into her demanding schedule. Candidly she shared that even though this was an important part of her work, her challenging schedule had unfortunately limited essential time for herself. She had a clear awareness of the loss, the potential dangers, and the need for renewal to more effectively lead by example. It was not difficult for me to identify with her struggle. Afterwards, I reflected on the description by Wheelis [4] of how we create and are able to change ourselves through a sequence of "suffering, insight, will, action, change." To do so, however, we must assume responsibility for prioritizing and managing what is important in our lives. What we do and how we do it are more important than who we are or what we say.

Underlying the question of the role of ongoing learning in complementary medicine is the need to identify the seemingly colossal obstacles physicians have in opening their own lives to change. In a recent presentation, Lee Lipsenthal (see Chapter 11) described the challenges physicians face in their training—challenges they must overcome in order to open ourselves to new methods and ideas. The basic elements of this presentation are discussed in the following section.

BECOMING A PHYSICIAN

The psychologic profile of a person predisposed toward heart disease includes type A behavior, hostility, anger, isolation, and depression. It also includes a sense of perceived responsibility without a sense of control. Physicians, in many ways, fit this profile, especially around responsibility and control. It is also true that physicians often enter medicine because it is a safe and stable profession. However, medicine is undergoing rapid change and is no longer stable.

In many ways, physicians are like siblings born into a dysfunctional system. The system that trained us to be doctors and facilitates our livelihood has also enhanced any dysfunctional behaviors we had coming into the system and taught us new ones. We have all experienced abuses in the transformation into this thing called "Doctor." We suffer the loss of ideals, of motivation, of compassion for patients, and of passion for our work. Fear holds us back from making change in our behaviors, and without changing these behaviors the system cannot begin to change.

The Idealist

What visions danced in your head when choosing a career in medicine? The desire to serve others, directly or through science? Was there an experience in your life that kindled an irresistible flame? Perhaps there was a healthy academic drive to learn and answer difficult questions. It is also likely that the prestige of the doctor's role had some influence. Many of us wanted to choose a career that would make our families proud and make us feel valuable. There was probably also the attraction of a career promising financial stability.

With these ideals we apply to medical school, competing with others for a limited number of spaces. This competition establishes a fear of failure and fuels competitive behavior. Self-interest predominates and empathy for colleagues takes a back seat. In the first years of medical school, academic knowledge assumes first priority. The role of creative thinker is supplanted by that of memorizing survivor, determined not only to pass but to excel. Relationships become less important, as evidenced by high divorce rates in this period. The process of isolation begins as trust becomes less important than survival.

Becoming a "Real" Doctor

When we graduate and move on to internship and residency, we feel that we are now "real" doctors with real responsibility.

Responsibility becomes real. We can stay up late, admit more patients than anyone else, and create long lists of unlikely diagnoses to prove our worth and support our pride. Failure is impossible, because you would disappoint everyone, especially yourself.

Finally, we accept a secure position with a large group, where we get an office, staff, and benefits. We see 20 patients a day, one patient every 15 minutes for 5 hours, plus an hour or two for charts and calls, an hour for rounds, a committee meeting or two and most days home for dinner. Soon we are seeing 25 patients, 30 patients, 35 patients, 40 patients, 50 patients, up to 60 patients a day. When does the reality of a sick system sink in? With our own illness? We need to step back from this routine and consciously decide how we can better serve ourselves and our patients. If we openly admit that there is a problem and look for ways to produce change, answers will come. None of us can do this alone. We need to talk in the cafeteria, at the preschools, tennis clubs, meetings, chat rooms—wherever and whenever we see each other. We need to take back what we have lost in the process of becoming a doctor so we can be healers for the first time.

THE DATA

To better understand and appreciate the impact and potential of complementary medicine, some data regarding physicians and current trends in medicine are essential. The total number of physicians in the United States is approximately 737,764. A high percentage of these (97.1%) are not federally employed. Most physicians are in patient care (81.2%), almost half are under 45 years of age (46.9%), and most are men (78.7%) [5]. Regarding average total hours worked per week, Table 16-1 shows statistics from 1996 demonstrating the increase and descrease in hours as related to physician age [6]. In addition, as of 1996, the average net income for all nonfederal physicians after expenses but before taxes and minus deferred compensation was $187,000 [7]. The mean age at death for all nonfederal physicians was 75.9 in 1996 (unpublished data, American Medical Association, 1998).

With so many physicians focused on patient care and most having long and productive careers, it is appropriate to ask which variables influence career satisfaction to better understand and improve work life. In a study that analyzed physician job satisfaction, results from a large group practice physician survey (n = 302) in 1988 were compared with data obtained from six focus groups (n = 26) in 1995 composed of underrepresented subgroups such as health maintenance organization (HMO), female, minority, and inner-city physicians [8]. Relationships with patients and colleagues were identified as a primary component of physician satisfaction. In addition, for the women in the focus groups, balance of work and family commitment was a concern, and being able to provide "total care" to their patients was a source of satisfaction. This is especially noteworthy because gender balance is becoming more prevalent in our medical schools and will clearly influence the future delivery of health care.

Many physicians are concerned about their ability to provide high-quality health-care relative to the effects of managed care on the physician–patient relationship [9••]. This focus on quality is indicative of significant paradigm shifts occurring in most organizations and systems. David Nash, Director of Health Policy and Clinical Outcomes for Thomas Jefferson University Hospital and Associate Dean for Jefferson Medical College, writes that "the next 20 years of medical practice will be characterized by medicine's first industrial revolution, one that pits the 'horse' of slavish adherence to professional autonomy against the 'steam engine' of public accountability..." [10]. After describing what he perceives as inevitable changes, Nash continues: "For those...who understand that public accountability is the essence of true professionalism, who are not deeply threatened by measures of individual performance, and who welcome a healthy self-evaluation, it is indeed the best of times" [10].

In their ongoing evaluations and strategic planning, most health-care systems have been grappling with how to pay for the high cost of specialized medical treatment. One response, managed care, has tended to challenge the integrity of physician–patient relationship by limiting services, mandating provider lists, and specifying financial expectations including, at times, the number of patients to be treated daily. This model has also redirected profits from medical institutions and doctors "toward those in the business of running medicine" [9••].

Another response has been to explore complementary medicine, which encompasses prevention, conventional, and alternative practices. It has also been referred to by some as *holistic medicine* because it embraces the whole system—body, mind, spirit and environment. Interestingly, this move toward complementary medicine is patient driven; health-care professionals have, for the most part, become interested because patients are using it in large doses [11]. For example, Americans spend $2 billion to $4 billion a year on massage therapy according to the American Massage Therapy Association in Evanston, Illinois [12]. Eisenberg *et al.* [13] published a follow-up survey in *JAMA* in late 1998 on the trends in alternative medicine use in the United States between 1990 and 1997. Total visits to practitioners of alternative medicine increased 47.3% (to 629 million), exceeding "total visits to all U.S. primary care physicians" [13]. In addition, the "total 1997 out-of-pocket expenditures relating to alternative therapies were conservatively estimated at $27 billion" [13].

TABLE 16-1. INCREASE AND DECREASE OF WORK HOURS BY PHYSICIAN AGE, 1996

Physician Age, y	Average Total Hours Worked Per Week
under 36	57.6
36 to 45	60
46 to 55	59.5
56 to 65	56.9
over 65	50.3

Data from Gonzalez and Zhang [6].

In the same issue of *JAMA*, which was devoted in large part to alternative and complementary medicine, Jonas [14] writes that the increasing popularity of complementary therapy practices

> reflects changing needs and values in modern society in general. This includes...an increase in public access to worldwide health information, reduced tolerance for paternalism...and an increased interest in spiritualism. In addition, concern about the adverse effects and escalating costs of conventional health care are fueling the search for alternative approaches to the prevention and management of illness. As the public's use of healing practices outside conventional medicine accelerates, ignorance about these practices by physicians and scientists risks broadening the communication gap between the public and the profession that serves them. [14]

The practices demonstrated by patients, coupled with data obtained from national surveys, have spurred many healthcare systems and providers to begin offering a menu of services and programs. Even some 60% of the medical schools have begun to teach aspects of alternative medicine practices.

Jonas [14], however, although acknowledging the many benefits of integration, warns of the potential risks in moving too quickly to integrate methods and practices that have not been critically assessed. He recommends caution, looking to effective research, and advancing with our wisdom and reason intact. Another concern expressed by Davis-Floyd and St. John [9••] is the practice by some HMO providers of offering low-cost alternative therapies to generate more profits. This practice, they write, "brings up the question of the co-option of holism by the hegemonic technomedical model" [9••].

RECOMMENDATIONS FOR CONTINUING EDUCATIONAL OPPORTUNITIES IN COMPLEMENTARY MEDICINE

How can physicians best learn about effective complementary medicine practices and avail themselves of ongoing learning opportunities? I recommend five primary methods, which, ideally, are employed in concert with each other. These are: 1) learning from colleagues and recognized experts, as well as respected medical institutions such as medical colleges; 2) learning from respected publications including books, journals, newsletters and websites; 3) attending selected regional and national conferences; 4) embracing healing partnerships; and 5) employing self-learning.

Learning from Colleagues and Recognized Experts

Many health-care systems today have a complementary or integrative medicine initiative with one or more experienced and knowledgeable physicians available for presentations and possibly even for consultation. Many medical colleges are also a valuable resource to explore. Another excellent source of physician programs in the United States offering complementary and alternative medicine education has been compiled by Bhaswati Bhattacharya [15]. In addition, one of the most notable programs in integrative medicine was initiated several years ago at the University of Arizona by Andrew Weil. Its vision is the redesign of medical education and the establishment of integrative medicine as a new medical discipline. Professional development and continuing medical education are primary elements of their mission.

In New York City, Mehmet Oz, a respected and accomplished cardiothoracic surgeon at Columbia-Presbyterian Medical Center, became involved with alternative therapies in early 1994 through a study designed to see how hypnosis changed the quality of life for patients after surgery. Since then, he has explored other areas including energy medicine [16]. Similar interest and expertise in a variety of medical practices are emerging in many areas of the country. See Russek and Schwartz [17] for additional information.

Learning from Respected Publications

There are many publications readily available that address complementary medicine, and new ones emerging regularly. *The New England Journal of Medicine* and *JAMA* are two highly respected and insightful sources of information, especially regarding current research. Of the many newsletters on the market, Andrew Weil's newsletter, *Self Healing*, as well as his website (http://www.drweil.com) are both very popular and highly influential. Books are more plentiful and, therefore, perhaps more challenging as sources of valuable information. (In addition to those already cited in this chapter, Table 16-2 lists a number of additional references.)

Attending Selected Regional and National Conferences

Two primary conferences for physicians and health care professionals with a national scope are Marc Micozzi's *World Med* (888-748-9800) and Jim Gordon's *Comprehensive Cancer Care* (202-966-7338). Both typically provide CME credits. Additional CME programs are listed in Table 16-3.

Embracing Healing Partnerships

It is not uncommon for many physicians to request and strongly encourage—even require—their patients to comply with their treatment prescription. The assumption is that the physician knows what will "work" best for the patient. This model, however, rings of paternalism. Jim Gordon writes that:

> Demands for, or expectations of, compliance—no matter how qualified—are not only disrespectful and inappropriate but, as the literature shows, ineffective. They work poorly for chronic illness and indifferently in acute situations. Equally important, even when they do work—when the patient does do what she is told—they can help maintain her in an enduring state of passivity and dependence, which is itself likely to be unhealthy in the long run. It would be far better

and healthier for everyone concerned if we abandoned the very concepts of compliance and adherence and regarded the doctor-patient relationship as a full collaboration, a genuine healing partnership. [25]

Chris Northrup concurs. "As doctors, we must move into a partnership model where the patient is taking responsibility for health and the doctor as a consultant. That will transform health care. It will never be transformed as long as we give over our bodies and souls and minds to experts" [9••].

This is a new paradigm of health care that respects the experience, knowledge, and intuition of patients. It also requires a certain level of maturity on the part of the physician. Letting go of control may be one of the most difficult aspects of the transition. But, as with their own children, physicians must recognize that this process of growth is inevitable if health care is to evolve to its full potential.

Employing Self-Learning

At Harvard's Mind/Body/Medical Institute, Herbert Benson [19] bases his work as well as his vision for the future of medicine on the model of a three-legged stool, "balanced and supported by…three components: self-care, medications, and procedures." He believes that "health and well-being can be maximized with the balanced application of pharmaceuticals, surgery and procedures, and self-care. In medical practice today, the stool is unbalanced because we rely far too much on pharmaceuticals and surgery and procedures." He advocates self-care among physicians "to optimize medicine, health, and well-being as well as to balance the stool" [19].

Physicians are trained to be independent thinkers and operators. They are active in medicine for a long period of time during which they can exert their influence. In recent years, however, most have become members of systems and teams for which they have had little training. In fact, in my experience, many physicians have had minimal learning (*see* Schmeling [44]) (experientially and knowledge based) in leadership and communication skills, group and team dynamics, effective listening and negotiating skills, and a host of other socialization dynamics. And yet by most standards, physicians are perceived to be leaders. However, as Gary Wills [45] writes, "It is one of the major disservices of the 'superman' school of leadership that suggests a leader can command all situations with the same basic gifts." Rather, ". . .leadership must differ from situation to situation." He continues:

> . . .and even those who are leaders must also be followers much of the time. This is the crucial role. Followers judge leaders. Only if the leaders pass that test do they have any impact. The potential followers,

TABLE 16-2. RECOMMENDED READING

Gesundheit! [18]
Timeless Healing: The Power and Biology of Belief [19]
Whole Healing: A Step-by-Step Program to Reclaim Your Power to Heal [20]
Meaning & Medicine: Lessons form a Doctor's Tales of Breakthrough and Healing [21]
Prayer Is Good Medicine [22]
Recovering the Soul: A Scientific and Spiritual Search [23]
The Four Pillars of Healing [24]
Manifesto For a New Medicine: Your Guide to Healing Partnerships and the Wise Use of Alternative Therapies [25]
Full Catastrophe Living: Using the Wisdom of Your Body and Mind to Face Stress, Pain and Illness [26]
Fundamentals of Complementary and Alternative Medicine [27]
Stress, Diet & Your Heart [28]
Dr. Dean Ornish's Program for Reversing Heart Disease [29]
Love & Survival: The Scientific Basis for the Healing Power of Intimacy [30]
Roots of Healing: The New Medicine [31]
Spontaneous Healing [32]
8 Weeks to Optimum Health: A Proven Program for Taking Full Advantage of Your Body's Natural Healing Power [33]
Doctor, What Should I Eat? [34]
Dr. Rosenfeld's Guide to Alternative Medicine: What Works, What Doesn't—and What's Right for You [35]
Healing Yourself: A Step-by-Step Program for Better Health Through Imagery [36]
Retreat: Time Apart for Silence and Solitude [37]
Healing Centers and Retreats: Healthy Getaways for Every Body and Budget [38]
Wounded Healers [39]
Encounters with Chi [40]
Complementary/Alternative Medicine: An Evidence-Based Approach [41]
Choices in Healing [42]
Essentials of Complementary and Alternative Medicine [43]
Healing Visualizations: Creating Health Through Imagery [44]

TABLE 16-3. CONFERENCES AND CONTINUING MEDICAL EDUCATION PROGRAMS

World Med (888-748-9800)
Comprehensive Cancer Care (202-966-7338)
Body & Soul (303-444-0202, http://www.naropa.edu/index.html)
Healing the Whole Self (800-944-1001, http://www.omega-inst.org/)
NCCAM-sponsored conferences (http://altmed.od.nih.gov/nccam/)
Harvard Medical School (617-432-1525, http://www.med.harvard.edu/conted/)
Columbia University (212-781-5990)
University of Arizona (http://www.ahsc.arizona.edu/integrative_medicine/cme.html)
NCCAM-sponsored conferences (http://altmed.od.nih.gov/nccam/)
Alternative Therapies Symposium and Exposition (800-899-1712)

if their judgement is poor, have judged themselves. If the leader takes his or her followers to the goal, to great achievements, it is because the followers were capable of that kind of response. [45]

Healing partnerships require such a model of balance and respect [46].

CONCLUSIONS

Stephan Rechtschaffen [47] believes that the advancement of mind–body medicine has developed in large part due to the accelerating pace of life. He writes, "the faster we go, the more likely we are to separate mind from body, and thus the more susceptible we become to a variety of diseases that have the lack of communication between mind and body as their root cause." With more than 40% of Americans seeking out alternative methods of self-care or alternative practitioners, it seems wise for physicians to become familiar with and attentive to the various alternative practices and their implications for the full complement of health care today. This is especially important because a majority of patients, more than 60%, are not revealing their alternative therapy use to their physicians.

Openness and interest, as well as receptivity to and encouragement of healing partnerships on the part of physicians will help to ameliorate this potentially dangerous chasm. This new paradigm of health care also has the potential to have a dynamic impact on physicians themselves, as they become more attentive to their own experiences, mind–body insights, intuition, daily practices, and general health. Then, from a position of greater insight and wisdom, they will more fully appreciate the words of Albert Schweitzer: "Example is not the main thing in influencing others. It is the only thing."

To lead by example in the area of integrative medicine will be a significant change for many physicians, and could have a profound impact on health care practice today. Historian Arnold Toynbee [48], in his book *A Study of History*, outlines a model of withdrawal and return that has the potential to help initiate this process. Toynbee moves through the ages of recorded history, giving numerous examples of how change and progress have come from creative and courageous individuals willing to step from the familiar and the secure into the unknown. Seminal advances have come about when these individuals—Peter the Great of Russia, Jesus, Mohammed, Buddha, Confucius, Kant, and Ibn Khaldun, to name a few—return to share their wisdom with others. (Some religious sects might argue the degree of awareness or nature of some of those mentioned here. Nonetheless, their significant roles as agents of change is undeniable.) The process or movement is one of withdrawal and return, and each creative person motivated in such a way becomes, in his or her own way, an agent of change.

Pulling back, even withdrawing for short periods of time, to reflect on their own stories and challenges, and the important stories of their families, physicians might well initate the renewal process that van der Post [1] believed is essential to our meaningful evolution. Certainly, it could have a profound impact on the physicians themselves as well as the patients/partners with whom they are learning to enrich the healing process. Cameron [49], Rechtschaffen [47], Moran [50], and Levy [51] have significant insights toward encouraging and guiding this process as does Fox [52], whose "Spirituality of Work Questionnaire" appears in Table 16-4. What is clear is that none of us can give what we do not have. At this time in our history, in the domain of complementary and integrative medicine, physicians have the opportunity to be wise and effective healers and leaders. Perhaps a respected health food store is a good place to start.

Table 16-4. A Spirituality of Work Questionnaire*

1) Do I experience joy in my work? When, and under what circumstances? How often? How can the joy be increased? How does this joy relate to the pain and difficulties at work?
2) Do others experience joy as a result of my work? Directly? Indirectly? How can this joy be increased?
3) Is my work actively creating good work for others? How? How might this be improved? How does my work prevent others' working?
4) When did I first feel drawn to the kind of work I am doing? What did it feel like? Has this feeling increased or decreased over the years? Have I lost touch with this feeling over the years? How can this feeling be regenerated?
5) Is my work smaller than my soul? How big is my soul? How big is my work? What can I do to bring the two together?
6) How can I simplify my work? Can I simplify my getting to and from work? How is my work play? How can I learn to confuse work and play?
7) Is my work real work or a job? Is it a vocation, calling, or role that the universe is asking of me? How do I know the answer to this question? How can I increase my awareness of the mystery and role my work plays in the world?
8) How does my work connect to the Great Work of the Universe? How is it contributing to the one work, the ongoing work of the universe? When am I most aware of this connection?
9) How is my work a blessing to generations to come? In what way is my work connected to the needs of young people today? How am I participating in "fashioning a gift for the young"?
10) How am I emptied at work? How does nothingness happen at my work? What is my response to nothingness at work?
11) What inner work have I been involved in over the last five years? What inner work do I expect to be involved in over the next five years? How is this inner work affecting my outer work? How does my outer work affect my inner work?
12) Could my work be more creative than it is? If so, how? What is holding me back? How does my work encourage the creativity of others? What is the most creative work I do?
13) Who profits from my work? Where does the money that my work generates go? Where does the money that I am paid in my work come from?
14) What does my work "interfere with"? How effective is this interference? How can this interference be more effective?
15) What allies have I made within my work world? How do I sustain my vision through base communities and in other ways outside my work world?
16) What enemies do I make because of my work? Whom does my work disturb? What do I learn if certain groups or persons are disturbed by my work?
17) How does my work affect the environment? How is it a gift to the animals that are not two-legged? How does it contribute to bringing about the environmental revolution? How can I improve environmental consciousness in my workplace?
18) Which of the ecological virtues (*eg*, vegetarianism, recycling, bicycling) am I practicing the most? Which of the ecological virtues have I paid the least attention to? How can I spread the word about the need for ecological virtues in our time?
19) What do I learn at work? In what ways is work a learning experience for me? In what ways is it a leaning experience for others?
20) Are awe and wonder experienced in my work? If so, when? If so, by whom? If not, why not?
21) Am I growing younger every day? Why? Why not? What can I do to stay young in heart and spirit? Am I emptying myself of bitterness, resentment, and self-pity?
22) If I were to leave my work today, what difference would it make to my spiritual growth? to the spiritual development of my colleagues at work? to the spiritual development of my family or significant others?
23) If I suddenly received an inheritance of $300,000, would I immediately cease my work? What would I do instead of the work I am doing? What would I do with the money itself?
24) What ways of doing Sabbath—of resting and letting go of work—do I engage in? What rituals do I engage in? What rituals do I most need to participate in?
25) What am I doing to reinvent the profession in which I work? How am I bringing justice, compassion, and celebration to the world by way of my work? How am I returning my profession to its origins as a sacred or sacramental work?
26) Which of the classical seven sacraments most characterizes the work that I do? Does this mean that I am a priest and midwife, bringing into being the grace of the sacrament of the universe?
27) What is the funniest thing about my work?
28) Am I afraid of time off? What do I do with leisure time? If I had a year off every seven years what would I do with that year?
29) How can my family and I lead a simpler lifestyle, get along on less, and enjoy life more? Do I work in order to spend? Why do I do the work I am doing?
30) What is sacred about the work I do? Were any references to the sacredness of my work made in my education or training for the work? How might the dimension of the sacred be included in the training for the work I do?

*Several of these questions may be difficult to fully understand or appreciate without referring to the original text [52].
From Fox [52]; with permission.

Acknowledgement

The author wishes to thank Dr. Lee Lipsenthal and Dr. Bhaswati Bhattacharya for their contributions and insight during the preparation of this chapter.

References and Recommended Reading

Recent publications of particular interest have been highlighted as:
- Of interest
- Of outstanding interest

1. Van der Post L: *Patterns of Renewal.* CITY:Pendle Hill; 1961.
2. •• Remen RN: *Kitchen Table Wisdom: Stories That Heal.* New York: Riverhead Books; 1996.

    This is a profoundly simple and wise book that inspires through stories of love, vulnerability, and healing.
3. •• Johnson RA: *Balancing Heaven and Earth: A Memoir of Visions, Dreams, and Realizations.* New York: Harper Collins; 1998.

    This is an excellent and insightful exploration of balance and its importance in our lives, a memoir and personal guide that emphasizes that "...there is one right thing and only one right thing to do at every moment."
4. Wheelis A: *How People Change.* New York: Harper Row; 1973.
5. Randolph L: *Physician Characteristics and Distribution in the U.S. 1997–1998.* Chicago: American Medical Association; 1997.
6. Gonzalez ML, Zhang P: *Socioeconomic Characteristics of Medical Practice 1997.* Chicago: American Medical Association; 1997.
7. Gonzalez ML, Zhang P: *Physician Marketplace Statistics 1997/98.* Chicago: American Medical Association; 1998.
8. McMurray JE, Williams E, Schwartz MD, *et al.*: Physician job satisfaction: developing a model using qualitative data. *J Gen Intern Med* 1997, 12:711–714.
9. •• Davis-Floyd R, St. John G: *From Doctor to Healer: The Transformation Journey.* New Brunswick, NJ: Rutgers University Press; 1998.

    This book is very important to physicians interested in better understanding the limitations of our current technomedicine and two major paradigms working to expand its narrowness—the humanistic and holistic models of medicine. It also includes interviews with numerous physicians and their transformational experiences that have profoundly changed their practice of medicine.
10. Nash D: Being held accountable. *New Physician* 1996, 45:6–8.
11. Durso C: Something old, something new. *New Physician* 1998, 47:12–15.
12. Perloff S: Here's the rub. *The Philadelphia Inquirer* January 22, 1999:20 [Weekend section].
13. Eisenberg DM, Davis RB, Etner SL, *et al.*: Trends in alternative medicine use in the United States, 1990–1997. *JAMA* 1998, 280:1569–1575.
14. Jonas WB: Alternative medicine: learning from the past, examining the present, advancing to the future. *JAMA* 1998, 280:1616.
15. Bhattacharya B: M.D. programs in the United States with complementary and alternative medicine education: an ongoing listing. *J Altern Complement Med* 1998, 4:325–335.
16. Brown C: The experiments of Dr. Oz. *The New York Times Magazine.* July 30, 1995:20–23.
17. Russek LG, Schwartz GE: Energy cardiology: a dynamical energy systems approach for integrating conventional and alternative medicine. *Adv J Mind–Body Health* 1996, 12:4–45.
18. Adams P: *Gesundheit!* Rochester, VT: Healing Arts Press; 1993.
19. Benson H: *Timeless Healing: The Power and Biology of Belief.* New York: Scribner; 1996.
20. Dacher ES: *Whole Healing: A Step-by-Step Program to Reclaim Your Power to Heal.* New York: Penguin Books; 1996.
21. Dossey L: *Meaning & Medicine: Lessons form a Doctor's Tales of Breakthrough and Healing.* New York: Bantam Books; 1992.
22. Dossey L: *Prayer Is Good Medicine.* New York: Harper Collins; 1996.
23. Dossey L: *Recovering the Soul: A Scientific and Spiritual Approach.* New York: Bantam Doubleday Deli; 1989.
24. Galland L: *The Four Pillars of Healing.* New York: Random House; 1997.
25. Gordon JS: *Manifesto For a New Medicine: Your Guide to Healing Partnerships and the Wise Use of Alternative Therapies.* Reading, MA: Addison-Wesley; 1996.
26. Kabat-Zinn J: *Full Catastrophe Living: Using the Wisdom of Your Body and Mind to Face Stress, Pain, and Illness.* New York: Dell Publishing; 1990.
27. Micozzi M: *Fundamentals of Complementary and Alternative Medicine.* New York: Churchill Livingstone; 1996.
28. Ornish D: *Stress, Diet, and Your Heart.* New York: Penguin Books; 1982.
29. Ornish D: *Dr. Dean Ornish's Program for Reversing Heart Disease.* New York: Random House; 1990.
30. Ornish D: *Love and Survival: The Scientific Basis for the Healing Power of Intimacy.* New York: Harper Collins; 1998.
31. Weil A, Remen RN, Goleman D, *et al.*: *Roots of Healing: The New Medicine.* Carson, CA: Hay House; 1997.
32. Weil A: *Spontaneous Healing.* New York: Ballantine Books; 1995.
33. Weil A: *8 Weeks to Optimum Health: A Proven Program for Taking Full Advantage of Your Body's Natural Healing Power.* New York: Alfred A. Knopf; 1997.
34. Rosenfeld I: *Doctor, What Should I Eat?* New York: Warner Books; 1995.
35. Rosenfeld I: *Dr. Rosenfeld's Guide to Alternative Medicine: What Works, What Doesn't—and What's Right for You.* New York: Random House; 1996.
36. Rossman ML: *Healing Yourself: A Step-by-Step Program For Better Health Through Imagery.* New York: Pocket Books; 1987.
37. Housden R: *Retreat: Time Apart for Silence and Solitude.* San Francisco: Harper San Francisco; 1995.
38. Miller J: *Healing Centers and Retreats: Healthy Getaways for Every Body and Budget.* Santa Fe: John Muir Publications; 1998.
39. *Encounters with Qi: Exploring Chinese Medicine* New York: WW Norton & Co; 1995.
40. Spencer JW, Joseph JJ: *Complementary/Alternative Medicine: An Evidence-Based Approach.* St. Louis: Mosby Books; 1999.
41. Lerner m: *Choices in Healing.* Cambridge, MA: MIT Press; 1994.
42. Jonas W, Levin JS: *Essentials of Complementary and Alternative Medicine.* Philadelphia: Lippincott, Williams & Wilkins; 1999.
43. Epstein G: *Healing Visualizations: Creating Health Through Imagery.* New York: Bantam Books; 1989.
44. Schmeling W: *Facing Change in Health Care: Learning Faster in Tough Times.* Chicago: American Hospital Publishing; 1996.
45. Wills G: *Certain Trumpets: The Call of Leaders.* New York: Simon & Schuster; 1994.
46. Easwaran E: *Take Your Time: Finding Balance in a Hurried World.* Tomales, CA: Nilgiri Press; 1994
47. Rechtschaffen S: *Time Shifting: Creating More Time to Enjoy Your Life.* New York: Doubleday; 1996.
48. Toynbee AJ: *A Study of History: The Growths of Civilizations* vol 3, edn 8. London: Oxford University Press; 1963.
49. Cameron J: *The Artist's Way: A Spiritual Path to Higher Creativity* New York: Tarcher/Putnam; 1992.
50. Moran V: *Shelter for the Spirit: How To Make Your Home A Haven in a Hectic World.* New York: Harper Collins; 1997.
51. Levy N: *To Begin Again: The Journey Toward Comfort, Strength, and Faith in Difficult Times.* New York: Alfred A. Knopf; 1998.
52. Fox M: *The Reinvention of Work: A New Vision of Livelihood for Our Time.* New York: Harper Collins; 1994.

Surveys of Complementary and Alternative Medicine

17

Jacqueline C. Wootton and Andrew G. Sparber

An interesting aspect of the survey literature on complementary and alternative (CAM) medicine over the past decade is changing terminology. Toward the end of the 1980s, when surveys of the field first started to appear, the tone was cautious if not alarmist. Authors referred therapies as *unproven, nonproven,* or *questionable.* In the early 1990s, the mood became defensive, reflected in the literature by terms such as *unorthodox, non-orthodox, unconventional, nonconventional,* and even (misleadingly) *nontraditional* medicine (all terms are relative, but the widely accepted convention is to reserve the term *traditional* for indigenous or ancient traditional systems of medicine, such as Ayurveda, Tibetan, or Chinese medicine. These systems of medicine usually also encompass a whole cosmology or world view. The relatively more recent Western system is referred to as *Western conventional biomedicine* or as any one of these three terms used alone). The founding of the U.S. National Institutes of Health's (NIH) Office of Alternative Medicine (OAM) in 1992 was a watershed event, conferring some legitimacy to the area. The more challenging and assertive term *alternative medicine* became current, later softened by adding or substituting the terms *complementary* or *adjunct* therapies, which are favored in Europe and other English-speaking parts of the world outside the United States. The newly elevated National Center for Complementary and Alternative Medicine (NCCAM) reflects this trend, but it ignores the current mainstreaming connoted by the concept of *integrated* or *integrative* medicine. The abbreviation CAM is used in this chapter unless some further refinement of the concepts is needed, and the limitations of this acronym are discussed.

The researcher may call into question the validity of any survey. However, despite the changing orientation of CAM surveys investigators, the findings and trends have been remarkably consistent throughout the past decade in the United States. Surveys from other parts of the world are excluded from this chapter because history of use varies considerably from continent to continent; the United States trails behind most other Western societies in its acceptance of CAM. Few investigations have studied patterns of use among minorities, and overreporting of the relatively affluent population is common. Little research exists on CAM practitioners and their patients; most surveys focus on patients in a conventional medical setting. There is a need for longitudinal, multidimensional research in favor of, or in addition to, the convenient snapshot view of cross-sectional data. This is expressed well in the following quote:

> Health is a process which needs to be captured at different points over a long period of time. We need to know, for example, the views of patients who have left practitioners they were consulting, and how they compare to the views of those who stayed and those who have moved back and forth, between and among practitioners. In the same vein, research on only one dimension, such as individual determinants of CAM use, explains only one part of the larger picture. (Summary Report of an

International Symposium on Why People Use Alternative and Complementary Medicine: Social Science Perspectives. University of Toronto, April 16–18, 1998 [unpublished])

The issue of objective effectiveness of therapies is not addressed here. Scientific investigation of all medical interventions is a separate topic of considerable current interest. The Cochrane Collaboration [1] has popularized the concept of evidence-based medicine and set standards for meta-analyses and systematic reviews of clinical trials, whether conventional or alternative. The surveys are discussed under the headings of general social trends, disease areas and specific health topics, physicians' and practitioners' perceptions, and federal initiatives. Some relevant crosscutting themes become evident, including the subjective assessment of the effectiveness of CAM therapies and the experience of specific segments of the population, such as children, young people, women, and ethnic groups.

METHODOLOGY

The databases searched for this review were MEDLINE (National Library of Medicine, Bethesda, MD), BIOSIS (User Communications, Philadelphia, PA), Embase (Elsevier Science Publishers, New York, NY), IAC (Information Access Company, Foster City, CA), and Health and Wellness (Information Access Company), all accessed through a librarian-directed search using Dialog. Bibliographies from the surveys were checked. An independent search was made of the publicly available version of MEDLINE, known as PubMed (http://www.ncbi.nlm.nih.gov/PubMed), accessed via the World Wide Web. The latter search, using search terms and the related articles feature, was particularly useful for retrieving the most recent relevant publications.

The overview of CAM national surveys in each section covers primarily the period of 1990 to the present. For the cancer section, surveys dating from the late 1970s have been included because they are relevant to the history of use. Speculative or small-scale studies and those with a response rate lower than 60% were rejected unless they were considered exploratory studies indicating an important area for further study. Other general concerns about survey design exist that are often drawn retrospectively by the authors themselves. For instance, many surveys rely on convenience or cross-sectional samples; this can be assumed unless indicated otherwise. In each section, common features of surveys have been systematically compared and put in tabular form but no attempt has been made to perform a meta-analysis because the studies are not sufficiently congruent. Not every survey that appears in the tables is discussed in the text.

It is not difficult to catalog the inconsistencies and faults with the surveys: unspecific definition; no operational definition; inappropriate sampling frame; investigator bias; discrepancies of secondhand reporting; and invalid conclusions drawn from nonrandom samples. These flaws can all be either found or suspected. Being overcritical destroys the objectivity of the review. Stepping back, watching the general trends, and assuming some cancelling by random error enables the researcher to view a fascinating composite picture.

Most recent surveys use the definition of CAM therapies from the first Harvard study by Eisenberg et al. [2]: "Medical interventions not taught widely at U.S. medical schools or generally available at U.S. hospitals." This definition has provided some consistency in the surveys, although it is difficult to assess how far it has been used as an operational definition. It has proved an evolving definition because, in the interim, medical school curricula has been rapidly changing, and some CAM therapies have already been integrated into the practice of certain U.S. hospitals. Although the Eisenberg et al. [2] 1993 study was pivotal, this chapter demonstrates that there have been many important surveys of the field and the composite picture that emerges from categorizing, comparing, and analyzing them is rich and informative.

GENERAL SOCIAL TRENDS IN THE USE OF COMPLEMENTARY AND ALTERNATIVE MEDICINE

The 1993 Harvard survey conducted by Eisenberg et al. [2] has become the most frequently cited study in the literature. The much-quoted figures on prevalence, use, and out-of-pocket expenditure encouraged researchers, practitioners, and patients, paved the way for commercial expansion into the area, gave incentive to insurance companies and health maintenance organizations (HMOs) to consider coverage of therapies, and compelled state legislatures to reconsider recognition and licensure of practitioners.

The study reported that, in 1990, a projected one third of the adult, English-speaking general population used unconventional health practices and found that 72% of these respondents did not inform their conventional physicians [2]. One third of users saw an unconventional medical practitioner an average of 19 times per year, for a total of 425 million visits. The typical user was found to be white, aged 25 to 49 years, with higher than average income and more years of formal education. Therapies were primarily used for chronic conditions. Of 16 therapies listed, the most commonly reported were relaxation, chiropractic, and massage. Costs of therapies, generally paid out of pocket, were estimated to be $13.7 billion per year.

A follow-up survey also by Eisenberg et al. [3] found increased prevalence of CAM use. Use of at least one alternative therapy increased from 33.8% in 1990 to 42.1% in 1997. The therapies with increased popularity included herbal medicine, massage, megavitamins, self-help groups, folk remedies, energy healing, and homeopathy. Visits to alternative medicine practitioners increased from 36.3% to 46.3%. In both surveys, the reason most frequently given for using alternative therapies was a chronic condition, including back problems, anxiety, depression, and headaches. No significant change was found in the likelihood of patients disclosing alternative therapy use to their conventional physician. The extrapolated figure for all out-of-pocket expenditures for products and services was estimated at $27 billion, a figure comparable with the 1997 projected out-of-pocket expenditure for *all* physician services in the United States.

In both surveys, the study design was a simple, cross-sectional, randomized telephone interview using comparable key questions, a technique widely used in market research. In 1991, 1539 adults were interviewed, and in 1997, 2055 adults were interviewed. The response rates were 67% and 60%, respectively. Limitations of methodology included confining responses to the English-speaking general public and only to those in households with telephones; individuals with cognitive or "physical impairment" were excluded.

Independent market research by Landmark Health Care [4] was in remarkable accord with the findings of the Eisenberg study. A randomized telephone survey of 1500 adults currently covered by some type of health insurance or healthcare plan found that 42% of respondents had used some form of alternative health care in the preceding year. Of these, 74% used CAM alongside their conventional care, whereas 15% used it in place of conventional care. The message to insurers from the public was very clear—31% reported that coverage of alternative care in selecting a health plan was very important, and 36% reported it to be somewhat important. Attitudes toward alternative care had become more positive during the previous 5 years in 40% of respondents.

A survey by Elder *et al.* [5] of a small convenience sample of 113 general practice patients in Portland, Oregon, found that 50% were using some form of alternative health care and that 53% had informed their family physician. This greater proportion may partly reflect the higher incidence of CAM use in the western United States but may also result from small sample size. The study used the same list of CAM therapies as Eisenberg's papers [2,3] and also a self-report design. Patients were asked which therapies they used, for what problem, and whether they had told their family practitioner. By contrast, another study of a local population of military personnel using a family practice center revealed that 28.2% were using some form of alternative medicine [6].

A national survey by Astin [7] performed in 1994 found that 40% of the general public had reported using CAM therapies during the previous year. A 1998 report by Astin *et al.* [8] that reviewed 25 international surveys (conducted between 1982 and 1995) examining the practices and beliefs of physicians about CAM came to a similar conclusion. From the responses on referrals and discussions with patients, it was inferred that between 30% and 50% of the general adult population in industrialized nations uses some form of CAM.

Assessing these findings is similar to the technique of triangulation used in land surveys. By coming from different directions, a reasonably consistent picture emerges. A national replication study reaches the same conclusion as a national market research study. An independent national survey, a local replication, and a review of international surveys from a physician perspective point to possible degrees of freedom around the figure of 42% found by two of the latest surveys [3,4]. A large national survey conducted by Paramore [9] in 1996 provides some confirmation of the Eisenberg findings. A sample of 3450, taken from a general probability sample of the 1994 Robert Wood Johnson National Access to Care Survey, were asked only about their use of CAM practitioners. The finding that 10% consulted practitioners is consistent with the Eisenberg estimate that one third of the 34% of users in 1990 consulted practitioners but is considerably lower than the estimated 19% Eisenberg found in 1997. Table 17-1 provides an overview of these surveys [2–7,9,10].

We know which therapies people are using, and we know that women are more likely to use CAM therapies than men, although this difference is seldom or only marginally significant and is usually proportional to the gender balance of people seeking treatment for conventional care. Women generally are greater users of health care and tend to suffer from chronic ailments more than men. The consistently most popular therapies from the recent surveys are depicted in Table 17-1 (*see* column heading "Types of CAM"). These therapies are used most often for chronic ailments and chronic pain. A study by Bullock *et al.* [11] of 760 clinic patients with 248 different complaints found that the largest category of health problems was musculoskeletal, followed by those related to addictions and psychiatric disorders. What is less clear is which health problems people are self-medicating.

Several anomalies and areas of ignorance remain. As outlined in the introduction, surveys tend to be skewed toward the more affluent end of the consumer market and generally find little or no significant difference in the sociodemographic characteristics of users and nonusers of alternative therapies. Astin [7] concluded that, of the socioeconomic variables, only educational level predicted use of CAM; a consistent positive correlation runs throughout the studies. A study by Cassidy [12] finds the predominant users of Chinese medicine in the United States are middle-aged, well-educated, middle-income people who expressed a high degree of satisfaction with their care.

Little is still known about patterns of use among less affluent or ethnic minority groups in society. It is possible that the actual pattern of use of CAM therapies is bimodal, with peaks of usage at the more affluent and the less affluent end. It is also possible that, in the United States, those without health insurance and those members of an ethnic community with their own healers and health workers have long incorporated an alternative system of health care into their communities. Traditional or folk systems of medicine are thus ingrained into the subculture.

This hypothesis is partly confirmed by a few small-scale surveys. A 1998 survey by Krastins *et al.* [10] found that only 27% of a sample of 199 lower-income, middle-aged patients in a family health center clinic used CAM therapies. By contrast, in a 1998 study, 70% of homeless young people in a Street Clinic Youth Program in Seattle, Washington, reported using CAM [13]. A 1996 study of 213 Mexican Americans found 44% had used an alternative medicine practitioner one or more times during the previous year [14]. Surveys on the use of Curanderos among Mexican-Americans estimated use to be 4% between 1982 and 1984 [15] and 21% in 1996 [16] for that one form of therapy alone. More anthropologic research is needed on these and other ethnic groups.

No doubt remains that people are turning toward CAM therapies, but little is known about why. The 1998 Astin *et al.* survey [8] provides some important leads and is consistent with the bimodality model. The study found that CAM users are not dissatisfied with conventional care but are shifting toward health care that is "more congruent with their own values, beliefs, and philosophical orientations towards health and life." This conjecture seems to fit the predilections of the baby boom generation and is also consistent with the belief systems of ethnic communities and the dissent of homeless youth.

Use of Cancer Therapies

The efforts of "cancer activists" led to the creation of the NIH OAM in 1992. The OAM was mandated to investigate alternative cancer therapies and conduct field investigations on their efficacy. No other topic has aroused so much ire and controversy; the debate over alternative cancer therapies continues to rage. Therapists' offices have been raided, their licenses have been revoked, and they have been taken to court. Two of the physician pioneers of alternative cancer therapies died in 1997. Dr. Josef M. Issels, who died at age 90, had developed cancer treatments based on diet and immunotherapy. Dr. Emanuel Revici, who lived just long enough to see his license restored at age 101, was known as an innovator in nontoxic cancer chemotherapy. Their obituaries [17,18] illustrate the mixture of mystique and outrage surrounding their lives.

TABLE 17-1. GENERAL SOCIAL TRENDS IN THE USE OF COMPLEMENTARY AND ALTERNATIVE MEDICINE

Author [ref]	Sample Size and Description	Response/Refusal Rate	Focus	Types of CAM	General Findings
Eisenberg et al. [2]	1539; Randomized, national, general population	67% Response	Prevalence, costs, usage patterns, physician disclosure	Relaxation Chiropractic Massage Imagery	34% used conventional therapy at least once in past 12 months; $13.7 billion spent; 72% did not disclose use to physician
Paramore [9]	3450; National, general population	75% Response	CAM use with professionals, (4 CAM therapies)	Chiropractic Massage Relaxation	10% saw CAM professional
Elder et al. [5]	113; Local, general populations	87% Response	Family practice patients	Chiropractic Massage Herbal Megavitamins	53% use; 50% disclosed use to physician
Landmark Health Care [4]	1500; National, general market survey	—	Adults covered by health insurance plan	Herbal Chiropractic Massage Megavitamins	42% use in past year
Krastins et al. [10]	199; Low-income population	10% Refusal	Prevalence and use	Prayer Chiropractic Meditation	29% use
Drivdahl and Miser [6]	250; Local military population	71% Response	Use by family practice population	Chiropractic Massage Herbal Acupuncture	28% use; less than half satisfied with alternative care
Astin [7]	1035; National, general population	69% Response	Reasons for seeking alternative medicine	Not applicable	Predictors were education, poorer health status, holistic orientation, change in word-view, various health problems
Eisenberg et al. [3]	1539 (1991) and 2055 (1997); National repeat study of trends in use 1990–1997	67% Response	Prevalence, costs, usage patterns, physician disclosure	Herbal Massage Megavitamins Self-help groups Folk remedies	Use increased from 33.8% in 1990 to 42.1% in 1997

CAM—complementary and alternative medicine.

The jury is still out. This chapter cannot comment on efficacy based only on patients' perceptions. The change in terminology noted in the introduction is most evident in cancer surveys. It is important to recognize that many of the early surveys were conducted from a highly skeptical, even antagonistic, viewpoint. Clinicians must maintain a healthy skepticism when conducting a scientific survey. However, many early investigators believed that alternative therapies were quackery and that the patients were being duped. This bias does not make for good science.

Nonetheless, findings from all of these surveys provide a useful research history. The initial focus of all CAM surveys was child safety; the studies showed a consistent proportion of patients, both adult and pediatric, trying alternative therapies to treat their cancer. The political stance of the investigators is inconsequential to these results. It is reflected, however, in the call to educate the public about the dangers of using "unproven" cancer remedies and to warn physicians that a proportion of their patients are likely experimenting with "fraudulent" cures.

These early surveys do not have the consistency and reliability needed for a systematic review, as illustrated in the review by Ernst and Cassileth [19] of 26 surveys from 13 countries. Their investigation dismisses most previous work as lacking reliable data and thus declares that no reliable conclusions can be reached given the inadequacy of the studies. The approach in this chapter is to present a constructive overview. However, these surveys provide a faithful testimonial to the trends of the past decade (Table 17-2) [20–29] and open up discussion.

The survey by Cassileth et al. [23] in 1984 takes the survey method to a new level. The authors attempted to understand motivation from the patient's perspective and thus describe the growing appeal of an antimedicine—a lifestyle-oriented natural approach to treatment. This large-scale survey focused on a population of 660 cancer patients, 304 from a conventional cancer center and 356 under the care of "unorthodox" practitioners. Participants were recruited through a consecutive recruitment convenience sampling frame. Patients of alternative practitioners were reassured that the investigation would not attempt to evaluate or discredit the therapies. Anonymity was guaranteed, and the ensuing interviews determined that 54% of patients receiving conventional therapy also sought unconventional therapies, on average 24 months after being diagnosed. Of those patients, 40% abandoned mainstream medical care entirely after adopting alternative methods of treatment. The other 60% continued with both. In addition, 14% had never undergone conventional treatment. The most frequently used therapies included metabolic therapy, diet therapies, megavitamins, mental imagery for antitumor effect, spiritual or faith healing, and immune therapy. Patients who used these therapies were well educated, frequently asymptomatic, and in the early stages of disease. One limitation of the study was that regional preferences may have skewed use preferences.

The papers by Mooney [24] and Goldstein et al. [25] reflect this new approach to understanding motivation. They report that users of unconventional therapies tend to be more action-oriented and informed [24] or better educated and decisive [25]. The papers follow Cassileth et al.'s [23] typology for cancer treatments, which has been used widely in later surveys and is expressed in Table 17-3. Another major survey was performed by Lerner and Kennedy [26] in 1992, who reported on a national 1998 telephone survey. Random-digit dialing was used to identify a group of 5047 cancer patients or former cancer patients. Of these, 2743 patients and 2304 family members or friends were interviewed to assess their use of "questionable" cancer treatments. Only 10% refused to be interviewed. Some form of alternative therapy had been used by 9%, or 452 patients. This low figure may reflect the censorious tone of the article; patients may have been unwilling to disclose their use of therapies.

Abu-Realh et al. [27] further refined the classification of cancer therapies by pointing out that many of the newer self-healing and psychosocial therapies are used as adjuncts to conventional care and thus can be clearly distinguished from alternatives to biomedical treatments. They reanalyzed data from a 1992 National Health Interview survey that compared the use of adjunct therapies before and up to 5 years after 1987. The sample of 2970 patients was divided into two groups, those diagnosed before and those diagnosed after 1987. The authors found that use of complementary therapies as an adjunct to conventional cancer treatments increased by 63.9% after 1987 (13.9% of patients versus 8.3 %). Limitations of this study include the failure to define self-healing and the loss of data from patients who did not survive cancer.

A recent, small-scale study by Friedman [28] updates earlier work on children with cancer and reflects the changing climate since those early studies. Parents of 81 pediatric patients were interviewed. Researchers found that cancer patients were not significantly more likely to use alternative therapies than other pediatric patients (65% versus 53%, respectively). Prayer, exercise, and spiritual healing were favored by the cancer group; prayer, massage, and spiritual healing were preferred by the control subjects. A survey by Coss [29] found that 16% of interview subjects had considered using alternative therapy for cancer but only 6% actually went to an alternative therapist; the therapists visited most frequently were nutritionists, counselors, herbalists, and massage therapists.

Overview of the cancer surveys highlights the importance of clarifying terminology, a factor glossed over in general surveys and masked by the currently convenient but misleading acronym CAM. Much of physicians' concern in the 1970s and 1980s was about pharmacologically active drug therapies used as alternatives to conventional treatment. The 1984 study by Cassileth et al. [23] found that patients are using radical alternatives to conventional treatment. Specific cancer treatments are still used as alternatives to conventional biomedicine but the extent is unclear from the existing surveys. The rising popularity of lifestyle and self-healing therapies, such as spirituality, exercise, humor, meditation, self-hypnosis, music, aromatherapy, and color therapy, are usually entirely compatible with conventional care. Healing touch, widely used by nurses, is similarly accordant. These therapies are used as adjuncts or complementaries to conventional treatment but are often misleadingly labeled "alternatives." The distinction between adjunct or complementary therapies and alternative therapies needs further delineation in a new, refined survey.

USE OF THERAPIES FOR HIV/AIDS

A new dynamic in the patient–physician–researcher relationship entered the scene with the diagnosis of AIDS in the 1980s. The AIDS community has long been highly vocal in demanding not just more from the research effort but more information about novel treatments used in other countries that are not yet available in the United States. Community resources and buyers' clubs sprang up to create a legitimate avenue for importing these therapies. The HIV/AIDS community is very well informed. Publications such as *AIDS Treatment News* are now

TABLE 17-2. USE OF CANCER THERAPIES

Author [ref]	Sample Size, Description, and Response	Focus	Types of CAM	General Findings
Faw et al. [20]	69; Children and parents	Tried or considered "unproved cancer remedies"	Laetrile Faith healers Diet therapies	6 (8.7%) used; 4 (5.8%) considered trying; 11 (24.6%) use recommended
Pendergrass and Davis [21]	106; Children and parents; 64% response	Knowledge and use	Faith healing Megavitamins Laetrile Greek cure Mind control Hoxey method	50% knew about alternatives; 16% used; 93.4% comfortable discussing use with physician
Copeland et al. [22]	66; Children and parents, multicultural pilot study	Use, parent attitudes, physician awareness	Chaparral Herbs Curanderos	6% use; 61% did not want information; physician not aware of use
Cassileth et al. [23]	660 (304 conventional medicine, 356 CAM)	Use and reasons for use	Metabolic Diet Megavitamins Imagery Spiritual Immune	54% use; 40% abandoned conventional care after adopting CAM
Mooney [24]	71; Adult	Use and reasons for use	Not applicable	18% use
Goldstein et al. [25]	82; Adults receiving radiation	Use	Selenium Mental imagery Garlic Herbal tea	5 (12%) used adjunct therapies
Lerner and Kennedy [26]	5047; Adults, national telephone survey	Use of "questionable" cancer therapies	"Mind" therapies Diet Drugs	9% use
Abu-Realh et al. [27]	2970; Adults, reanalysis of 1992 survey	Use of self-healing and psychosocial techniques before and after 1987	Not applicable	Complementary therapy use increased by 63.9% after 1987 (8.3% before, 13.9% after)
Friedman et al. [28]	161; Parents of children	Comparison of CAM use by cancer patients and general medicine patients	Prayer Exercise Spiritual healing Massage	65% use by cancer patients; 51% use by controls
Coss et al. [29]	503; Adults, local survey	Attitudes and preferences for potential use at medical center	Nutrition Herbal Massage	16% considered use

CAM—complementary and alternative medicine.

freely available online (http://www.immunet.org/atn) as is a number of excellent, informative websites.

Individuals infected with HIV have typically assumed the management of their own treatment, advised their own physicians, and engineered their own entry into clinical trials. Tales of selling and swapping blood and urine samples to get onto the desired clinical trials are legion. Once accepted into trials, patients have even contrived to pool their pills to ensure that everyone receives at least a half dose of the experimental drug. This has posed new problems for biomedical researchers who find that this sharing of information interferes with the conduct of randomized controlled trials. It has also raised new bioethical issues about using patients as controls to assess the efficacy of new drugs, when such seriously ill patients need access to any treatment that may prolong their life. A patient who may not survive to participate in another clinical trial wants to be sure that he or she is receiving the active treatment. The patient may drop one trial to enroll in another more promising one, covertly participate in more than one, help a friend get into a trial, or share the treatment.

With this noncompliant, unpredictable patient group, the validity of surveys is questionable as well as the validity of the trials. This is a new problem completely unrelated to questions of sample size, skewed questions, or low response rate. The sheer inventiveness of this group and their intolerance of what they may perceive as time- and energy-wasting activities means their attention and cooperation in studies is not likely to be engaged.

No large surveys of HIV/AIDS patients and their use of alternative or complementary therapies have yet been undertaken. The AIDS community probably has a far clearer idea of what occurs among patients than do researchers. The small-scale surveys that are available show a pattern similar to the cancer studies. Early surveys concentrate on alternative, unapproved drug therapies, whereas more recent surveys, published since 1993, concentrate on lifestyle-complementary therapies, such as relaxation, touch, diet, humor, and imagery. The latest of the surveys, by Carwein and Sabo [30], claims 100% use of CAM therapies among HIV/AIDS patients. The emphasis in treatment has changed from cure to quality of life. Research summaries are presented in Table 17-4.

The study by Rowlands and Powderly [31] of 79 HIV-positive patients demonstrates the desperation and independent spirit of these patients. From a list of 22 categories of therapies, 44 patients had tried at least one; 11 patients had tried non–FDA-approved drug therapies and nine patients were taking experimental medications. One had taken high doses of oral acyclovir and another had obtained parenteral interferon from a friend. Most of the patients questioned had not informed their doctor of their self-medication. Kassler et al. [32] conducted a telephone survey on the use of medicinal herbs by 114 randomly selected HIV-positive patients participating in a longitudinal study of health services use. The purpose of the survey was to assess the use of herbs and to identify the existing toxicity literature. Of those surveyed, 22% reported using one or more herbal products in the past 3 months. Of those using herbs, 20% stated that their primary physician was unaware of herb use; 16% of respondents were currently involved in clinical trials. Symptoms possibly caused by herbal products were experienced in 28%.

Greenblatt et al. [33] conducted a longitudinal telephone survey of 197 randomly selected HIV-positive patients to study polypharmacy use, in particular, the use of prescribed, unorthodox, and investigational treatments and participation in multiple trials. Of those surveyed, 29% had used an unorthodox treatment prior to the 3-month study, use of which was associated with later stages of illness. Simultaneous enrollment in multiple research trials was reported in 18%. Anderson et al. [34], Bandy et al. [35], and Dwyer et al. [36] all conducted self-administered surveys of similar size. Estimates of patient use of alternative therapies ranged from 30% to 70%, whereas the study by Nokes et al. [37] of 145 patients and their use of alternative therapies found all participants (100%) had used at least one therapy.

A different approach was used by Singh et al. [38]. This prospective, longitudinal study was designed to assess the demographic and psychologic characteristics of 56 patients who sought "nontraditional" remedies. A self-administered questionnaire was given at baseline and every 6 months thereafter in a U.S. Veterans Administration medical center. Laboratory results, medical status, and various standardized tools were used to assess psychologic functioning. Use of nontraditional therapies was reported by 30% of interview subjects. These users were significantly older than 35 years of age, used more support groups, and perceived a greater level of social support than nonusers.

Carwein and Sabo [30] used a mail survey to study patterns of use, types of alternative therapies used, and issues related to patient care in 127 patients from three clinical settings. Of respondents, 16% percent had used an alternative therapy prior to diagnosis, with 100% use after being infected. Laughter/humor and relaxation therapies were used most often for increasing well-being, treating infections, and delaying disease progression. The study produced an algorithm for assessing use of alternative therapies and their possible interactions; as with cancer therapy categories, grouping the interventions as lifestyle/relaxation/self-help therapy, diet-related therapy, or "ingested (pharmacologic)" therapy is significant when calculating potential reaction to prescription or trial medications.

A 1998 study by Fairfield et al. [39] follows the same questionnaire format as the Eisenberg et al. [2,3] studies of

TABLE 17-3. TYPOLOGY FOR CANCER TREATMENTS

Metabolic therapy
Dietary therapy
Megavitamins
Mental imagery
Spiritual or faith healing
"Immune therapy"

Table 17-4. Use of CAM Therapies for HIV/AIDS

Author [ref]	Sample Size, Description, and Response Rate	Focus	Types of CAM	General Findings
Rowlands and Powderly [31]	79; HIV-positive patients attending a clinic	Patients in clinical-trials. Use, effect on well-being, costs, how learnt, physician disclosure	Vitamins Herbal Nonapproved drugs Imagery	44 (56%) used 1 or more therapies; 11 (13.9%) had tried non–FDA-approved drug therapies
Kassler *et al.* [32]	114; HIV-positive patients randomly selected from another study	Use of medicinal herbs and adverse effects	Single herbs and Asian combinations	22% used herbs in past 3 months; 48% used for more than 90 d; 20% no physician disclosure
Greenblatt *et al.* [33]	197; HIV-positive patients; 81% response	Use of prescribed unorthodox and investigational treatments	Mega C AL 721 Riboflavin	29% use of "unorthodox" treatments
Anderson *et al.* [34]	184; HIV/AIDS patients; 86% response	Conventional clinics, clinical trials	Immune enhancement agents Diet Supplements Religious healing Imagery Body work	40% overall CAM use; 42% in clinical trials used CAM
Bandy *et al.* [35]	122; HIV-positive volunteers	Use of "unproven" nutritional therapies; attitudes and practices	Herbal Wheat grass Enzymes Lecithin	30% use of 1 or more unproven nutritional therapy; 61% use of vitamin or mineral supplements
Dwyer *et al.* [36]	63; HIV-positive men living in California	36 patients in trials, 27 in community clinic	Diet Acupuncture Herbal	70% overall use (more common with clinic patients)
Nokes *et al.* [37]	145; HIV-positive patients (72 in New York, 73 in Boston)	Use of CAM for 1 year	Vitamins Relaxation Humor Prayer Meditation	100% use
Singh *et al.* [38]	56; HIV-positive patients, prospective, longitudinal study	Psychosocial characteristics, impact on disease progression and mortality	Meditation Herbal Diet Imagery Vitamins	33% use
Carwein and Sabo [30]	127; HIV-positive patients	Use, implications for care	Relaxation Touch Diet Ingestion Spiritual	100% use
Fairfield *et al.* [39]	289; HIV-positive respondents to telephone survey	Use, expenditure, perceived efficacy	Several categories	67% used herbs, vitamins, dietary supplements; 45% visited CAM provider; 23.9% used marijuana; $938/y, mean expenditure

CAM—complementary and alternative medicine.

general CAM usage. This small-scale survey of use patterns, expenditures, and perceived CAM therapy efficacy concludes that HIV positive patients make extensive use of CAM (including marijuana), make frequent visits to CAM practitioners, incur substantial costs, and believe that the treatments help their conditions. The question of alternative drug therapies still has not been addressed. This study demonstrates the need for research methodology that varies according to the group and perspective being studied. The HIV-positive population is clearly a difficult group to characterize and study. An approach far more inventive than the detached rigor advocated by Ernst [40] or the formulaic approach of the Eisenberg studies is needed.

Use of Complementary and Alternative Medicine for Miscellaneous Health Categories

No large scale studies in the United States have assessed CAM use for specific health problems other than cancer and HIV/AIDS. A review of the literature reveals a miscellany of health categories and a patchwork of information on prevalence, choice of therapy, use of practitioners, and self-medication/self-help measures; there are no reliable projections as to cost. Table 17-5 attempts to assemble and illustrate this patchwork of information. The existing studies are of variable quality; most are convenience samples drawn from a clinic population. What information emerges confirms the assessment of the studies on cancer and HIV/AIDS. Patients with chronic ailments increasingly are turning to complementary and lifestyle practices for palliative measures, such as using massage for relief of pain. A problem of terminology arises; categorization varies from health problem to health problem. Use of a chiropractor for a back problem may well be categorized as an alternative treatment to conventional surgery. Use of megavitamins may be considered an adjunctive therapy for arthritis but an alternative therapy for psoriasis. Megavitamins may also be used as a preventive or wellness measure rather than a complementary or alternative treatment.

Use of CAM therapies is becoming so widespread that, before collecting more data, it is imperative to separate the

TABLE 17-5. COMPLEMENTARY AND ALTERNATIVE MEDICINE USE FOR MISCELLANEOUS HEALTH CATEGORIES

Author [ref]	Sample Size, Description, and Response Rate	Focus	Types of CAM	General Findings
Kronenfeld and Wasner [41]	98; Arthritis patients	Use	Topical lotions Diet Megavitamins Jewelry, trips	94% use of at least one therapy
Coleman et al. [42]	101; Alzheimer's patients	Caregiver's use for patient's memory	Diet Herbal Yoga Meditation	55% of caregivers had given at least one unproven therapy
Fleischer et al. [43]	317; Psoriasis patients	Past or present use	Diet Herbal Sunlight or tanning devices Vitamins	62% use (including sunlight/tanning equipment); 51% no sunlight/tanning equipment
Ai et al. [44]	151; Coronary artery bypass graft patients	Use of CAM after surgery; psychosocial recovery	Prayer Exercise Diet Herbal	85% use
Crone and Wise [45]	323; Organ transplant patients	Herbal medicines and health food supplements	Nutritional supplements	64% use
Wainapel et al. [46]	103; Rehabilitation unit outpatients, random cross-sectional survey	Prevalence, patterns of use, perceived effectiveness	Massage Chiropractic Vitamins Nutritional supplements Acupuncture	29% use in the past 12 months

CAM—complementary and alternative medicine.

complementary/adjunct therapies from the alternative therapies and general preventive or wellness uses. Physicians are increasingly willing to incorporate or recommend many lifestyle practices, such as exercise and changes of diet for heart patients and yoga, *tai chi*, or meditation for Alzheimer's patients. Further research must be fine tuned by experts in the field, physicians and other members of the health-care team, and alternative medicine practitioners to assess how to categorize therapies in a meaningful way for particular groups of patients.

PHYSICIAN INVOLVEMENT IN COMPLEMENTARY AND ALTERNATIVE MEDICINE

In a call for papers for the alternative medicine issue of the *Journal of the American Medical Association* (*JAMA*), the editors urged members to regard alternative medicine more seriously because of the increase in questions from patients. In November 1998, *JAMA* published its alternative medicine issue, and of the five clinical trials reported, two were positive, one was neutral, and two were negative with respect to CAM. A preliminary report and a review were also positive. Clearly there has been a large shift in the attitudes of physicians and the medical establishment over the past decade regarding attention to this field. This change is most likely due to increased patient demand. A further appeal is the association of CAM with autonomy and control, not only for the patient but also for the physician; many physicians are uneasy about centralized health-care management.

Astin's [8] international review of studies of physician attitudes toward CAM found that large numbers of physicians are either referring patients to CAM practitioners or are practicing a range of therapies themselves. Most data were outside the scope of this national review, but it does point to important widespread trends in the Western world. Alternative practice in the West may be mainstream practice in many other parts of the world and, conversely, mainstream practice in the United States is seen as alternative in areas where traditional systems of medicine are still predominantly practiced.

Two surveys of physicians in the United States were conducted in the wake of the study by Eisenberg *et al.* [2]. Blumberg *et al.* [47] conducted a national survey mailed to 572 primary care internists. The results indicated that physician interest and participation in alternative medicine is increasing considerably. The researchers found that 93% of physicians surveyed accepted at least one CAM therapy; 94% were willing to refer patients for at least one CAM therapy; 57% were willing to refer patients for six or more therapies; and 36% practiced at least one CAM therapy.

The second survey, an exploratory study by Berman *et al.* [48], used a convenience sample from three conferences of family physicians (a total of 295 physicians). These researchers similarly found a high degree of interest in CAM and that many of the physicians were practicing alternatives and desired further training. This study, despite its formal limitations as a survey, provided a greater in-depth analysis and discussion of the trends. More than 90% of respondents felt that lifestyle therapies were already legitimate medical practices and more than 50% considered acupuncture, massage therapy, and hypnotherapy to be legitimate medical practices. However, herbal medicine, homeopathy, Native American medicine, traditional Asian medicine, and electromagnetic applications were only acceptable to 27%. Table 17-6 outlines these studies.

Some surveys have been conducted into the practices and beliefs of physicians in various specialties. These are summarized in Table 17-7. There is little methodologic comparability, but results show physician interest in incorporating CAM therapies into their general practice is increasing. More outcomes studies are needed on which to base scientific decisions about treatment; however, in practice, most physicians have already decided to give CAM serious consideration and to find ways to integrate CAM therapies into conventional clinical care. The survey evidence seems to indicate a desire among physicians to return to the art of healing.

Concentration on shifting attitudes in the medical establishment has drawn attention away from the practitioners themselves. Commensurate with increased interest and activity among conventional physicians, the numbers of CAM practitioners who are practicing independently or who have patients referred to them for their services is also growing. Table 17-8 reviews two published studies of practitioners. The study by Calabrese *et al.* [53] identifies 117 providers who offer CAM therapies to HIV-infected individuals. The investigators attempted to identify all providers nationally through their professional associations and conferences. The study by McPartland and Soons [54] concentrates on the state of Vermont to gain a realistic assessment of the number of practitioners. These researchers located 897 practitioners that derived most of their income from practicing at least one of 97 different types of CAM. Extrapolating from this local study, they estimate that more than 403,000 full-time alternative healers are practicing in the United States.

A survey from the Harvard School of Public Health on malpractice claims [55] found that claims against chiropractors, massage therapists, and acupuncturists in the period from 1990 to 1996 occurred less often and typically involved less severe forms of injury than claims against conventional physicians during the same period. Conventional physicians may soon have to guard against claims of malpractice for *not* advising patients on alternative forms of care.

Medical school students provide another area of interest. The Rosenthal Center at the Columbia University College of Physicians website (http://cpmcnet.columbia.edu/dept/rosenthal/guide.html) has charted the growing number of CAM courses taught at medical schools in the United States for several years. The complete list appears periodically in the *Journal of Alternative and Complementary Medicine* [56]. Surveys demonstrate a dramatic rise in recent years in the number of institutions teaching CAM courses; 33 (34%) medical schools offered CAM electives in 1995 [57] compared with 75 (64%) in a 1997 to 1998 survey [58]. In the

Table 17-6. Surveys of Physician Involvement in Complementary and Alternative Medicine

Author [ref]	Sample Size, Description, and Response Rate	Focus	Types of CAM	General Findings
Berman et al. [48]	180; 61% response	Family physician's knowledge of, use of, training in CAM	Categorized	Over 90% considered lifestyle therapies and counseling legitimate medical practices
Blumberg et al. [47]	572; Internists, national mailed survey; less than 25% response	Internists' attitude toward CAM	All	57% willing to refer patients for CAM
Astin et al. [8]	Not applicable	Review of 25 international surveys	Referrals for Acupuncture (43%) Chiropractic (40%) Massage (20%) Most often practiced by physician Chiropractic (19%) Massage therapy (19%) Least often practiced by physician Homeopathy (9%)	Large numbers of physicians refer or practice CAM therapies

CAM—complementary and alternative medicine.

Table 17-7. Specialist Physician Involvement in Complementary and Alternative Medicine

Author [ref]	Sample Size, Description, and Response Rate	Focus	Types of CAM	General Findings
King et al. [49]	594; Physicians, mailed survey, seven states; 59% response	Physician attitudes toward and experience with faith healing	Faith healing	55% disapproved; 20% approved; 23% believed faith healers could heal
Diehl et al. [50]	312; Acupuncturist-physicians; 44% response	Characteristics	Acupuncture	Mainly used for pain therapy; age group 35 to 54 years; nonspecialists in private practice
Jacobs et al. [51]	27; Physicians and osteopaths	Physicians using homeopathy	Homeopathy	Much lower use of testing and conventional medications; primarily chronic conditions; patients were younger, affluent
Sikand and Laken [52]	348; Physicians, members of AAP; 40.5% response	Attitudes toward CAM in pediatrics	General	55.2% would use CAM; 50.3% would refer patients

CAM—complementary and alternative medicine.

latter study, 84 of 123 CAM-related courses were stand-alone electives or, in one case, part of an elective; 38 were part of a required course.

FEDERAL SURVEYS AND INITIATIVES

The changing status of CAM over the past decade has been largely due to consumer pressure and government action. In 1986, John Dingell, then Chairman of the U.S. House of Representatives' Committee on Energy and Commerce, wrote to the Office of Technology Assessment requesting a study of "out of mainstream" cancer treatments. An advisory panel was set up and a series of studies were made of "unconventional cancer treatments."

The National Cancer Institute (NCI) reported on a range of therapies in 1990, all of which were found to have produced inadequate evidence to justify further research. Patients were advised to consult their medical doctor for advice before using any of the treatments in place of conventional care. Public dissatisfaction with the report provoked the U.S. Congress into mandating the formation of an office in the NIH for the purpose of investigating and validating alternative therapies. The OAM was created in 1992 in the office of the NIH Director with an initial budget of $6 million.

In 1998, OAM was raised to the status of a National Center within the NIH, with a $50 million budget. Also in 1998, the NCI reports on unconventional cancer treatments were withdrawn [59]. NCI continues to investigate potential new treatments from alternative practitioners, provided that the methods can be evaluated according to the standards of orthodox scientific criteria. One laboratory specializes in the assessment of anticancer botanicals in conjunction with field researchers throughout the world.

In addition to funding both small experimental research projects and large clinical trials, OAM funded several surveys in 1997 at a number of research centers in the United States. These are shown in Table 17-9. Three NIH intramural surveys are currently in progress; these are outlined in Table 17-10. Within the Department of Health and Social Services generally, the National Center for Health Statistics is conducting investigations into CAM usage and the Centers for Disease Control and Prevention provide consultation services for questionnaire design for CAM surveys.

CONCLUSIONS AND RECOMMENDATIONS

The main emphasis in survey research is on fact finding. If a survey is well structured, the sample randomly drawn, and the questions carefully worded and tested in a pilot study, it can be an effective way to find out *What, Where, When,* and *How.* Surveys are not, however, a suitable method for finding out *Why.* Complex causal relationships cannot be investigated this way. The surveys presented here, despite, or even because of, their defects as scientific survey tools, provide a vivid account of the changes that have occurred in medicine in the United States during the past two decades. They constitute a documentary record of the development of the field and the changing visions and concerns of investigators. They also provoke discussion points and highlight ethical issues in biomedical research and clinical practice.

Largely due to these surveys of patient use and physician attitudes, alternatives to conventional biomedicine are now openly discussed at the NIH and at other medical institutions. Greater acceptance has opened up a dialogue with patients and has broken down denial. Case conferences and seminars are held frequently on such ethical issues as whether the health-care team should break the commitment to confidentiality if a patient's life may be endangered by mixing incompatible treatments. Concern is also increasing about the lack of evidence for efficacy and data on toxicity and safety, particularly in the area of herbal therapies.

Widespread use of therapies has raised questions about their potential impact on research. Research protocols typically seek to isolate particular variables that cure or provide relief from specific symptoms. Patients, in contrast, frequently use complementary therapies as a palliative to manage a disease, symptom, or side effect more efficaciously. Treatment has become an open and changing concept. Problems remain in clinical trial design if patients use complementary therapies to support their participation in trials or to maximize their chances of cure. Reporting of drug toxicities, particularly in phase 1 studies, is critical for later escalation of dosages. If a

TABLE 17-8. PRACTITIONER INVOLVEMENT IN COMPLEMENTARY AND ALTERNATIVE MEDICINE

Author [ref]	Sample Size, Description, and Response Rate	Focus	Types of CAM	General Findings
McPartland and Soons [53]	Not applicable	Practitioners in Vermont	All; 97 listed	897 practicing; extrapolates to 153 per 100,000 population
Calabrese et al. [54]	117; CAM providers	Providers of CAM for HIV-positive patients	HIV/AIDS	Practitioners claim effectiveness for methods

CAM—complementary and alternative medicine.

TABLE 17-9. OFFICE OF ALTERNATIVE MEDICINE COMPLEMENTARY AND ALTERNATIVE MEDICINE SURVEYS FOR 1997

Institution	Principal Investigator	Survey Focus	Survey Description
Bastyr University—OAM Center for HIV/AIDS	Leanna J. Standish	Alternative medicine practitioners	Implemented to gather information on the practice of alternative forms of health care among professionals who treat HIV-positive patients
Beth Israel Hospital—OAM Center for General Medicine	David Eisenberg	Follow-up of national survey of alternative medicine prevalence, costs, and patterns of use	Follow-up exploration of topics left unanswered in original survey, including use of alternative medicine in the pediatric population, using a sample of the U.S. population
Columbia University—OAM Center for Women's Health	Fredi Kronenberg	Pilot survey of CAM users for women's health conditions	Random telephone survey of women in New York city to determine the use of CAM among urban women in three ethnic groups: white, black, and Hispanic
		Women-to-women Prevention Magazine menopause survey	Women will be surveyed on their use of conventional and CAM therapies for the management of menopause symptoms; data will assist in determining efficacy of the treatments used
Stanford University—OAM Center for Aging	William Haskell	Survey of CAM use by older persons	Documents the use of CAM by enrollees of the Blue Shield of California Medicare suppplement plan, "Shield 65," which includes coverage of acupuncture and chiropractic therapies
University of Texas Health Sciences Center—OAM Center for Cancer	Mary Ann Richardson	Survey of CAM use for treatment of cancer	Investigators are surveying patients in eight clinics at MD Anderson Cancer Center to determine prevalence of use and interest in CAM therapies among cancer patients in large, comprehensive cancer centers

CAM—complementary and alternative medicine; OAM—Office of Alternative Medicine.

TABLE 17-10. NATIONAL INSTITUTES OF HEALTH INTRAMURAL STUDIES IN PROGRESS

Institution	Principal Investigator	Survey Focus
National Cancer Institute—Bethesda Naval Hospital	Mary Quinn	Use of alternative medicine therapies in adult cancer patients enrolled in phase 1 clinical trials
NIH Clinical Center	Eunice Johnson	Use of herbal therapies by adults seen in an ambulatory care research setting
Clinical Center	Andrew Sparber	Use of complementary medicine by adult patients participating in cancer clinical trials
		Use of complementary medicine by adult patients participating in HIV/AIDS clinical trials

potential toxicity, such as nausea, is reduced through relaxation or acupuncture, this may affect the standard measures for establishment of safety parameters.

The next phase of survey research should aim to build on previous knowledge, not repeat it. A more systematic approach to designing future surveys is desirable but this should not be overengineered or it will not capture the dynamics and nuances of changing values. The physician–patient relationship is overemphasized in the current studies, which thus lack insight into the wider environment of health-care relationships. Patients need to be seen within their social context of family, friends, and community. A specific focus could be the underrepresented groups, such as ethnic minorities and lower income families, who are less likely to participate in the clinical trials from which most samples are currently drawn. A more versatile approach to research design would help, such as involving medical anthropologists in the survey team. Health-care team members generally are not also experts in social survey design; however, they often can detect trends. They may have a hunch for what is changing in the patient population or may draw out a new perspective that is important when building a composite picture of a complex phenomenon.

Conventional physicians are relatively new to the CAM field, and yet already more is known about their relationship to CAM than about the practitioners who have been practicing it for many years. Physicians operate in a clinical context of nurse practitioners, physician's assistants, and pharmacists. They refer patients to practitioners or supervise eclectic practices. The role of midlevel professionals is an important part of the picture. They bring fresh insights and different perspectives. Nurses, for example, incorporated some adjunct treatments into professional practice many years ago, and therapies such as healing touch have been widely taught in college courses.

Increased integration of therapies into mainstream care tends to favor relatively uncontroversial lifestyle changes while marginalizing actual medical alternatives to conventional care. Perhaps mainstreaming is sanitizing the field, or perhaps this simply reflects a need to clarify terminology. The acronym CAM may have a use when ambiguity exists as to whether a therapy is complementary or alternative, a distinction that varies between diseases. Conversely, the acronym can mask important differences and nullify survey findings. Acceptance of "alternatives" is now so widespread that the situation will soon arise in which nearly 100% of the population will answer "yes" when asked if they have used any of a long, inclusive list of therapies during the past year, as is now the case for the HIV/AIDS population.

REFERENCES AND RECOMMENDED READING

Recently published papers of particular interest have been highlighted as:
- Of interest
- Of outstanding interest

1. Berman B: The Cochrane Collaboration and evidence-based complementary medicine. *J Altern Complement Med* 1997, 3:191–194.
2. Eisenberg DM, Kessler RC, Foster C, *et al.*: Unconventional medicine in the United States: prevalence, costs, and patterns of use. *N Engl J Med* 1993, 328:246–252.
3. Eisenberg D, Davis RB, Ettner SL, *et al.*: Trends in alternative medicine use in the United States, 1990–1997: results of a follow-up national survey. *JAMA* 1998, 280:1569–1575.
4. Landmark Health Care: *The Landmark Report on Public Perceptions of Alternative Care.* Sacramento, CA: Landmark Healthcare, Inc; 1998.
5. Elder NC, Gillcrist A, Minz R: Use of alternative health care by family practice patients. *Arch Fam Med* 1997, 6:181–184.
6. Drivdahl C, Miser W: The use of alternative health care by a family practice population. *J Am Board Fam Pract* 1998, 11:193–199.
7. Astin J: Why patients use alternative medicine. *JAMA* 1998, 279:1548–1553.
8. Astin JA, Marie A, Pelletier KR, *et al.*: A review of the incorporation of complementary and alternative medicine by mainstream physicians. *Arch Intern Med* 1998, 158:2303–2310.
9. Paramore LC: Use of alternative therapies: estimates from The Robert Wood Johnson Foundation National Access to Care Survey. *J Pain Symptom Manage* 1997, 13:83–89.
10. Krastins M, Ristinen E, Cimino JA, *et al.*: Use of alternative therapies by a low income population. *Acupunct Electrother Res* 1998, 23:135–142.
11. Bullock M, Pheley AM, Kiresuk TJ, *et al.*: Characteristics and complaints of patients seeking therapy at a hospital-based alternative medicine clinic. *J Altern Complement Med* 1997, 3:31–37.
12. Cassidy CM: Chinese medicine users in the United States, Part 1: utilization, satisfaction, medical plurality. *J Altern Complement Med* 1998, 4:17–27.
13. Breuner CC, Barry PJ, Kemper KJ: Alternative medicine use by homeless youth. *Arch Pediatr Adolesc Med* 1998, 152:1071–1075.
14. Keegan L: Use of alternative therapies among Mexican Americans in the Texas Rio Grande Valley. *J Holist Nurs* 1996, 14:277–294.
15. Higginbotham JC, Trevino FM, Ray LA: Utilization of curanderos by Mexican Americans: prevalence and predictors. Findings from HHANES 1982–1984. *Am J Public Health* 1990, 80(suppl):32–35.
16. Skaer TL, Robison LM, Sclar DA, *et al.*: Utilization of curanderos among foreign born Mexican-American women attending migrant health clinics. *J Cult Divers* 1996, 3:29–34.
17. Cohen M: Emanuel Revici, MD: Innovator in nontoxic cancer chemotherapy, 1896–1997. *J Altern Complement Med* 1998, 4:140–145.
18. Hildenbrand G: An appraisal of the life and work of Dr. Josef Maria Issels, 1907–1997. *J Altern Complement Med* 1998, 4:137–140.
19. Ernst E, Cassileth B: The prevalence of complementary/alternative medicine in cancer. *Cancer* 1998, 83:777–782.
20. Faw C, Ballentine R, Ballentine L, vanEys J: Unproved cancer remedies: a survey of use in pediatric outpatients. *JAMA* 1977, 238:1536–1538.
21. Pendergrass TW, Davis S: Knowledge and use of "alternative" cancer therapies in children. *Am J Pediatr Hematol Oncol* 1981, 3:339–345.
22. Copeland DR, Silberberg Y, Pfefferbaum B: Attitudes and practices of families of children in treatment for cancer: a cross-cultural study. *Am J Pediatr Hematol Oncol* 1983, 5:65–71.
23. Cassileth BR, Lusk EJ, Strouse TB, Bodenheimer BJ: Contemporary unorthodox treatments in cancer medicine: a study of patients, treatments, and practitioners. *Ann Intern Med* 1984, 101:105–112.
24. Mooney K: *Unproven Cancer Treatment Usage in Cancer Patients Who Have Received Conventional Therapy* [thesis]. Salt Lake City, UT: University of Utah College of Nursing; 1987.

25. Goldstein J, Chao C, Valentine E, *et al.*: Use of unproved cancer treatment by patients in a radiation oncology department: a survey. *J Psychosoc Oncol* 1991, 9:59–66.
26. Lerner IJ, Kennedy BJ: The prevalence of questionable methods of cancer treatment in the United States. *Cancer J Clinicians* 1992, 42:181–191.
27. Abu-Realh MH, Magwood G, Narayan MC, *et al.*: The use of complementary therapies by cancer patients. *Nursing Connections* 1996, 9:3–12.
28. Friedman T, Slayton WB, Allen LS, *et al.*: Use of alternative therapies for children with cancer. *Pediatrics* 1997, 100:E1 (*electronic format*).
29. Coss RA, McGrath P, Caggiano V: Alternative care: patient choices for adjunct therapies within a cancer center. *Cancer Pract* 1998, 6:176–181.
30. Carwein VL, Sabo CE: The use of alternative therapies for HIV infection: implications for patient care. *AIDS Patient Care STDs* 1997, 11:79–85.
31. Rowlands C, Powderly WG: The use of alternative therapies by HIV+ patients attending the St. Louis AIDS Clinical Trials Unit. *Missouri Med* 1991, 88:807–810.
32. Kassler WJ, Blanc P, Greenblatt R: The use of medicinal herbs by human immunodeficiency virus-infected patients. *Arch Intern Med* 1991, 151:2281–1188.
33. Greenblatt RM, Hollander H, McMaster JR, Henke CJ: Polypharmacy among patients attending an AIDS clinic: utilization of prescribed, unorthodox, and investigational treatments. *J Acquir Immune Defic Syndr* 1991, 4:136–143.
34. Anderson W, O'Connor BB, MacGregor RR, Schwartz JS: Patient use and assessment of conventional and alternative therapies for HIV infection and AIDS. *AIDS* 1993, 7:561–566.
35. Bandy CE, Guyer LK, Perkin JE, *et al.*: Nutrition attitudes and practices of individuals who are infected with human immunodeficiency virus and who live in south Florida. *J Am Diet Assoc* 1993, 93:70–72.
36. Dwyer JT, Salvato-Schille AM, Coulston A, *et al.*: The use of unconventional remedies among HIV-positive men living in California. *J Assoc Nurses AIDS Care* 1995, 6:17–28.
37. Nokes KM, Kendrew J, Longo M: Alternative/complementary therapies used by persons with HIV disease. *J Assoc Nurses AIDS Care* 1995, 6:19–24.
38. Singh N, Squier C, Sivek C, *et al.*: Determinants of nontraditional therapy use in patients with HIV infection. *Arch Intern Med* 1996, 156:197–201.
39. Fairfield KM, Eisenberg DM, Davis RB, *et al.*: Patterns of use, expenditures, and perceived efficacy of complementary and alternative therapies in HIV-infected patients. *Arch Intern Med* 1998, 158:2257–2264.
40. Ernst E: Complementary AIDS therapies; the good, the bad and the ugly. *J STD AIDS* 1997, 8:281–285.
41. Kronenfeld JJ, Wasner C: The use of unorthodox therapies and marginal practitioners. *Soc Sci Med* 1982, 16:1119–1125.
42. Coleman LM, Fowler LL, Williams ME: Use of unproven therapies by people with Alzheimer's disease. *J Am Geriatr Soc* 1995, 43:747–750.
43. Fleischer AB Jr, Feldman SR, Rapp SR, *et al.*: Alternative Therapies Commonly used within a Population of Patients with Psoriasis. *Cutis* 1996, 58:216–220.
44. Ai AL, Peterson C, Bolling SF: Psychological recovery from coronary artery bypass graft surgery: the use of complementary therapies. *J Altern Complement Med* 1997, 3:343–353.
45. Crone CC, Wise TN: Survey of alternative medicine use among organ transplant patients. *J Transplant Coord* 1997, 7:123–130.
46. Wainapel SF, Thomas AD, Kahan BS: Use of alternative therapies by rehabilitation outpatients. *Arch Phys Med Rehabil* 1998, 79:1003–1005.
47. Blumberg DL, Grant WD, Hendricks SR, *et al.*: The physician and unconventional medicine. *Altern Ther Health Med* 1995. 1:31–35.
48. Berman BM, Singh BK, Lao L, *et al.*: Physicians' attitudes toward complementary or alternative medicine: a regional survey. *J Am Board Fam Pract* 1995, 8:361–366.
49. King DE, Sobal J, Haggerty J III, *et al.*: Experiences and attitudes about faith healing among family physicians. *J Fam Pract* 1992, 35:158–162.
50. Diehl DL, Kaplan G, Coulter I, *et al.*: Use of acupuncture by American physicians. *J Altern Complement Med* 1997, 3:119–126.
51. Jacobs J, Chapman EH, Crothers D: Patient characteristics and practice patterns of physicians using homeopathy. *Arch Fam Med* 1998, 7:537–540.
52. Sikand A, Laken M: Pediatricians' experience with and attitudes toward complementary/alternative medicine. *Arch Pediatr Adolesc Med* 1998, 152:1059–1064.
53. Calabrese C, Wenner CA, Reeves C, *et al.*: Treatment of human immunodeficiency virus-positive patients with complementary and alternative medicine: a survey of practitioners. *J Altern Complement Med* 1998, 4:281–287.
54. McPartland JM, Soons KR: Alternative medicine in Vermont, a census of practitioners: prevalence, patterns of use, and national projections. *J Altern Complement Med* 1997, 3:337–342.
55. Studdert DM, Eisenberg DM, Miller FH, *et al.*: Medical malpractice implications of alternative medicine. *JAMA* 1998, 280:1610–1615.
56. Bhattacharya B: Programs in the United States with complementary and alternative medicine education: an ongoing listing. *J Altern Complement Med* 1998, 4:325–335.
57. Carlston M, Stuart MR, Jonas W: Alternative medicine instruction in medical schools and family practice residency programs. *Fam Med* 1997, 29:559–562.
58. Wetzel MS, Eisenberg DM, Kaptchuk TJ: Courses involving complementary and alternative medicine at U.S. medical schools. *JAMA* 1998, 280:784–787.
59. Moss RW: Big changes at National Cancer Institute [letter]. *J Altern Complement Med* 1998, 4:267.

Herbs or Homeopathy: What's the Difference?

Joyce C. Frye

18

Many people confuse homeopathy with herbal medicine. This is not surprising, because at least 750 of the 2000 or so homeopathic remedies are derived from herbs and are called by their botanical names. For example, aloe is aloe in both its herbal and homeopathic forms. How should the consumer distinguish between them and learn the appropriate use for each form? Three distinctions are crucial: indications for use, method of preparation, and dosage schedules are different in homeopathy than they are in traditional botanical medicine. Understanding these differences is important for both the practitioner and the consumer to maximize potential benefit and minimize risk in the use of these substances.

BACKGROUND

As a background to understanding the distinction between homeopathy and herbal medicine, it is useful to review the concept of *hormesis*. *Dorland's Medical Dictionary* defines hormesis as "the stimulating effect of subinhibitory concentrations of any toxic substance on any organism" [1]. Thus, normally toxic substances or effects are believed to be beneficial when used in low doses. A current major topic of controversy in this arena concerns the effect of ionizing radiation, which is well known to be damaging in excessive amounts but has been demonstrated to prolong life in a number of species when they are exposed to low doses [2].

In the realm of medicinal herbs, Charaka, who wrote the first treatise on Ayurvedic medicine during the first century [3], tells his readers "plants powerful enough to cure disease are often the very plants which are most poisonous when used by those who do not understand their properties." Among Western medicinal herbs, *Digitalis purpurea*, commonly known as foxglove, provides an example of hormesis. *The Physicians' Desk Reference* [4], describing one brand of digitoxin that is identical in action to the whole leaf of the plant, gives as indications for its use "the treatment of heart failure, atrial flutter, atrial fibrillation, and supraventricular tachycardia." It adds under the Warning section, "Many of the arrhythmias for which digitalis is advised are identical with those reflecting digitalis intoxication."

An elegant series of experiments by Jonas [5] demonstrates this principle in a more general way. She sprouted seeds under extremely well-controlled conditions in varying concentrations of herbicide and in water. Not surprisingly, increasing concentrations of herbicide created more unfavorable growth conditions. In an extremely diluted concentration of herbicide, however, improved growth was noted. The sprouts grew better than they did in water, and the herbicide actually acted as a fertilizer under this condition.

One theory for explaining these different actions at different concentrations compares herbal activity with the three states of matter. Just as a substance may be present in a solid, liquid, or gaseous state, it is proposed that three levels of action are possible for botanical substances—a toxic state, a tonifying or nutritional state, and a homeopathic state. The concentration that is determined to be therapeutic varies with the desired effect. Just as some forms of matter do not readily exist in every state (eg, carbon dioxide sublimates from its solid state, "dry ice," to its gaseous state without existing as a liquid) some botanical substances may not readily act in every state. The therapeutic state of *Digitalis* appears to be its homeopathic action, which with increasing concentration transitions to its toxic state without any intervening state.

In many cases, we may recognize only one state because the substance maintains that state over a wide range of conditions or concentrations, or one state will be predominant under usual conditions or at usual concentrations. For example, it is difficult to think of a toxic action of lettuce, which seems to exist primarily in its nutritional state. However, for other leafy plants, such as jimsonweed (*Datura strimonium*), the toxic components change seasonally, with the plant being edible in one season and toxic in another. In chemistry, the terms *melting point* and *boiling point* identify transitions from one material state to another. In pharmacology, the LD_{50} (lethal dose) marks the dose of a substance at which it becomes lethal for 50% of the population. At the other end of the continuum, however, an HD_{50} (homeopathic dose) could mark the concentration at which it acts homeopathically for 50% of the population.

INDICATIONS FOR USE
The Law of Similars

Homeopathy uses the practical therapeutic implication of the hormesis phenomenon. Although Hippocrates may have been the first to suggest that medicinal substances should be chosen according to their ability to produce symptoms similar to those of the sick person, homeopathy, as a system of medicine, was formalized by a German physician, Samuel Hahnemann (1755–1843). Through a series of observations and experiments, Hahnemann derived the law of similars, which states that any substance that creates symptoms in a healthy person can be used to treat similar symptoms in a sick person.

Hahnemann's initial observation was that quinine, extracted from the bark of the cinchona tree and in use in his lifetime to treat malaria, caused malaria-like symptoms when he took it himself. Subsequently, he carried out *provings* in which a substance was given to a group of healthy individuals to observe which symptoms it induced. The complex of observed symptoms then became the indication for the therapeutic use of that substance in sick persons. Thus, the first and chief distinction between the homeopathic and conventional use of herbs is in the therapeutic selection of the herb according to the law of similars.

Some additional examples illustrate this point. Internal consumption of aloe vera juices, gels, or capsules is recommended by many herbalists for "colon cleansing" as well as for its other nutritional benefits. In excess, aloe vera causes diarrhea. In homeopathy, aloe vera is used to treat diarrhea. Another example is found in the use of ipecac, a syrup made from the plant *Cephaelis ipecacuanha*. Most parents and physicians are familiar with the emergency use of syrup of ipecac as an emetic. Its therapeutic value in conventional medicine comes from the herb's toxic action of inducing vomiting. According to the law of similars, the homeopathic use of ipecac is the relief of vomiting. Thus, potential indications for the homeopathic use of ipecac include the treatment of nausea and vomiting due to pregnancy, gastroenteritis, motion sickness, or after anesthesia or chemotherapy.

Treating the Whole Person

As important as choosing the remedy is considering the totality of symptoms demonstrated by the sick individual. In treating nausea and vomiting, many other substances (eg, tabacum [a derivative of tobacco]), are also used. Any substance that includes nausea and vomiting as toxic or side effects is a potential candidate. To choose a substance, the physician must consider the entire complex of symptoms demonstrated by the individual. These would include *general* symptoms, such as fever or chill, as well as *mental and emotional* symptoms, such as lethargy or irritability, and *local* symptoms, such as excess salivation or abdominal cramping. The therapeutic goal is to find a substance that matches the individual's symptoms in as many characteristics as possible.

PREPARATION OF THE HOMEOPATHIC REMEDY

The second important distinction between homeopathic and botanical medical use of herbs is the preparation and concentration of the substance used. In homeopathy, extremely minute doses of the medicinal substance are used to minimize the potentially toxic effects of the herb. Homeopathic remedies are all prepared under careful pharmaceutical conditions. And unlike herbs in the United States, these preparations are approved for use by the U.S. Food and Drug Administration (FDA).

The preparation process requires starting with an amount of herbal tincture and serially diluting it either ten- or 100-fold, a number of times, with water. The final product is labeled with its herbal name followed by a number and letter indicating which dilution (tenfold (X) or 100-fold (C)) was used and the number of times it was diluted. For example, a 6C would have been diluted 100-fold six times.

This dilution process is somewhat mysterious because vigorous shaking known as succussion between each dilution seems to be critical in giving the substance, or remedy as it is known in homeopathy, its medicinal power. Substances that are serially diluted without succussion do not provide the same therapeutic effect [6]. Even more mysteriously, remedies seem to become more potent with increasing numbers of dilutions. Thus, a 6C is more potent than a 6X, and a 30C is more potent than a 6C. It is this anomaly, difficult to explain in terms of conventional molecular scientific theory, that causes many skeptics to question the plausibility of homeopathy.

DOSAGE

Taking a remedy is easy. Although some practitioners prefer dosing with the liquid form, most often the final dilution is sprayed onto small pellets of milk sugar, which may be purchased in vials or tubes in health-food stores. A few of these pellets are simply dissolved under the tongue when a dose is required.

A major difference between herbs and conventional medicines is in the dosing schedule. Homeopathic remedies are believed to catalyze the body's own healing powers rather than to have a direct effect on bacteria, viruses, organs, or pain centers. In acute illnesses, the onset of response to the remedy is often startlingly rapid. If no response is noted, it usually is an indication that the wrong remedy was chosen, and further consideration is needed.

Redosing a homeopathic remedy should continue on an as-needed basis only for as long as symptoms persist. The instructions on a bottle or tube of homeopathic remedy are confusing in this regard because of FDA regulations concerning labeling of over-the-counter products. Inclusion of a specific indication and dosing schedule is required by law. However, in contrast to conventional dosing schedules that require repetition at regular intervals for a specific period of time, the indication for the next dose of a homeopathic remedy is a return of the symptoms or a slowing of the healing response. Depending on the severity and the pace of the illness, this might occur after a few minutes, a few hours, or perhaps not at all.

To simplify the process of choosing a remedy, some manufacturers have created *combination remedies*. These low-potency remedies combine several substances typically thought to be helpful for a specific condition. They are labeled by the condition, such as allergy, menstrual cramps, insomnia, and nausea, rather than being chosen for their specificity to the totality of symptoms of the individual. However, when access to classical homeopathic prescribing information is limited, these combinations can be used safely and are often helpful for self-limited and acute conditions, with minimal side effects.

More Information

More information about homeopathy is available in many popular books available in the health or alternative medicine section of your local bookstore or library. Or contact The National Center for Homeopathy. They can be reached by phone at 703-548-7790, by Email at nchinfo@igc.org, or on the World Wide Web at http://www.homeopathic.org.

References and Recommended Reading

Recently published papers of particular interest have been highlighted as:
- Of interest
- • Of outstanding interest

1. *Dorland's Illustrated Medical Dictionary* edn 28. Philadelphia: WB Saunders; 1994.
2. Luckey TD: *Radiation Hormesis.* Boca Raton, FL: CRC Press; 1991.
3. Patnaik N: *The Garden of Life: An Introduction to the Healing Plants of India.* New York: Doubleday; 1993.
4. *Physician's Desk Reference* edn 50. Montvale, NJ: Medical Economics; 1996.
5. Jonas L: Paper presented at the 52nd Congress of the Liga Medicorum Homeopathica Internationalis. Seattle, Washington, May 1997.
6. Davenas E, Beauvais J, Amara M, *et al.*: Human basophil degranulation triggered by very dilute antiserum against IgE. *Nature* 1998, 333:816–818.

Index

Page numbers in italics indicate figures; *t* indicates tables.

A

Abortion, from red clover, 22
Accreditation Commission for Acupuncture and Oriental Medicine, 58, 61
Acquired immunodeficiency syndrome *see* AIDS
Active treatment, in therapeutic touch, 81
Acupuncture, 57–66
    background on, 57–58
    biological effects of, 60–61
    communication among professionals on, 61
    economic access to, 61
    in fibromyalgia and chronic fatigue/immune dysfunction syndrome, 49
    history of, 57–58
    individualization of protocols in, 65
    insurance coverage of, 108
    licensing of, 61, 112
    mechanisms of, 63
    National Institutes of Health Consensus Report on, 58–59
    other methods *versus*, 59–60, 65
    patient education about, 61
    physicians' acceptance of, 148, *149t*
    research issues in, 64–65
        future, 62
        new, 62–63
    sham, 64
    tolerance to, 60
Acute low back pain, 72, *72t*
    chronic *versus*, 72–73
Acute myocardial infarction, anger and, 95
Acyclovir, in fibromyalgia and chronic fatigue/immune dysfunction syndrome, 52
Adaptogen, ginseng as, 12, 37
Additives, food intolerance to, *40t*
Adjunct treatment, in cancer therapy, 143–144
Adjustment disorder with depressed mood, in depression classification, 30, *30t*
Adrenal function, in fibromyalgia and chronic fatigue/immune dysfunction syndrome, 50
Adrenocorticotropic hormone, ginseng and, 13
Aerobic exercise, in fibromyalgia and chronic fatigue/immune dysfunction syndrome, 52
    in HIV/AIDS, 103–104
Affinity products, defined, 112
    insurance coverage of, 112–113, *113t–114t*
Agency for Health Care Policy and Research, on HIV/AIDS pain, 101–102
    on low back pain, 69–70, 74
AIDS *see also* HIV/AIDS
    Saint John's wort for, 36
AIDS Treatment News, as resource, 144–145
Air pollution, indoor, 128, *128t*
Alameda County Study, of coronary artery disease, 95
Alcohol, kava and, 15
Aldosterone, in fibromyalgia and chronic fatigue/immune dysfunction syndrome, 50
Aletris vulgare see Unicorn root
Alfalfa sprouts, as phytoestrogens, 22
Allergy, in chronic fatigue/immune dysfunction syndrome treatment, 51, *53t*
    to Echinacea, 10
    in fibromyalgia treatment, 51, *53t*
    food, 39–42 *see also* Food allergy
Allicin, as active garlic ingredient, 11
Allium sativum see Garlic
Allopathic medicine *see also* Conventional medicine
    alternative medicine *versus*, 79–80
Aloe, in formulary, 4–5
    in homeopathy, 156
    in wound healing, 26
Aloe vera see Aloe
Alprazolam, kava and, 15
Alternare Health Services, alternative medicine offered by, 112, *114t–115t, 117t*
Alternative and Allied Medicine Database, *5t*
Alternative medicine, business plan in, 125
    changing terminology of, 139
    continuing educational opportunities in, 131–136
    defined, 45, 121
    insurance coverage for, 107–118
    in integrated practice, 121–123
    office design in, 125–128
    overview of, 79–80
    physicians' perceptions of, 109–110, 121, 131
    surveys of, 139–152
        in Alzheimer's disease, *147t*, 148
        in arthritis, 147, *147t*
        in cancer therapy, 142–144, *144t–145t*
        in coronary artery disease, *147t*
        federal, 150, *151t*
        in HIV/AIDS, 144–145, *146t*, 147
        methodology of, 140
        in organ transplantation, *147t*
        physician involvement and, 148, *149t–150t*, 150
        prevalence in, 140
        in psoriasis, 147, *147t*
        in rehabilitation, *147t*
        social trends in, 140–142, *142t*
Alternative Medicine Referral Services, affinity products offered by, *114t–115t*
Alzheimer's disease, ginkgo for, 11
    surveys of alternative medicine in, *147t*, 148
AMED database, *5t*
Amenorrhea, herbs for, 22
American Academy of Medical Acupuncture, 58, 61
American Board of Chelation Therapy, 88
American Cancer Society, on dietary fiber, 94
American College for Advancement in Medicine, chelation therapy training by, 88
American College of Cardiology, on coronary artery disease, 96
American College of Rheumatology, fibromyalgia classification of, *46t*
American College of Sports Medicine, on exercise in HIV/AIDS, 105
American coneflower *see* Echinacea
American Heart Association, coronary artery disease diet of, 93
    Secondary Prevention Panel of, 96
American Herbal Products Association, standards of, 37
American Massage Therapy Association, 133
American Medical Association, on acupuncture, 60
    on chiropractic, 70
American Society of Heating and Refrigeration and Air Conditioning Applications, 128
American WholeHealth, in integrated practice, 122–123
Amitriptyline, in fibromyalgia and chronic fatigue/immune dysfunction syndrome, 49, 52
Anaphylaxis, in food allergy, 40, *40t*
Androgen receptors, saw palmetto and, 12
Angelica *see also* Dong quai
    in fibromyalgia and chronic fatigue/immune dysfunction syndrome, 50
Angelica sinensens see Dong quai
Anger, in coronary heart disease, 95
Angina pectoris, chelation therapy for, 86–87
Angioedema, in food allergy, 40, *40t*
Anthem Blue Cross Blue Shield, affinity products offered by, 112
Antibiotics, intolerance to, *40t*
Anticoagulants *see also* Warfarin
    chelation therapy and, 87
    ginger and, 14
Antidepressants, fatal overdosage of, 36
    in fibromyalgia and chronic fatigue/immune dysfunction syndrome, 49, 52
    Saint John's wort as, 13–14, 29–37 *see also* Saint John's wort
    side effects of, 35
    transition to Saint John's wort from, 36
Antifungal agents, in fibromyalgia and chronic fatigue/immune dysfunction syndrome, 52
Anti-infective herbs, in women's health care, 24–26
Antioxidants, in coronary heart disease diet, 94
    garlic as, 11
    ginkgo as, 11
Antithrombotics, garlic as, 11

Antiviral agents, lemon balm as, 26
Anxiety, in coronary heart disease, 95
  in fibromyalgia and chronic
      fatigue/immune dysfunction
      syndrome, 52
  kava for, 14–15, 37
  Saint John's wort in, as cause of, 35
    as treatment for, 13, 31
    from selective serotonin reuptake
      inhibitors, 35
Anxiolytics, interactions of kava with, 15
  kava as, 14–15
  Saint John's wort as, 13, 31
Applied kinesiology testing, in food allergy, 41
Aquinas, attributes of art of, 125–126
Arabinogalactan, in Echinacea, 9
Arbutin, sources of, 25
Arctostaphylos uva ursis see Bearberry
Arizona Center for Health and Medicine,
    design of, *127*, 128
Arnica, in formulary, 5
Aromatherapy, in office environment, 127
Art, in office design, 126–127
Arthritis, in food allergy, *40t*
  ginger for, 14
  survey of alternative medicine in, 147, *147t*
Asian medicine *see also* Chinese medicine;
    specific therapies
  physicians' acceptance of, 148
Assessment, in therapeutic touch, 81, 103
Asthma, in food allergy, 40, *40t*
  ginkgo for, 11
Astragalus, in fibromyalgia and chronic
    fatigue/immune dysfunction
    syndrome, 52
Atherosclerosis, chelation therapy for, 85–87
  lifestyle modifications and, 93
Atopic dermatitis, in food allergy, *40t*
Autonomic function, in chronic
    fatigue/immune dysfunction
    syndrome treatment, 50, *53t*
  in fibromyalgia treatment, 50, *53t*

B

Bache, Franklin, 57
Back pain, acute *versus* chronic, *72t–73t*, 72–73
  compensation in, 70–71
  leg pain with, 74, *74t–75t*
  spinal adjustment for, 69–76 *see also*
    Chiropractic
  subluxation in, 70, *71t*
  surveys of alternative medicine in, 147, *147t*
Bacterial infections, urinary tract, 24–25
  vaginal, 25
Bacterial toxins, food intolerance to, *40t*
Balance of elements, in office design, 125–127
Balick, Michael, *2t*
Baptist Saint Vincent Health System,
    consumer survey of, 108, 110
Barbiturates, kava and, 15
Bean sprouts, as phytoestrogens, 22
Bearberry, dosage of, 25
  for urinary tract infections, 25
Becker, Robert, 80
Beinfeld, Harriet, *2t*
Benign prostatic hypertrophy, saw palmetto
    and, 12, *12*
Benzodiazepines, kava *versus*, 15, *15*
  Saint John's wort as similar to, 34

valerian *versus*, 14
Bergson, Henri, 80
Beth Israel Medical Center, holistic medicine in, 1
BIOSIS, as survey source, 140
Bipolar disorder, in depression classification,
    30t, 31
Black cohosh, dosage of, 23
  estrogen *versus*, 23
  indications for use of, 22–23
  mechanism of action of, 23
Bladder infections, in women, 25
Blood pressure, acupuncture and, 63
  garlic and, 11
Blue Cross Blue Shield of Colorado, alternative medicine covered by, *116t*
  consumer survey of, 108, *108t*
Blue Cross of California, affinity products
    offered by, 112
Blue Shield of California, affinity products
    offered by, 112
Blumenthal, Mark, *2t*
Body weight, in coronary artery disease, 91
Botanical Influences on Illness, *6t*
Botanical Medicine in Modern Clinical Practice, 6
Bove, Mary, *2t*
Breast cancer, black cohosh and, 23
  red clover and, 22
British Medical Journal, on low back pain, 73–74
  on Saint John's wort, 31–32
Bronchitis, herbs for, 4
Bureau of Primary Health Care, on alternative
    medicine, 109
Burns, herbs for, 4–5
Burr, Harold Saxton, 80
Bursae pastoris see Shepherd's purse
Business and Health, on alternative medicine, 118
  consumer survey of, 109

C

Caffeine, intolerance to, *40t*
Calabrese, Carlo, *2t*
Calcium EDTA, in chelation therapy, 85, *86*
Cancer, alternative medicine in, 142–144,
    144t–145t
Candidiasis, in fibromyalgia and chronic
    fatigue/immune dysfunction
    syndrome, 52
Carbidopa, in receptor model, 6
Cardiac effects, of valerian, 14
Cardiopulmonary function in HIV/AIDS,
    exercise and, 103
Cardiovascular disease, chelation therapy for,
    85–86
Catalogs, herbal, 4, *4t*
Catecholamines, in coronary artery disease, 95
Cauda equina syndrome, in low back pain, 74
CD4+ cells in HIV/AIDS, exercise and, 104–105
Celiac disease, in food allergy, *40t*
Cell-mediated immunity, Echinacea in, 10
Center for Health Design, patient criteria
    studied by, 128
Center for Integrative Health Care, holistic
    medicine in, 1
Centering, in therapeutic touch, 81
Centers for Disease Control and Prevention,
    chronic fatigue syndrome criteria of, *47t*
Centralized Information Service for
    Complementary Medicine, *5t*
Cephalis ipecacuanha, in homeopathy, 156

Cervical disk herniation, chiropractic care in, 74
Chamaelirium luteum see False unicorn root
Chamomile, in formulary, 4
Charaka, on herbs, 155
Chasteberry, dosage of, 24
  in fibromyalgia and chronic
      fatigue/immune dysfunction
      syndrome, 50
  mechanism of action of, 24
  in menstrual disorders, 24
Chelation therapy, 85–88
  clinical applications of, 87
  contraindications to, 87–88, *88t*
  history of, 85–86
  mechanism of action of, 86–87
  protocol for, 88
Cherry bark, in formulary, 4
Chicago Holistic Center, as integrated
    practice center, 122–123
Children, alternative cancer therapy in, 143
  bearberry contraindicated in, 25
Chinese medicine, acupuncture in, 57–66 *see
    also* Acupuncture
  demographics of consumers of, 141
  dong quai in, 23
  energy in, 80
Chiropractic, contemporary practice of, 69–70
  in fibromyalgia and chronic
      fatigue/immune dysfunction
      syndrome, 49
  insurance coverage of, 70, 109
  licensing of, 112
  for low back pain, 70–71
    acute *versus* chronic, *72t–73t*, 72–74
    choice of practitioner for, 76
    contraindications to, 71
    cost-effectiveness of, 75–76
    diagnosis of, 71
    with leg pain, 74, *74t–75t*
    patient screening in, 71–72
    research on, 72
    safety issues in, 74–75
  primary care physicians and, 70
Cholecystokinin, acupuncture and, 60
Cholesterol, chelation therapy and, 86
  in coronary artery disease, 91
    dietary intake of, 93
  garlic and, 11
Cholesterol-lowering therapy, in coronary
    artery disease, 93
Chronic fatigue/immune dysfunction
    syndrome, diagnosis of, 46–47, *47t*
  fibromyalgia *versus*, *48t*
  integrative treatment of, 45–53
    allergies in, 51, *53t*
    autonomic function in, 50, *53t*
    coping in, 52, *53t*
    digestion in, 50–51, *53t*
    energy in, 49, *53t*
    exercise in, 52
    healing path in, 48
    hormone balance in, 49–50, *53t*
    immune function in, 51–52, *53t*
    mood in, 52, *53t*
    nutrition in, 51, *53t*
    pain in, 49, *53t*
    patient interview in, 47–48
    sleep in, 49, *53t*
  Saint John's wort for, 31
Chronic illness, alternative medicine in, 140–141

Chronic low back pain, 72–73, *73t*
  acute *versus*, 72
Ciguatera poisoning, *40t*
Cimicifuga racemosa see Black cohosh
Circle of Design process, in office design, 126, *126t*
Circulation, acupuncture and, 63
  ginkgo in, 11, 24, 37
Cirrhosis, milk thistle for, 15
CISCOM database, *5t*
Civil War, acupuncture used in, 57
  Saint John's wort used in, 30
Clinical Global Impressions Scale, in Saint John's wort trials, 33
Cochrane Collaboration, 140
Cochrane Collaboration Database of Systematic Reviews, *5t*
Cognitive therapy, in fibromyalgia and chronic fatigue/immune dysfunction syndrome, 52
Colitis, in food allergy, *40t*
Common cold, Echinacea in, 10, *10*
Compensation, chiropractic care in, 70–71
Complementary medicine *see also* Alternative medicine; Integrative medicine
  changing terminology of, 139
  continuing educational opportunities in, 131–136
  defined, 45
  surveys of, 139–152
    social trends in, 140–142, *142t*
Comprehensive Cancer Care, in continuing education, 134
Coneflower *see* Echinacea
Congestive heart failure, EDTA and, 87
Consensus Health, affinity products offered by, 112, *114t–115t*
Consortium Center for Chiropractic Research, 69
Consumers of alternative medicine, insurance coverage and, 107–109, *108t*
Continuing medical education, in complementary medicine, 131–136
  conferences for, 134, *135t*
  readings for, 134, *135t*
Conventional medicine, alternative medicine in, medical schools and, 148, 150
  alternative medicine *versus*, 79–80
  costs of, 133
    alternative medicine *versus*, 134
  in integrated practice, business aspects of, 122–123
    rationale for, 121
  integrative medicine *versus*, 45–47
  rediscovery of herbs by, 30
Cook, Captain James, 14
Cook-Medley Hostility Scale, in coronary heart disease, 94
Coping and support, in chronic fatigue/immune dysfunction syndrome treatment, 52, *53t*
  in fibromyalgia treatment, 52, *53t*
Coronary artery bypass grafting, in coronary artery disease, 92
Coronary artery disease, chelation therapy for, 86–87
  cholesterol-lowering therapy for, 93
  lifestyle interventions for, 91–96
    diet in, 93–94
    exercise in, 94
    psychosocial risk factors and, 94–95
    stress management in, 95–96
  prevalence of, 91
  revascularization procedures for, 92–93
  surveys of alternative medicine in, *147t*
Coronary Artery Surgery Study, 92
Coronary stenting, in coronary artery disease, 92–93
Cortisol, in fibromyalgia and chronic fatigue/immune dysfunction syndrome, 50
  Saint John's wort and, 34
Costs, of alternative medicine, 134, 140
  of medical care, 133
  of spinal manual therapy, 75–76
Council on Chiropractic Education, 69
Counseling, in fibromyalgia and chronic fatigue/immune dysfunction syndrome, 52
Craniosacral therapy, in HIV/AIDS, 102
Crataegus see Hawthorn
Credentialing, of alternative medicine providers, 112
Crustaceans, allergy to, 39
Cumulative Index for Nursing and Allied Health, *5t*
Curanderos, as alternative medicine practitioners, 141
Cyclobenzaprine, in fibromyalgia and chronic fatigue/immune dysfunction syndrome, 49
Cytotoxic food testing, in food allergy, 41

D

Dandelion, as diuretic, 24
Databases, herbal, *5t*
Datura strimonium, effects of, 156
Dehydroepiandrosterone, in fibromyalgia and chronic fatigue/immune dysfunction syndrome, 50
Dementia, ginkgo for, 11
Demographics, in alternative medicine, 140–141
Dental pain, acupuncture and, 59, 63
Depression, 30–31
  causes of, 31
  in chronic fatigue/immune dysfunction syndrome, 47, 52
  classification of, *30t*, 30–31
  in coronary heart disease, 95
  in fibromyalgia, 47, 52
  prevalence of, 30
  Saint John's wort for, 13–14, 29–33 *see also* Saint John's wort
  symptoms of, *30t*
Dermatitis, in food allergy, *40t*
  from ginseng, 13
  from kava, 15
Dermatology, herbs used in, 4–5
Dermopathy, kava, 15
Design, of healthy buildings, 127–128
  office, 125–128, *126t*, *127*, *128t*
Diabetes, milk thistle and, 15
Diagnostic and Statistical Manual of Mental Disorders, depression classification of, *30t*, 30–31
Diarrhea, from garlic, 11
Diascorea villosa see Wild yam
Diet, in coronary artery disease, 93–94
  in food allergy testing, 40–41
  Saint John's wort and, 37
Digestion, in chronic fatigue/immune dysfunction syndrome treatment, 50–51, *53t*
  in fibromyalgia treatment, 50–51, *53t*
Digestive enzymes, in fibromyalgia and chronic fatigue/immune dysfunction syndrome, 51
Digitalis purpura, effects of, 155–156
Digitoxin, effects of, 155
Dihydroxytestosterone, saw palmetto and, 12
Dilution, in homeopathy, 156
Dimenhydrinate, ginger *versus*, 14
Dioscorides, Saint John's wort mentioned by, 30
Diosgenin, in wild yam, 24
Disease-centered medicine, patient-centered medicine *versus*, 46
Disk herniation, chiropractic care in, 74
Diuretics, dandelion as, 24
  goldenrod as, 24
Dong quai, contraindications to, 23
  indications for, 23
Double-blind placebo-controlled food challenges, in food allergy, 40
Drug side effects, in HIV/AIDS, 101
Duke, James A., *2t*
Dutch East India Company, acupuncture and, 57
Dyes, intolerance to food, *40t*
Dysmenorrhea, black cohosh for, 23
  raspberry leaf infusion for, 4
Dysthymia, in depression classification, *30t*, 30–31
  Saint John's wort for, 31

E

Eating disorders, food intolerance in, 40
Echinacea, 9–11, *10*
  contraindications to, 10, 25
  dosage of, 11, 25
  drug interactions with, 10–11
  in formulary, 5
  for genital herpes, 25
  for vaginal yeast infections, 25
Economic bias, in alternative medicine surveys, 141
Eczema, herbs for, 4–5
EDTA, chelation therapy with, 85–88
  dosage of, 88
  structure of, 85, *86*
  toxicity of, 87
Education, of alternative medicine consumers, 141, 143
  continuing, in complementary medicine, 131–136
  in herbal formulary, 5–6
    databases in, *5t*
    texts in, *6t*
Egb 761, as ginkgo extract, 11–12, 24
Eggs, allergy to, 39
Electrodermal testing, in food allergy, 41
Electromagnetic therapy, physicians' acceptance of, 148
Elimination, in chronic fatigue/immune dysfunction syndrome treatment, 50–51, *53t*
  in fibromyalgia treatment, 50–51, *53t*
Elimination diet, in food allergy, 40
Embase, as survey source, 140

Emesis *see also* Vomiting
    acupuncture in prevention of, 59, 62
Emotional flatness, from selective serotonin reuptake inhibitors, 35
Emotions, acupuncture and, 66
    in coronary artery disease, 94–95
Endogenous opioids, acupuncture and, 60
Endogenous toxins, food intolerance to, *40t*
Endothelial function, chelation therapy and, 86
Energy, in acupuncture, 57, 61, 65–66
    as alternative medicine principle, 80
    in chronic fatigue/immune dysfunction syndrome treatment, 49, *53t*
    in fibromyalgia treatment, 49, *53t*
Energy efficiency, in building design, 127–128
Energy medicine, in HIV/AIDS, 102–103
    therapeutic touch as, 79
Enterocolitis, in food allergy, 40, *40t*
Enteropathy, gluten sensitive, *40t*
Environment, creation of healing, 125–128
    healthy buildings in, 127–128
    in integrated practice, 122–123
Enzymes, in fibromyalgia and chronic fatigue/immune dysfunction syndrome, 51
Eosinophilic gastroenteritis, in food allergy, *40t*
Epidural hematoma, from garlic, 11
Epinephrine, in food allergy treatment, 39, 42
Epitome of Practical Surgery, on acupuncture, 57
Ergil, Kevin, *2t*
Estrogen, black cohosh *versus*, 23
    in fibromyalgia and chronic fatigue/immune dysfunction syndrome, 50
    in ovarian cycle, 22
    phytoestrogens and, 22
Estrogen receptors, black cohosh and, 23
    phytoestrogens and, 22
    red clover and, 22
    saw palmetto and, 12
Estrogen-like herbs, in women's health care, 22–24
Ethnic minorities, alternative medicine in, 141, 152
Exercise, in chronic fatigue/immune dysfunction syndrome treatment, 52
    in coronary artery disease, 94
    in fibromyalgia treatment, 52
    in HIV/AIDS, 103–104
Experimental drugs, for HIV/AIDS, 145
Eye disorders, acupuncture for, 63

F

Faith healing, in cancer therapy, 143
    physicians' acceptance of, 148, *148t*
False unicorn root, in women's health care, 23–24
Farnsworth, Norman, *2t*
Fat intake, in coronary heart disease, 93–94
Fatal allergic reactions, to food, 39
Fatigue, ginseng and, 12–13
Fatty acids, in coronary heart disease, 94
Fennel, in women's health care, 23
Fever, from Echinacea, 10
Fiber, in coronary heart disease diet, 94
Fibromyalgia, chronic fatigue/immune dysfunction syndrome *versus*, *48t*
    diagnosis of, *46t–47t*, 46–47
    integrative treatment of, 45–53
        allergies in, 51, *53t*
        autonomic function in, 50, *53t*
        coping and support in, 52, *53t*
        digestion and elimination in, 50–51, *53t*
        energy in, 49, *53t*
        exercise in, 52
        healing path in, 48
        hormone balance in, 49–50, *53t*
        immune system function in, 51–52, *53t*
        mood in, 52, *53t*
        nutritional deficiencies in, 51, *53t*
        pain in, 49, *53t*
        patient interview in, 47–48
        sleep in, 49, *53t*
    Saint John's wort for, 31
Financial aspects, of herbal therapy, 7
    of integrated practice, 123
Finasteride, saw palmetto *versus*, 12
First World Conference on Academic Exchange of Medical Qigong, 104
Fish, allergy to, 39
Flavonoids, in Saint John's wort, 13
Flaxseed, in formulary, 4
    as phytoestrogens, 22
Fludrocortisone, in fibromyalgia and chronic fatigue/immune dysfunction syndrome, 50
Flulike illness, Echinacea in, 10, *10*
Fluoxetine, Saint John's wort as similar to, 34
    side effects of, 35
    transition to Saint John's wort from, 36
Foeniculum vulgare see Fennel
Folic acid, in coronary heart disease diet, 94
Follicle-stimulating hormone, in hot flashes, 23
    in ovarian cycle, 22
Food additives, intolerance to, *40t*
Food allergy, defined, 39
    evaluation of, 39–41, *40t*
    in fibromyalgia and chronic fatigue/immune dysfunction syndrome, 51
    myths and realities of, 39–42
    unproven methods in diagnosis of, 41
Food and Drug Administration, on acupuncture, 58
    on chelation therapy, 85
    homeopathic remedies approved by, 156–157
Food aversion, *40t*, 41
Food challenges, in food allergy, 40
Food diaries, in food allergy, 40
Food dyes, intolerance to, *40t*
Food hypersensitivity, food intolerance *versus*, 39, 41–42
Food immune complex assay, in food allergy, 41
Food intolerance, defined, 39
    etiologic factors in, 39, *40t*
    food hypersensitivity *versus*, 39, 41–42
Formulary, herbal *see also* Herbal formulary
    creation of, 1–7
Fountains, in office design, 127, *127*
Four-day rotation diet, in food allergy, 41
Foxglove, effects of, 155–156
Freud, Sigmund, 80
Frontier Cooperative Herbs, *4t*
Fungal infections, vaginal, 24–25
Fungal toxins, food intolerance to, *40t*

G

Gallstones, ginger and, 14
Gamma aminobutyric acid, valerian and, 14
Gardens, in office design, 127, *127*
Garlic, 11
    dosage of, 11
    in formulary, 4
    for vaginal infections, 26
Gastric motility, acupuncture and, 63
Gastroenteritis, in food allergy, 40, *40t*
Gastrointestinal disorders, from kava, 15
    from Saint John's wort, 35
Gender, in alternative medicine usage, 141
Genetics, in depression, 31
Genitourinary tract, herbs in infections of female, 24–26
    saw palmetto and male, 12, *12*
Georgia Blue Cross Blue Shield, affinity products offered by, 112
German Commission E Monographs, on bearberry, 25
    on black cohosh, 23
    on chasteberry, 24
    on common herbs, 9
    on Echinacea, 10–11, 25
    on garlic, 11, 26
    on ginger, 14
    on ginkgo, 11
    on ginseng, 13
    on goldenrod, 24
    on kava, 15, 37
    on milk thistle, 15
    on Saint John's wort, 13
    on saw palmetto, 12
    on shepherd's purse, 24
    on valerian, 14
    as valuable resource, 22
Ginger, 14
Gingerol, in ginger, 14
Ginkgo, 11–12
    dosage of, 12, 24
    drug interactions with, 11–12
    in formulary, 5
    Saint John's wort and, 37
    in sexual dysfunction, 24
Ginkgo biloba see Ginkgo
Ginseng, 12–13
    dosage of, 13
    drug interactions with, 13
    Saint John's wort and, 37
    species of, 12
Ginsenosides, in ginseng, 12
Glucocorticoids, in fibromyalgia and chronic fatigue/immune dysfunction syndrome, 50
Glucose, ginseng and, 13
Glucose levels, garlic and, 11
Gluten sensitive enteropathy, in food allergy, *40t*
Glycogen, ginseng and, 13
Glycosides, in Echinacea, 9
    in ginkgo, 11
Glycyrrhiza glabra see Licorice
Glycyrrhizin, in licorice, 23
Goldenrod, as diuretic, 24
    dosage of, 24
    for premenstrual syndrome, 24
Green buildings, characteristics of, 127–128
Gut, in fibromyalgia and chronic fatigue/immune dysfunction syndrome, 51
Gynecology, herbs in, 21–26

H

Hahnemann, Samuel, 156
Hamilton Anxiety Scale, kava and, 15, *15*

Hamilton Depression Index, depression
  measured by, 31
  in Saint John's wort trials, *32–33, 32–34*, 36
Harmony, in office design, 125–127
Harvard School of Public Health, survey of, 148
Harvard's MindBody Medical Institute,
  alternative medicine covered by, 116
Hatha yoga, in coronary artery disease, 95–96
Hawthorn, in formulary, 4
Headache, in food allergy, 40–41
  from ginseng, 13
  from selective serotonin reuptake
    inhibitors, 35
Headaches, acupuncture for, 63
  from valerian, 14
Healing path, in fibromyalgia treatment, 48
Healing spaces, office design in creation of,
  125–128
Health and Healing Card, affinity products
  offered by, *114t–115t*
Health and Healing Trust, affinity products
  offered by, *114t–115t*
Health and Wellness database, as survey
  source, 140
Health Care Financing Administration, on
  alternative medicine, 109
Health maintenance organizations *see also*
  Insurance coverage of alternative
  medicine
  insurance coverage of, 108
    chiropractic care as, 70
    low-cost alternative medicine in, 134
Health plans *see* Insurance coverage of
  alternative medicine
Healthy buildings, characteristics of, 127–128
Heart disease *see also* Coronary artery disease;
  other disorders
  chelation therapy for, 85–87
  lifestyle interventions for, 91–96
  prevalence of, 92
Heart rate, acupuncture and, 63
Heiner's syndrome, in food allergy, *40t*
Helonius opulus *see* False unicorn root
Heme iron, in coronary heart disease, 94
Hemorrhage, shepherd's purse for uterine, 24
Hepatic disease, chelation therapy
  contraindicated in, 87
Hepatitis C, milk thistle for, 15
Hepatotoxicity, of Echinacea, 11
Hepatotoxins, milk thistle against, 15
Herb Research Foundation Library, *5t*
Herbal formulary, contents of, 4–5
  creation of, 1–7
  current examples of, 1
  education and, 5–6
    databases in, *5t*
    texts in, *6t*
  evaluation of, 6
  herb suppliers to, 4, *4t*
  hospital pharmacy and, 3
  implementation of, 3–4
  legal aspects of, 6–7
  outpatient pharmacy and, 3
  preparation of, 4
  purpose of, 2
  reassessment of, 3
  research into, 2–3, 6
  specialists to consult for, *2t*
Herbal medicine *see also* Herbs; specific herbs
  homeopathy *versus*, 155

Herbalists, credentials for, 112
Herbicide, as fertilizer, 155
Herbs *see also* Herbal formulary; specific herbs
  contraindications to, patient handouts on, 4
  in homeopathy, 155–157
  most commonly used, 9–17
    advice to patients on, 16, *17t*
    Echinacea as, 9–11, *10*
    garlic as, 11
    ginger as, 14
    ginkgo as, 11–12
    ginseng as, 12–13
    kava as, 14–15, *15*
    milk thistle as, 15
    panaxoside content of, 16, *16t*
    Saint John's wort as, *13*, 13–14
    sales of, *10*
    saw palmetto as, 12, *12*
    valerian as, 14
  physicians' acceptance of, 148
  potential drug interactions with, 21
  principles of therapy with, 21
  public acceptance of, 9
  suppliers of, *4t*
  in women's health care, 21–26
    anti-infective, 24–26
    estrogen-like, 22–24
    as menstrual cycle aids, 24
    other hormonal, 24
Herpes lesions, Echinacea for, 25
  lemon balm for, 26
Hippocrates, Saint John's wort mentioned by, 30
Histamine, intolerance to, *40t*
HIV/AIDS, clinical problems in, 102, *102t*
  complementary therapy in, 101–105
    energy-based, 102–103
    movement-based, 103–105
    for pain, 101–102
    surveys of, 144–145, *146t*, 147
  conventional therapy of, 101
Holism, reductionism *versus*, 45
Holistic medicine *see also* Alternative medicine
  in medical schools, 1
Homeopathy, dosages in, 156–157
  herbal medicine *versus*, 155
  law of similars in, 156
  physicians' acceptance of, 148, *149t*
  principles of, 155–156
  remedy preparation in, 156
Homeostasis, as energy balance, 80
Homocysteine, in coronary heart disease, 94
Honest Herbal, *6t*
Hops, in formulary, 4
Hormesis, defined, 155
Hormonal cycle, physiology of female, 22
Hormonal effects of herbs, in women's health
  care, 24
Hormone balance, in chronic fatigue/immune
  dysfunction syndrome treatment,
  49–50, *53t*
  in fibromyalgia treatment, 49–50, *53t*
Hospital pharmacy, herbal formulary and, 3
Hostility, in coronary heart disease, 94–95
Hot flashes, black cohosh for, 23
  dong quai for, 23
  physiology of, 23
  red clover for, 22
Human immunodeficiency virus *see*
  HIV/AIDS
Humulus lupulus see Hops

Hydromorphone, acupuncture *versus*, 62
Hyperemesis gravidarum, ginger for, 14
Hyperforin, in Saint John's wort, 34, 37
Hypericin, in Saint John's wort, 13, 32
Hypericum see Saint John's wort
Hypermobility of joints, chiropractic care in, 71
Hypersensitivity reactions, to food, 39–42, *40t*
Hypertension, acupuncture for, 63
  from ginseng, 13
Hyphema, from ginkgo, 11
Hypnotherapy, physicians' acceptance of, 148
  study of, 134
Hypocalcemia, from chelation therapy, 87
Hypoglycemia, from chelation therapy, 87
Hypoglycemic agents, ginger and, 14
Hypotension, from antidepressants, 35
  in fibromyalgia and chronic
    fatigue/immune dysfunction
    syndrome, 50
  in food allergy, *40t*
Hypothalamic-pituitary-adrenal axis, ginseng
  and, 12–13
Hypothalamus, menstrual cycle and, 22
Hypothyroidism, in fibromyalgia and chronic
  fatigue/immune dysfunction
  syndrome, 49–50
Hyssop, in formulary, 4
Hyssopus officinalis, 4

I

IAC database, as survey source, 140
IBIS, as herbal database, 5, *5t*
IgE, in food allergy, 39, *40t*, 42
Imidazole, Echinacea *versus*, 25
Imipramine, Saint John's wort *versus*, *32, 32*
Immune dysfunction syndrome, diagnosis of,
  46–47, *47t*
  integrative treatment of, 45–53
Immune function, in chronic fatigue/immune
  dysfunction syndrome treatment,
  51–52, *53t*
  in fibromyalgia treatment, 51–52, *53t*
Immunoglobulin E, in food allergy, 39, *40t*, 42
Immunoglobulin G testing, in food allergy, 41
Immunostimulants, Echinacea as, 9–10, 25
  in formulary, 5
Infancy, food allergy in, 39
Infections *see also* specific infections and types
  of infection
  in food intolerance, *40t*
  herbs in women's health care for, 24–26
  in HIV/AIDS, 101
Infinite Health, affinity products offered by,
  112, *114t–115t*
Insomnia, from ginseng, 13
  kava for, 14–15, 37
  Saint John's wort for, 31
Insurance coverage of alternative medicine,
  107–118
  acupuncture as, 61
  benefit selection in, 111–118
    affinity and, 112–113, *113t–114t*
    core or add-on, *117t*, 117–118
    other benefits and, 116–117
    providers and, 112
    riders for, 113, 114–116, *115t–116t*
  chiropractic care as, 70
  consumer interest in, 107, *108t*
    choice of policy and, 108

Insurance coverage of alternative medicine, *continued*
    health plan views on, 108–109
    mandates for, 109
    current extent of, 110–111, *111t*
    as grafting or health creation, 118
    herbal, 7
    motivators and obstacles to, 110
    physician perceptions of, 109–110
    plan purchasers and, 109
Integrative medicine, benefits and risks of, 133–134
    business aspects of, 121–123
        environmental, 122
        financial, 123
        personnel, 122
    in chronic fatigue/immune dysfunction syndrome, 45–53
    continuing medical education in, 131–132
    conventional medicine *versus*, 45–47
    defined, 45
    evolution of, 139
    in fibromyalgia, 45–53
    future of, 123
Integrator for the Business of Alternative Medicine, on insurance riders, 113
Interactive BodyMind Information System, 5, *5t*
Internal medicine, acupuncture in, 62–63
International Prostate Symptom Score, saw palmetto and, 12
Internet *see also* Websites
    herbal databases on, 5, *5t*
Intestinal hyperpermeability test, in fibromyalgia, 51
Intestines, in fibromyalgia and chronic fatigue/immune dysfunction syndrome, 51
Ionizing radiation, effects of, 155
Ipecac, in homeopathy, 156
Irritable bowel syndrome, acupuncture for, 63
Isoflavone, in red clover, 22

J

JAMA, on alternative medicine, 148
    therapeutic touch as, 82–83
    trends in, 133–134
Jimsonweed, effects of, 156
Joint dysfunction, chiropractic care of, 71–72
Journal of Alternative and Complementary Medicine, as resource, 148
Journal of Geriatric Psychiatry and Neurology, on Saint John's wort, 31

K

Kaiser North California, consumer survey of, 108, *108t*
K'an Herb Company, *4t*
Kaptchuk, Ted, *2t*
Kava, 14–15, *15*
    dermopathy from, 15
    dosage of, 15, 37
    drug interactions with, 15
    Saint John's wort and, 37
Kavalactones, in kava, 14–15, 37
Ketoconazole, garlic *versus*, 26
Kidney disorders, in women, 25
Kinesiology testing, in food allergy, 41
Kira, as Saint John's wort preparation, 32

Kligler, Benjamin, 1
Krieger, Delores, 80–81, 102–103
Kronenberg, Fredi, *2t*
Kunz, Dora, 80–81, 102
Kupperman's Menopause Index, black cohosh and, 23

L

Lactase deficiency, food intolerance in, *40t*
Lactation, bearberry contraindicated in, 25
Landmark Healthcare, alternative medicine covered by, *116t–117t*
    consumer survey of, 107–108, *108t*, 111, 141, *142t*
Laryngoedema, in food allergy, 40, *40t*
Latent prolactinemia, chasteberry in, 24
Law of similars, in homeopathy, 156
Lead intoxication, chelation therapy for, 85
Lectins, intolerance to, *40t*
Leg pain, spinal manual therapy for, 74, *74t–75t*
Legal aspects, of acupuncture, 58
    of herbal formulary, 6–7
Lemon balm, as antiviral agent, 26
Levodopa, in receptor model, 6
LI160, as Saint John's wort preparation, 32
Libido decrease, ginkgo for, 24
Licensing, of alternative medicine providers, 112
    in acupuncture, 61, 112
Licorice, in formulary, 4
    in women's health care, 23
Lifestyle, cancer therapy and, 143
    Saint John's wort and, 37
Lifestyle Heart Trial, 93, 96
Lifestyle therapy, physicians' acceptance of, 148, *149t*
Light therapy, for seasonal affective disorder, 33–34
Linum usitatissimum see Flaxseed
Liver, disorders of, chelation therapy contraindicated in, 87
    milk thistle for, 15
    in fibromyalgia and chronic fatigue/immune dysfunction syndrome, 51
Lotus Development, alternative medicine covered by, 115, *116t*
Louis XVI of France, Mesmer's techniques and, 80
Lovelace Health System, alternative medicine pilot project of, 110
Low back pain, acute *versus* chronic, *72t–73t*, 72–73
    compensation in, 70–71
    in HIV/AIDS, 102
    leg pain with, 74, *74t–75t*
    spinal adjustment for, 69–76 *see also* Chiropractic
    subluxation in, 70, *71t*
Low density lipoprotein, chelation therapy and, 86
    in coronary artery disease, 91
Lumbar disk syndrome, chiropractic care in, 74
Luteinizing hormone, black cohosh and, 23
    in hot flashes, 23
    in ovarian cycle, 22

M

Magnesium therapy, in chelation therapy, 88
    in fibromyalgia and chronic fatigue/immune dysfunction syndrome, 31, 49
Major depressive disorder, in depression classification, 30, *30t*
Malic acid therapy, in fibromyalgia and chronic fatigue/immune dysfunction syndrome, 49
Malingering, in chronic fatigue/immune dysfunction syndrome, 47
    in fibromyalgia, 47
Managed care, physician-patient relationship and, 133
Mandragora autumnalis see Mandrake
Mandrake, in women's health care, 23–24
Manic depression, ginseng and, 13
Manual therapy, in HIV/AIDS, 101–103
Maprotiline, Saint John's wort *versus*, 33
Massage therapy, in cancer therapy, 143
    in fibromyalgia and chronic fatigue/immune dysfunction syndrome, 49
    in HIV/AIDS, 102
    licensing of, 112
    money spent on, 133
    physicians' acceptance of, 148, *149t*
Mastalgia, from ginseng, 13
Matricaria recutita see Chamomile
McCaleb, Rob, *2t*
Medalia Healthcare, consumer survey of, 110
Median homeopathic dose, defined, 156
Median lethal dose, defined, 156
Medicaid, acupuncture covered by, 61
Medical history, in chronic fatigue/immune dysfunction syndrome, 47–48
    in fibromyalgia, 47–48
Medical schools, alternative medicine taught in, 148, 150
    lack of herbal training in, 1
Medicare, acupuncture covered by, 61
    chiropractic care covered by, 70
Meditation, in HIV/AIDS, 104
Meditation garden, in office design, *127*
MEDLINE, as herbal database, 5, *5t*
    as survey source, 140
Megavitamins, as alternative medicine or adjunct therapy, 147
Melatonin, in fibromyalgia and chronic fatigue/immune dysfunction syndrome, 49
    Saint John's wort and, 34
Melissa officinalis see Lemon balm
Memoir on Acupuncturation, 57
Menopause, black cohosh in, 23
    red clover in, 22
Menorrhagia, shepherd's purse for, 24
Menstrual disorders, black cohosh for, 23
    chasteberry for, 24
    dandelion for, 24
    dong quai for, 23
    ginkgo for, 24
    goldenrod for, 24
    red clover for, 22
    shepherd's purse for, 24
    wild yam for, 24
Menstruation, herbal aids in, 22–24
    physiology of, 22
Mental functioning, ginkgo and, 37
    ginseng and, 12–13
Mesmer, Franz, 80–81
Metabolic disorders, food intolerance in, *40t*

Metagenics, *4t*
Metal chelate, defined, 85
Mexican-Americans, alternative medicine in, 141
Midwives, licensing of, 112
Migraine, acupuncture for, 63
   in food allergy, 40–41
   valerian for, 14
Milk, allergy to, 39
Milk thistle, 15
   dosage of, 15
   in formulary, 5
Minnesota's Health Partners, affinity products offered by, 112
Minority groups, alternative medicine in, 141, 152
Mitochondrial resuscitant factors, in fibromyalgia, 49
Monoamine oxidase inhibitors, Saint John's wort as, 13–14, 34
   transition to Saint John's wort from, 37
Monosodium glutamate, intolerance to, *40t*
Montefiore Medical Center, holistic medicine in, 1
Mood, in chronic fatigue/immune dysfunction syndrome treatment, 52, *53t*
   in fibromyalgia treatment, 52, *53t*
Morand, on acupuncture, 57
Motion sickness, ginger for, 14
Movement therapy, defined, 104
   in HIV/AIDS, 103–105
Mullein, in formulary, 4
Multi-Center Lifestyle Heart Trial, 96
Murray, Michael, *2t*
Muscle energy technique, in HIV/AIDS, 102
Muscle stimulants, ginseng as, 12
Musculoskeletal disease, in HIV/AIDS, 102
Musculoskeletal pain, acupuncture in treatment of, 60
Music, in office environment, 127
Mutual of Omaha, alternative medicine covered by, 116
Myocardial infarction, anger and, 95
Myofascial release techniques, in HIV/AIDS, 102

N

NAPRAlert database, *5t*
Narcotics, in fibromyalgia and chronic fatigue/immune dysfunction syndrome, 49
National Blue Cross Blue Shield Association, on affinity products, 112
National Cancer Institute, studies of alternative therapy by, 150, *151t*
National Center for Complementary and Alternative Medicine, 3, 6, 139
National Center for Health Statistics, studies on alternative medicine by, 150
National Center for Homeopathy, 157
National Certification Commission for Acupuncture and Oriental Medicine, 61
National Council Against Health Fraud, 82–83
National Institute of Arthritis and Musculoskeletal Disease, center for chiropractic research of, 69
National Institutes of Health, Consensus Report on acupuncture of, 58–59, 62
   Consortial Center for Chiropractic Research of, 69
National Center for Complementary and Alternative Medicine of, 3, 6
   studies on alternative medicine by, 150, *151t*
National Managed Health Care Congress, on alternative medicine, 111
Native American medicine, physicians' acceptance of, 148
Natural killer cells, in fibromyalgia and chronic fatigue/immune dysfunction syndrome, 51–52
Nature's Way Herbs, *4t*
Naturopaths, licensing of, 112
Nausea, from Echinacea, 10
   in food allergy, 40, *40t*
   from garlic, 11
   ginger for, 14
   in homeopathy, 156
   from selective serotonin reuptake inhibitors, 35
Nephrotoxicity, of EDTA, 87
Neurology, acupuncture in, 63
Neuropathic pain, therapeutic touch for, 82, 102–103
Neurotransmitters, in depression, 31
   Saint John's wort and, 34
New England Journal of Medicine, on alternative medicine, 96
Nitrates, intolerance to, *40t*
Nitric oxide, ginseng and, 13
Nitrites, intolerance to, *40t*
Noncontact therapeutic touch, in HIV/AIDS, 102–103
Nonsteroidal anti-inflammatory drugs, in fibromyalgia, 49
   ginkgo and, 11–12
   ginseng and, 13
   for low back pain, 69
North Karelia Study, of coronary artery disease, 95
Nortriptyline, in fibromyalgia and chronic fatigue/immune dysfunction syndrome, 49, 52
Nursing, therapeutic touch in, 81, 152
Nutritional deficiencies, in chronic fatigue/immune dysfunction syndrome treatment, 51, *53t*
   in fibromyalgia treatment, 51, *53t*
Nuts, allergy to, 39

O

Ocular disorders, acupuncture for, 63
Office design, for healing environment, 125–128
Office of Alternative Medicine, acupuncture conference sponsored by, 58
   on cancer therapy, 142, 150
   Consortial Center for Chiropractic Research of, 69
   creation of, 139, 142, 150
Office of Medical Applications of Research, acupuncture conference sponsored by, 58
Office of Technology Assessment, alternative medicine surveys of, 150, *151t*
Opportunistic infections, in HIV/AIDS, 101
Oral contraceptives, in fibromyalgia and chronic fatigue/immune dysfunction syndrome, 50
   vaginal secretions and, 25
Organ transplantation, surveys of alternative medicine in, *147t*
Organic brain syndrome, ginkgo for, 11
Osler, William, 57
Outpatient pharmacy, herbal formulary and, 3
Ovarian cycle, physiology of, 22
Ovulation, vaginal secretions in, 25
Oxford Health Plans, affinity products offered by, 112
Oxidants, in coronary heart disease, 94
Oz, Mehmet, 134

P

Pain, acupuncture in treatment of, 59–60
   in chronic fatigue/immune dysfunction syndrome treatment, 49, *53t*
   in fibromyalgia, 46, *46t*
      treatment of, 49, *53t*
   in HIV/AIDS, 101–102
   low back *see* Chiropractic; Low back pain
   surveys of alternative medicine in, 147, *147t*
   therapeutic touch for, 82
Palmer Center for Chiropractic Research, 69
Panax see Ginseng
Panaxoside, in common herbs, 16, *16t*
Pancreatic insufficiency, food intolerance in, *40t*
Paracelsus, Saint John's wort mentioned by, 30
Parkinsonism, receptor model in, 6
Paroxetine, side effects of, 35
Patient satisfaction, with chiropractic, 70
Patient screening, for spinal manual therapy, 71–72
Patient-centered medicine, disease-centered medicine *versus*, 46
Patient-controlled analgesia, acupuncture *versus*, 62
Patients, acupuncture and, education about, 61
   satisfaction with, 63
   advice on herbs to, 16, *17t*
   assessment in therapeutic touch of, 81, 103
   with HIV/AIDS, 145
   interview in fibromyalgia treatment of, 47–48
   as physicians' partners, 134–135
PDR for Herbal Medicines, *6t*
Peanuts, allergy to, 39
Pediatrics, acupuncture in, 63
   alternative cancer therapy in, 143
Pelvic infections, in women, 25
Peptides, acupuncture and, 60
Percutaneous transluminal coronary angioplasty, in coronary artery disease, 92
Pericardium 6, in acupuncture, 59, 62
Peripheral neuropathy, in HIV/AIDS, 102–103
Peripheral vascular disease, chelation therapy for, 86–87
Personnel, in integrated practice, 122
Phagocytosis, Echinacea in, 9–10
Phantom pain, therapeutic touch for, 82
Pharmacologic receptor model, in herbal therapy, 6
Pharmacopsychiatry, on Saint John's wort, 34
Pharmacotherapy *see also* specific agents
   of coronary artery disease, 93
   rationale for, 91
   for low back pain, 69
Pharmacy, herbal formulary in, hospital, 3
   outpatient, 3
Pharyngitis, herbs for, 4
Phenylethylamine, intolerance to, *40t*
Phillips Family Practice/Institute for Urban Health, holistic medicine in, 1

Photosensitivity, from Saint John's wort, 14, 35–36
Phototherapy, for seasonal affective disorder, 33–34
Physical therapy, chiropractic care *versus*, 72–73
Physicians, acupuncturists and, 61
   in alternative medicine, credentials for, 112
      surveys of, 148, *149t–150t*, 150
   average income of, 133
   chiropractic for back pain and, 70
   creation of, 132
   in herbal formulary development, 2–3
   herbal training in, continuing medical education in, 5
      lack of, 1
   as idealists, 132
   licensing of, 6–7
   as patients' partners, 134–135
   perceptions of alternative medicine of, 109–110, 121, 131
   personal evolution of, 132–133
   personality types of, 132
   workload of, 133, *133t*
Phytoestrogens, in women's health care, 22–23
Phytosterols, in licorice, 23
Picker Institute, design criteria studied by, 128
Pituitary, menstrual cycle and, 22
Planetree Health Resource Center, *5t*
Platelets, in coronary heart disease, 93–94
Pliny, Saint John's wort mentioned by, 30
Pollution, indoor air, 128, *128t*
Polycystic ovary syndrome, black cohosh for, 22–23
Polysaccharides, in Echinacea, 9
Postoperative pain, acupuncture in treatment of, 59
Potatoes, intolerance to solanine in, *40t*
Prana, in energy medicine, 80
Prayer, in cancer therapy, 143
Preferred provider organization, chiropractic care covered by, 70
Pregnancy, contraindications in, bearberry as, 25
   chelation therapy as, 87
      dong quai as, 23
      Echinacea as, 11
      licorice as, 23
   ginger in, 14
Premenstrual syndrome, black cohosh for, 23
   chasteberry for, 24
   goldenrod for, 24
   Saint John's wort for, 31, 34
Preservatives, food intolerance to, *40t*
Primary care physicians, chiropractic care and, 70
Progesterone, in fibromyalgia and chronic fatigue/immune dysfunction syndrome, 50
   in ovarian cycle, 22
Prolactin, chasteberry and, 24
   in ovarian cycle, 22
Prostate, saw palmetto and, 12
Protein maldigestion, in fibromyalgia and chronic fatigue/immune dysfunction syndrome, 51
Providence GoodHealth Plan survey, 107, *108t*
Provocation/neutralization testing, in food allergy, 41
Prunus virginiana see Cherry bark
Pseudohypericin, in Saint John's wort, 13
Psoriasis, herbs for, 4–5
surveys of alternative medicine in, 147, *147t*
Psychologic factors, in food intolerance, *40t*, 41
Psycho-neuro-immunology, principles of, 79
Psychosocial risk factors, in coronary artery disease, 94–95
Purple coneflower *see* Echinacea

Q

Qi, in acupuncture, 57, 61, 65–66
   in energy medicine, 80
Qigong, in HIV/AIDS, 104
Quackwatch, Inc., 82–83
Quinine, in homeopathy, 156

R

Radicular syndromes, in low back pain, 74
Radioallergosorbent testing, in food allergy, 41
Raspberry leaf, in formulary, 4
Raynaud's syndrome, acupuncture for, 63
Receptor model, in herbal therapy, 6
Recycled material, in building design, 128
Red clover, for amenorrhea, 22
   as isoflavone source, 22
Reductionism, holism *versus*, 45, 79
Rehabilitation, surveys of alternative medicine in, *147t*
Reich, Wilhelm, 80
Relaxation, in fibromyalgia and chronic fatigue/immune dysfunction syndrome, 52
   in HIV/AIDS, 104
   kava for, 14–15, 37
Relaxation response, in alternative medicine, 79
Renal toxicity, of EDTA, 87
Research, on acupuncture, 62–65
   herbal formulary, 2–3, 6
      databases in, *5t*
   on spinal manual therapy, 72
   on therapeutic touch, 81–82
Respiratory tract, herbs useful for, Echinacea as, 10, *10*
   in formulary, 4
Revascularization procedures, in coronary artery disease, 92–93
Rhinitis, in food allergy, 40, *40t*
Rider, insurance, defined, 113
   as integrated benefit, 115–116
Rosenthal Center, as alternative medicine course resource, 148
Rotary diversified diet, in food allergy, 41
Rotation diet, in food allergy, 41
Rubus idaeus see Raspberry

S

Safety, of spinal manual therapy, 74–75
Saint John's wort, *13*, 13–14, 29–37
   background of, 29
   botanical description of, 30
   clinical research in, *13*, 13–14, *32–33*, 32–33, 36
   diet and lifestyle and, 37
   dosage of, 14, 31, 35
   drug interactions with, 14, 36
   in fibromyalgia and chronic fatigue/immune dysfunction syndrome, 49
   formulations of, 37
   indications for use of, in depression, 29–33, *31t*
      in premenstrual syndrome, 34
      in seasonal affective disorder, 33–34
   mechanism of action of, 13, 34–35
   other drugs *versus*, *32–33*, 32–33, 36, *36t*
   other herbs used with, 37
   recent popularity of, 13, 30
   side effects of, 35–36
Saponins, in ginseng, 12
Saw palmetto, 12, *12*
   dosage of, 12
Saxitoxin, intolerance to, *40t*
Scandinavian Simvastatin Survival Study, 93
Schweitzer, Albert, 136
Screening of patients, for chiropractic care, 71–72
Scromboid poisoning, *40t*
Scutellaria laterifolia see Skullcap
Seafood, intolerance to, *40t*
Seasickness, ginger for, 14
Seasonal affective disorder, in depression classification, *30t*, 31
   Saint John's wort for, 31, 33–34
Sedatives, kava as, 14–15
   valerian as, 14
Selective serotonin reuptake inhibitors, Saint John's wort as, 13
   side effects of, 35
   transition to Saint John's wort from, 36
Self Healing, as resource, 134
Self-regulation, in fibromyalgia and chronic fatigue/immune dysfunction syndrome, 50, 52
Serotonin, in fibromyalgia, 31
   Saint John's wort and, 34, 36
Serotonin receptors, selective serotonin reuptake inhibitors and, 35
Serotonin reuptake inhibitors *see* Selective serotonin reuptake inhibitors
Serotonin syndrome, Saint John's wort and, 14
Sertraline, side effects of, 35
Sexual dysfunction, ginkgo for, 24
   from selective serotonin reuptake inhibitors, 35
Sham acupuncture, in research, 64
Shapiro, Marcey, 1, *2t*
Shepherd's purse, dosage of, 24
   for menorrhagia, 24
Shogaol, in ginger, 14
Sick building syndrome, defined, 128
Sick euthyroid, in fibromyalgia and chronic fatigue/immune dysfunction syndrome, 49
Silybinin, in milk thistle, 15
Silymarin, in milk thistle, 15
Single-blind placebo-controlled food challenges, in food allergy, 40
Single-photon emission computed tomography, acupuncture and, 61
Skin testing, in food allergy, 39–40
Skullcap, in formulary, 4
Sleep, in chronic fatigue/immune dysfunction syndrome treatment, 49, *53t*
   in fibromyalgia, symptoms of, 31
      treatment of, 49, *53t*
   Saint John's wort and, 34–35
Small intestine, in fibromyalgia and chronic fatigue/immune dysfunction syndrome, 51
Social isolation, in coronary artery disease, 95
Social trends, in alternative medicine, 140–142, *142t*

Solanine, intolerance to, *40t*
Solidago see Goldenrod
Soy, allergy to, 39, 41
    as phytoestrogen, 22
Specialists, as herbal formulary consultants, *2t*
Spinal adjustment *see also* Chiropractic
    for low back pain, 69–76
Spinal manual therapy, for low back pain, 69–76
Spiritual healing, in cancer therapy, 143
    physicians' acceptance of, 148, *148t*
Spirituality of Work Questionnaire, 136, *137t*
Staffing, in integrated practice, 122
Stanford University, consumer survey of, *108t*, 110
Stanford/American Specialty Health Plans, alternative medicine survey of, 107, *117t*
Stenting, in coronary artery disease, 92–93
Stool analysis, in fibromyalgia and chronic fatigue/immune dysfunction syndrome, 51
Strain and counterstrain technique, in HIV/AIDS, 102
Stress, in coronary artery disease, 95
    management of, 95–96
    menstrual cycle and, 22
Stroke, acupuncture after, 62
Subdural hematoma, from ginkgo, 11
Subluxation, chiropractic care of, 70, *71t*
Subtle hypothyroidism, in fibromyalgia and chronic fatigue/immune dysfunction syndrome, 49–50
Succussion, in homeopathy, 156
Sunlight, seasonal affective disorder and, 31, 33–34
Suppliers of herbs, 4, *4t*
Support groups, in fibromyalgia and chronic fatigue/immune dysfunction syndrome, 52

T

Tai chi, in HIV/AIDS, 104
Taraxacum officinale see Dandelion
Tattleman, Ellen, 1
Terpene lactones, in ginkgo, 11
Testing, in food allergy, 41
Testosterone, saw palmetto and, 12
Texts, herbal, *6t*
Theobromine, intolerance to, *40t*
Therapeutic touch, 79–83
    as alternative medicine, 79
    clinical applications of, 82
    controversy in, 82–83
    energy in, 80
    history of, 80–81
    in HIV/AIDS, 102–103
    research into, 81–82
    technique of, 81
Thistle, milk *see* Milk thistle
Thrombocytopenia, milk-induced, *40t*
Thrombosis, in coronary artery disease, 93
Thromboxane, in coronary artery disease, 93–95
Thyme, in women's health care, 23
Thymus vulgaris, 23
Thyroid function, in fibromyalgia and chronic fatigue/immune dysfunction syndrome, 49
Tieraona Low Dog, 1, *2t*
Tieraona's Herbals, *4t*
Tinea, herbs for, 4–5
Tolerance, to acupuncture, 60
Touch, therapeutic, 79–83 *see also* Therapeutic touch
Toxicology manual, in herbal formulary, 4
Toxins, food intolerance to, *40t*
Toxline database, *5t*
Toynbee, Arnold, 136
Tracking systems, in herbal formulary, 6
Transcutaneous acupoint electrical stimulation, clinical trials of, 62
Trease and Evans' Pharmacognosy, *6t*
Tricyclic antidepressants, Saint John's wort versus, 32–33, *32–33*
    side effects of, 35
    transition to Saint John's wort from, 36
Trifolium pratense see Red clover
Trigger point therapy, in fibromyalgia and chronic fatigue/immune dysfunction syndrome, 49
    in HIV/AIDS, 102
Triglycerides, garlic and, 11
Triterpenoid saponins, in ginseng, 12
Tryptamine, intolerance to, *40t*
Tufts Health Plans, alternative medicine covered by, 115, *116t*
Turmeric, in formulary, 5
Tyler, Varro, *2t*
Tyramine, intolerance to, *40t*
Tyramine reaction, from Saint John's wort, 34

U

Unicorn root, in women's health care, 23–24
United States, acupuncture laws in, 58
    alternative medicine in, other countries *versus*, 148
    heart disease in, 92
    number of physicians in, 133
University of Arizona Program in Integrative Medicine, holistic medicine in, 1
Urinary tract, infections of, bearberry for, 25
    blueberry for, 25
    cranberry for, 25
    garlic for, 26
    in women, 24–25
    saw palmetto and, 12
Urticaria, in food allergy, 39, *40t*
Uva ursi see Bearberry

V

Vaginal infections, clinical features of, 25
    herbs for, 25–26
Vaginal secretions, cyclical changes in, 25
Valepotriates, in valerian, 14
Valerian, 14
    dosage of, 14
    in fibromyalgia and chronic fatigue/immune dysfunction syndrome, 49
Valeric acid, in valerian, 14
Vascular dementia, ginkgo for, 11
Vascular disease, chelation therapy for, 85–87
Vasospasm, in coronary artery disease, 93, 95
Vegetarian diet, in coronary heart disease, 93–94
Verbascum thapsus see Mullein
Vessel spasm, in coronary artery disease, 93, 95
Veterans Administration, on alternative medicine, 109
Viral infections, Saint John's wort for, 31
Visceral manipulation, in HIV/AIDS, 102
Vitality Access, affinity products offered by, *114t–115t*
Vitamin C, in asthma, 5
    in chelation therapy, 88
Vitamin E, in asthma, 5
Vitamins, as alternative medicine or adjunct therapy, 147
    in fibromyalgia and chronic fatigue/immune dysfunction syndrome, 49
    Saint John's wort and, 37
Vitex adnus-castus see Chasteberry
Vomiting, acupuncture in prevention of, 59, 62
    from Echinacea, 10
    in food allergy, 40
    from garlic, 11
    in homeopathy, 156

W

Warfarin, chelation therapy and, 87
    ginkgo and, 11
    ginseng and, 13
Washington state, insurance coverage of alternative medicine in, 109–110
Websites, of *AIDS Treatment News*, 145
    of herb suppliers, *4t*
    of National Center for Complementary and Alternative Medicine, 3
    of National Center for Homeopathy, 157
    of Rosenthal Center, 148
    Weil's, 134
Wege Center for Health and Learning, design of, 127
Weight, in coronary artery disease, 91
Weil, Andrew, 1, *2t*, 134
Wheat, allergy to, 39
Wild yam, in women's health care, 24
Women's health care, herbs in, 21–26
    anti-infective, 24–26
    estrogen-like, 22–24
    in formulary, 4
    as menstrual cycle aids, 24
    other hormonal, 24
    surveys of alternative medicine in, 141
Worker's compensation, chiropractic care covered by, 70
Workload, of physicians, 133, *133t*
World Health Organization, on acupuncture, 60
World Med, in continuing education, 134
Wound healing, aloe for, 26
    Echinacea for, 9

X

Xanthones, in Saint John's wort, 13

Y

Yeast infections, vaginal, clinical features of, 25
    Echinacea for, 25
Yellow Emperor's Classic of Internal Medicine, on acupuncture, 58
Yoga, in coronary artery disease, 95–96
    credentials for practitioners of, 112
    in HIV/AIDS, 104
Yuen, Jeffrey, *2t*

Z

Zolpidem, in fibromyalgia and chronic fatigue/immune dysfunction syndrome, 49